MW00436618

Replacing the Dead

Replacing the Dead

The Politics of Reproduction in the Postwar Soviet Union

MIE NAKACHI

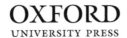

OXFORD

UNIVERSITY PRESS

OXFORD
UNIVERSITY PRESS

Oxford University Press is a department of the University of Oxford. It furthers
the University's objective of excellence in research, scholarship, and education
by publishing worldwide. Oxford is a registered trade mark of Oxford University
Press in the UK and certain other countries.

Published in the United States of America by Oxford University Press
198 Madison Avenue, New York, NY 10016, United States of America.

© Oxford University Press 2021

Library of Congress Cataloging-in-Publication Data
Names: Nakachi, Mie, author.
Title: Replacing the dead : the politics of reproduction in
the postwar Soviet Union / Mie Nakachi.
Description: New York, NY : Oxford University Press, [2021] |
Includes bibliographical references and index.
Identifiers: LCCN 2020026364 (print) | LCCN 2020026365 (ebook) |
ISBN 9780190635138 (hardback ; alk. paper) | ISBN 9780190635152 (epub) | ISBN 9780190635169
Subjects: LCSH: Abortion—Soviet Union. | Reproductive rights—Soviet Union. |
Women's rights—Soviet Union. | Women—Soviet Union—Social conditions.
Classification: LCC HQ767.5.S65 N35 2021 (print) | LCC HQ767.5.S65 (ebook) |
DDC 362.1988/800947—dc23
LC record available at https://lccn.loc.gov/2020026364
LC ebook record available at https://lccn.loc.gov/2020026365

DOI: 10.1093/oso/9780190635138.001.0001

For my family

Contents

Acknowledgments   ix
Glossary   xiii

Introduction   1

1. The Patronymic of Her Choice: Nikita S. Khrushchev
   and Postwar Pronatalist Policy   21

2. Abortion Surveillance and Women's Medicine   56

3. Postwar Marriage and Divorce: The New Single Mother
   and Her "Fatherless" Children   88

4. Who Is Responsible for Abortions? Demographic
   Politics and Postwar Studies of Abortion   123

5. Women's Reproductive Right and the 1955 Re-legalization
   of Abortion   153

6. Beyond Replacing the Dead: Women's Welfare and
   the End of the Soviet Union   186

   Epilogue: Reviving Pronatalism in Post-Socialist Russia   216

Notes   223
Bibliography   291
Index   313

Acknowledgments

Writing this book was a long journey. Without generous and persistent support and encouragement from many individuals and institutions, this project would have never been completed. First, I thank my interviewees who invited me to their homes and told me memories of postwar family life, including intimate episodes from the most difficult moments of their reproductive lives. These women inspired this book.

The project began as a dissertation at the University of Chicago. I would like to express my gratitude to Sheila Fitzpatrick who guided me at every step, always generously shared her knowledge, and inculcated in me her love for archival research. Her prolific work and diverse interests have been a great example and inspiration. David Ransel made me aware of the importance of the language of rights, which became a major theme of this book. Susan Gal introduced me to gender analysis of reproduction and politics under socialism. The late Richard Hellie taught me the importance of statistics in analyzing history.

I had many opportunities to present versions of various parts of this book and benefited from comments, guidance, and advice. Particularly I would like to thank the participants of the Chicago Russian History Workshop, the Berkeley Kruzhok, the Historian's Seminar at Harvard's Davis Center, Seminar at the Ukrainian Research Institute at Harvard University, the Russian History Seminar of Washington, DC, and the Shiokawa Seminar at Tokyo University. I am especially grateful to my hosts at these lively exchanges: the late Reggie Zelnik, Yuri Slezkine, Terry Martin, Catherine Evtuhov, Michael David-Fox, and Nobuaki Shiokawa.

Many individuals offered comments, guidance, and support. I can mention only a few here. Mark Edele has been a generous comrade and best critic, who commented on the entire manuscript. Charles Hachten shared a key set of archival documents with me. Chris Burton guided me through the Ministry of Health archive. Alan Barenberg, Ed Cohn, Brian LaPierre, and Ben Zajicek provided insightful comments on earlier versions of chapters. Their company brightened the otherwise lonely process of research and writing. Alain Blum gave me a lecture on the history of Soviet demography at a Paris café and introduced me to Russian demographers. Jennifer Utrata shared her expert knowledge on single mothers in post-Soviet Russia. Don Filtzer offered expertise on the postwar Soviet landscape. Rickie Solinger shared her deep knowledge of reproductive politics and energized an early version of Chapter 3. Tim Colton, Gzergorz Ekiert, and Liz Tarlow at the Davis Center and Lubomyr Hajda of the Ukrainian Research Institute welcomed me to Harvard as a postdoctoral fellow and provided me with many chances to present my work. Yasuhiro Matsui invited me to the group of Japanese historians working on social history of the Soviet Union. T. A. Listova helped me arrange oral interviews with doctors in Moscow.

Paula Michaels read the entire manuscript and strongly encouraged me to consider global perspectives. Michele Rivkin-Fish also took time to read the entire manuscript and provided me with detailed and expert comments. This book improved greatly because of their critical comments.

The research for this book was funded by the University of Chicago Overseas Research Grant, the Matsushita International Research Fellowship, the Mellon-Fitzpatrick Field Research Fellowship, and the Suzukawa Fellowship. The Robert C. Tucker and Stephen F. Cohen Dissertation Award of the Association for Slavic, East European, and Eurasian Studies provided me with a grant to turn my dissertation into this book.

My appreciation goes to archivists of Russian federal and local archives. Their dedication and warmth made research efficient and pleasant. I thank the members of Slavic-Eurasian Research Center of Hokkaido University for their support of my research. Hokusei Gakuen University supported completion of this book and publication. I thank Susan Ferber, my editor at Oxford University Press, for her patience, generosity, and professionalism. All mistakes found in this book are mine.

My friends helped me in various ways. Long friendship with Varya made my trips to Moscow always a homecoming. She made her extensive social network available to my interview project. I deeply regret that she did not live to see this book before her untimely death. Zhenya also helped organize interviews. Irina, Karlene, Kirsten, Ayako, Noriko, and Yumiko always welcomed me whenever I had a chance to travel to their homes around the globe.

I dedicate this book to my family. Without the enduring support of my parents, Masami and Toshio, I would never have been able to continue studies and research. Miho, Yutaka, and Yu always made sure that I didn't miss out on important and fun family events, even when I had to keep writing. Akira always brought me the greatest joy throughout this journey. David read the whole manuscript and insisted that these women's stories were too important not to be published. Without his loving support through a nuclear crisis, great flood, earthquake, and now pandemic, this book would have never been finished.

Glossary

Soviet Organizations appearing in this book

All-Union Central Council of Trade Unions (VTsSPS) the head of trade unions in the Soviet Union, tasked with protecting women as workers

Communist Party of the Soviet Union (CPSU) Ruling party between 1917 and 1991 dominating all government decision-making bodies

Gosplan the State Planning Committee

Komsomol Communist Youth League

MinFin Ministry of Finance. Narkomfin before 1946

MIu Ministry of Justice. NKIu before 1946

MVD Ministry of Internal Affairs, predecessor of the KGB. NKVD before 1946

MZ Ministry of Health. NKZ before 1946

People's Commissariats (NK) renamed Ministries in 1946

People's Court the lowest level court where most civil law cases were decided

Politburo Highest governing body of the CPSU meeting in the Moscow Kremlin, chaired by the General Secretary (called Presidium from 1952 to 1966)

Sovmin Council of Ministers (Council of People's Commissars before 1946)

TsSU Central Statistical Administration

ZAGS Office of Vital Records, documenting all marriages, births, and deaths

Soviet Terms and Events mentioned in this book

babka women healers, midwives, and abortionists who are not trained in modern Western medicine

blat a system of reciprocal favors, often financial or in kind

Court of Honor a postwar Stalinist institution for disciplining scientific workers and bureaucrats

Doctors' Plot conspiracy accusations concocted by Stalin and security organs in 1951–1953, according to which Kremlin doctors, mostly Jewish, were allegedly assassinating Soviet leaders

Great Terror Late 1930s mass executions and imprisonments under Stalin without going through proper legal procedure.

kolkhoz collective farm

Kliueva-Roskin affair (KR affair) the first Court of Honor case (1946), condemning medical researchers for handing over their secrets to foreign spies

krai region

militsiia police

oblast' region

patronymic Russian second name, usually formed from the father's first name; used together with the first name in all formal conversations

prikaz a governmental order

raion district (smaller than a region)

RSFSR Russian Soviet Federated Socialist Republic. Russian part of the Soviet Union, now the territory of the Russian Federation

sovkhoz state-owned farm

spravka informational note, often accompanying draft legislation or policies

SSSR Russian transliteration of USSR (Union of Soviet Socialist Republics)

Virgin Lands Khrushchev's campaign calling for Slavic people to settle northern Kazakhstan in order to transform the vast grasslands into an agricultural belt through mechanized farming

Replacing the Dead

USSR : abortion legal <u>1920</u> (first country in world)
why? commitment to utopian society ū equal rights
for men & women

Stalin : 1936 made it illegal again

post Stalin : 1955 (2 Y after death) again legal

Introduction

A woman should be given the right to decide herself.
Mariia D. Kovrigina, USSR Minister of Health (1955)

Lena, an unmarried, twenty-one-year-old village school teacher, became pregnant for the first time in 1946.[1] She was single and did not want to continue the pregnancy, but abortion was then illegal in the Soviet Union. With the help of a girlfriend, she found a gynecologist who was willing to terminate the pregnancy by curettage for an "outrageous amount of money" that she did not have. However, she knew she needed to hire a specialist in order to avoid hemorrhage or worse consequences that so many acquaintances had suffered. In desperation, she borrowed the money from an affluent male friend, telling him that one of her girlfriends needed money to get an abortion.

She scheduled the procedure during the day, when her parents, who knew nothing about her pregnancy, were out working. Everything happened in the kitchen, without painkillers or antiseptics. She experienced excruciating pain, but could not scream, fearing the neighbors might hear her and call the *militsiia*. As soon as the operation was over, the doctor left the apartment. Later in life, she married and gave birth to one child.

Like Lena, millions of Soviet women between 1936 and 1955 arranged illegal abortions through networks of friends, and many abortionists, both medically trained and untrained, performed operations for a large fee. Typically, abortionists did not have anesthesia or special instruments, and women experienced agonizing pain and anxiety. As modern contraception was never made widely available, Soviet women, married and unmarried, often went through this traumatic experience not once, but multiple times during their reproductive lives. Lena had several abortions after her marriage. Based on the registration record, Russian demographers estimate that the average woman living in the Soviet Union in the late 1950s had had four

Replacing the Dead. Mie Nakachi, Oxford University Press (2021). © Oxford University Press.
DOI: 10.1093/oso/9780190635138.003.0001

abortions. But Lena insisted that "women on average had five to ten abortions in their lives."[2] Like Lena, lucky women did not have complications and never got caught. Unlucky ones were caught, suffered medical complications, or died. Some had successful underground abortions, but could not conceive later in life.[3]

Underground abortion was hardly a new postwar phenomenon, but demographic chaos during the Great Patriotic War, as World War II is known in Russia, created many conditions for a postwar increase in abortions. During the war, a total of 34 million men and 600,000 women were mobilized into the armed forces. These numbers included those who worked as military administrators and those in training, so not all left immediately, but most were relocated to the front, military bases, and production units, leaving their families behind.[4] The process of family breakup was also accelerated by evacuation. Siberia, the Caucasus, and Central Asia became destinations for approximately 16.5 million evacuees from the western border regions of the Soviet Union.[5] In German-occupied areas, civilians were sorted and killed, most notably over 2 million Jews. Other able-bodied women and men were taken for labor.[6] In the midst of such demographic turmoil, many family members lost contact with each other.

Many wanted to wait for their partners until the end of the war. But not all could wait, nor could all who waited be reunited.[7] Most tragically, vast numbers of partners never came back, as the war took the lives of approximately 27 million Soviet citizens, of whom an estimated 20 million were male.[8] As a result, the postwar sex ratio in Russian society would be extremely skewed. In 1944, the average ratio of adult men to women of reproductive ages in rural areas was 28 men per 100 women, with great regional variation.[9] And high mobility among the wartime and immediate postwar population meant an increased chance of new liaisons in the military, on transportation, on the home front, and in the occupied areas. All of these conditions multiplied difficulties for the postwar development of families and women's reproductive lives.

The Soviet government did not know the exact number of deaths and casualties at that time, but leaders understood that the war's demographic damage was unprecedented.[10] They were aware that postwar conditions were far from ideal for families, but the country needed a labor force for reconstruction and development. To replace the dead, the government introduced an extreme pronatalist policy, the July 8, 1944, decree entitled "On increasing government support for pregnant women, mothers with many children, single mothers, and strengthening protection of motherhood and childhood; on the establishment of the honorary title 'Mother Heroine,' the foundation of the order 'Motherhood Glory,' and the medal 'Motherhood Medal' " (hereafter, the 1944 Family Law or the 1944 law).[11]

As the title of this law suggests, the government promised new state aid and material support for postwar mothers. More quietly, it introduced measures to encourage men to father children outside conjugal relationships. This idea of state promotion of out-of-wedlock births came from Nikita S. Khrushchev, who saw the war's effects firsthand as the head of the Ukrainian Communist Party. Like Lena, many women aborted to avoid giving birth to "out-of-wedlock" children, a legal status that the 1944 Family Law created for the first time in Soviet history. The clearest and most painful expression of this legal change dictated that mothers could no longer include the biological father's name in the birth certificate, leaving open the question of what patronymic to give to the child, instead of the one usually derived from the actual father's first name.[12] But many others also gave birth believing that the baby's father would marry them or having found out about the pregnancy too late to have a safe illegal abortion. The Central Statistical Administration recorded about 8.7 million children as out of wedlock between 1945 and 1954.

This book is about Soviet women struggling to create the best possible family life in difficult postwar conditions under the pronatalist regime, and the medical and legal professionals who tried to improve the welfare of postwar mothers and children. Policymakers considered the births of millions of out-of-wedlock children as success, but women from many walks of life complained about the difficulties of finding a marriage partner, disapproved of out-of-wedlock status, and expressed dissatisfaction with abortion's illegality. Female party activists reported on these conversations, but it was medical and legal professionals who would regularly hear from women at medical consultations and in legal meetings. Over time, women's collective pleas and demands convinced many educated professionals to advocate change in Soviet family and abortion policies, and this significant segment of public opinion evolved into a reform movement. Not surprisingly, it was the medical profession that focused most on the issue of abortion, as doctors witnessed thousands of deaths and crippling injuries every year from illegal abortions.[13]

The Soviet Union had initially legalized abortion in 1920, thereby becoming the first country in the world to provide legal abortion on demand.[14] But I. V. Stalin, who emerged as the successor to the Soviet Union's first leader Vladimir Lenin, recriminalized abortion in 1936, except for those with a very limited list of medical conditions. Criminalization continued throughout the 1940s, but gradual reform began in the early 1950s and finally, in 1955 the Soviet Union re-legalized abortion.

The primary reasons for the 1920 legalization were medical and paternalistic protection of women, not the acknowledgment of women's rights. After the 1917 Revolution, Bolshevik physicians wished to help working women, whom they considered to be still suffering from patriarchal exploitation and subjugation, by providing safe abortion, despite their belief that it was generally harmful for women's health. Physicians believed that legalization would be temporary, because once the communist system was firmly established, women would no longer need to worry about childbirth and childrearing.[15]

The 1955 re-legalization was different from the 1920 legalization, because the main motivation was not the medical protection of women's health but the recognition of a woman's right to abortion. Exemplifying this view was Mariia D. Kovrigina, the Soviet Union's only female minister of health. Taking advantage of the brief political interregnum, Kovrigina pushed for legalization based on the principle of women's rights.[16] Her opinion developed over many years of carrying out pronatalist policies as a medical administrator, witnessing the deleterious effects of unwanted pregnancies on women's health, and receiving letters directly from women asking for legal abortion.[17] The significant female presence in the medical and legal professions was also crucial as female participants at meetings and conferences eloquently spoke out about women's difficult situations and argued for reform.[18]

Undeniably, the recognition of women's reproductive rights was very limited, and a woman's right not to become a mother at all was not considered appropriate in the USSR, since the government considered motherhood a woman's obligation to the state, and women generally accepted this.[19] "Any normal woman wants to become a mother": this statement of Dr. A. I. Dmitrieva, chairwoman of the Moscow Central Abortion Committee, expressed this widespread normative idea.[20] Nonetheless, the 1955 law stands out as the world's first legalization that recognized woman's right to, rather than medical need for, abortion. Between the 1936 Soviet criminalization and the 1955 re-legalization, other countries, including England, Sweden, Finland, and Japan, made legal abortion available for women. But these were on medical, eugenic, and/or ethical grounds.[21] Only when women insisted on women's rights to abortion during the feminist movement of the 1960s and 1970s did England, the United States, and some European countries make abortion legal or available practically on demand.[22] In this sense, the 1955 USSR re-legalization broke new ground, as did the original 1920 legalization.[23]

Beyond professional circles, women's rights in the Soviet Union never received widespread discussion. Propaganda publications generally did not publicize a woman's right to abortion. Thus, even specialists on Russia did not think that women's rights were a decisive factor behind the 1955 re-legalization of abortion.[24] In fact, even the law used the word "possibility" instead of the "right" of women to "decide the question of motherhood by themselves."[25] In addition, after re-legalization, the newly instituted system of providing abortion was restrictive, involving anti-abortion propaganda campaigns and individual consultations aimed at dissuading women from the procedure.[26] However, after the 1954 cancellation of women's criminal responsibility for their abortions, legalization would not have been necessary if the primary goal had been medicalization. A significant expansion of criteria would have sufficed, as was done in Japan in 1949.

In the absence of a feminist movement, how did the idea of a woman's right to abortion emerge in the Soviet Union? And how was it suppressed? In order to answer these questions, this study analyzes the postwar politics of reproduction, a complex relationship among policymakers, experts, men, and women over their sometimes competing and other times overlapping political, economic, social, health, and family interests.[27] Policymakers were primarily interested in securing an adequate level of population growth while keeping women in the workforce. After the war, Soviet leaders desperately wanted to recover population to secure the future labor force needed to reconstruct economic and military strength to meet the multiplying conflicts of the Cold War. This required women to bear and raise as many children as possible. At the same time, the government needed to keep women in the workforce because of the dearth of surviving laborers. To achieve both goals, Soviet leaders adopted Khrushchev's pronatalist proposal of social engineering through repression, penalization, and incentivization. Importantly, the final law dropped repressive measures; instead, it introduced extremely gendered reproductive policies.

As policymakers had wished, postwar Soviet women remained in the labor force. In fact, they were always around half the labor force in the postwar Soviet economy, including agriculture.[28] They cultivated the land, worked in factories, drove tractors, and ran transport. In contrast to the West, where many middle-class women chose to or were forced to go back to domesticity after demobilized male soldiers reclaimed their prewar jobs,[29] most Soviet women had no choice but to remain in the workforce because so few men returned from the battlefields and many survivors were physically or mentally crippled. After returning home every day from full-time jobs, Soviet women were responsible for finding and preparing food, cleaning house, and taking care of children, the elderly, and often wounded and crippled demobilized family members.[30] These tasks at home were far from simple, especially since living space, food, clean water, and essential consumer products were scarce.[31] Furthermore, women often became the main tenders of the family vegetable plots, indispensable sources of nutrition for survival.[32] Even so, Soviet women generally desired a family and children. In this sense, women and the state had a shared interest. However, many women resisted the idea of becoming unmarried mothers. Their desire for motherhood within marriage was in direct conflict with the postwar pronatalist policy.

Soviet experts, such as medical and legal professionals and demographers, acted as mediators. They provided policymakers with data and analyses and recommended policies. For women, they gave consultation and advice and provided professional services. How they would do so depended on their professional interests and relationships with the leadership and women. Demographers and statisticians, who suffered heavily in the prewar purges, developed a culture of self-censorship and focused on supporting leadership opinions rather than presenting scientific analysis.[33] They avoided presenting analysis that potentially contradicted policymakers' statements.[34] In contrast, wartime experience of acting on their own decisions empowered other postwar specialists who did not experience severe repression in the prewar period. In the hope of improving postwar life in the Soviet Union, they were ready to address problems within their areas of expertise, criticize policies, and suggest alternative ideas.[35] Professionals of women's medicine, many of them women, and female party members were especially active in mediating between the state and women, since they had the most direct contact and conversations about reproduction and family.

To analyze the politics of Soviet reproduction, this book utilizes rich primary materials from former Soviet archives. Policymakers' discussions and documents generally come from the Central Party Archive and the State Archives and sometimes ministerial archives. Court cases and legal petitions emerge from central and local archives and provide fine-grained descriptions and analysis regarding marriage and divorce, on women's family problems, and on their interactions with the state. The Ministry of Health archive contained stenograms and reports in which professionals of women's medicine discussed abortion cases. Party activists also conducted independent investigations on unmarried mothers. In addition, I conducted fifteen interviews with women in Moscow who became mothers during the Soviet period. The Archive of the Economy and the archives of the Ministries of Justice and Health provide statistical data and professional discussions among statisticians/demographers, medical and legal professionals. These materials deepened analysis of the interactions among different actors and identify moments of change that shaped this politics.

Roots of 1944: Socialist Ideology and Soviet Reproductive Policies

The 1944 Family Law was not the first pronatalist policy in the Soviet Union. The first pronatalist policy was the 1936 Family Law, which, on the one hand, criminalized abortion, made divorce difficult, and set high child support requirements from fathers; on the other hand, it instituted state support for mothers with many children and expanded the childcare network. While the 1944 Family Law also included similar measures, it significantly departed from the prewar measures in its reconsideration of men's role.

The socialist ideologies of women and population development, to-gether with the changing course of reproductive policies before 1944, pro-vide important long-term historical contexts for the development of the 1944 Family Law.[36] Socialist thinkers of the nineteenth century argued that under socialism women would be completely equal to men, have full access to education, and contribute to the economy, society, and culture as workers. Equality would not be limited to the public sphere of law, education, and work, but it would also apply to the private sphere of family. Freeing women from "kitchen slavery" would become one of the key Bolshevik slogans. To realize this vision, the state would provide socialized childcare institutions and household services. In this ideal future, the state would ensure material well-being and take over household work and the task of raising children, while working women would happily bear many children. As the state would take over all of the functions of the family, family would eventually "wither away."[37]

Socialists took anti-Malthusian and anti-neo-Malthusian positions, coun-tering eighteenth-century English scholar Thomas Malthus's theory. Malthus argued that if the government provided minimum subsistence, this would actually increase poverty by raising wages, increasing unemployment, and encouraging indulgent practices, in particular, early marriage, childbearing, and drinking among the poor. Being an Anglican priest, he promoted late childbirth through moral strength and abstinence, not contraception.[38] Later in the century, neo-Malthusians advocated contraceptive methods to prevent high fertility among the poor. Karl Marx and Friedrich Engels rejected Malthusian and neo-Malthusian theories for masking class relations and creating unequal distribution of wealth under capitalism. In contrast, the socialist system could support a large population, and workers would be able to have as many children as they wished without material concerns.[39] In this way, socialism saw population growth as a natural development and reflection of workers' well-being and satisfaction with the socialist state.

Some socialist thinkers reluctantly addressed the theoretical possibility of future fertility decline. Both Engels and August Bebel, the socialist leading lights on issues of women and family, suggested that well-educated, politically conscious socialist working women might want to regulate fertility at some point in the future. However, neither advocated specific methods of prevention. Engels refused to specify the method of regulation,[40] while Bebel simply proscribed "any injurious abstinence or any repellant preventive measures."[41] At the time neo-Malthusians were promoting preventive measures for curtailing rapid population growth among the poor, socialists did not want to appear to support these methods. Bolshevik leader Vladimir Lenin also believed that workers wanted many children and considered contraception a bourgeois practice.[42] What else would happen after women started regulating fertility was never addressed.

The socialist theory of sex also implied high fertility and negated the necessity of contraception or abortion. Alexandra Kollontai, one of the few early female Bolshevik leaders and a theoretician of love and sex under socialism, advocated "free love." It was not taken seriously by other Bolshevik leaders, but it became popular among a small circle of urban youth.[43] But she did not advocate fertility control, as she saw motherhood as a social obligation and believed that under socialism women and men in love should freely follow their sexual instincts because the socialist state would raise children.[44]

Thus, socialist ideology generally insisted on growing the population and took a negative stance on any form of fertility control, since workers under fully developed socialism should not need it.[45] Conversely, contraceptive practices could be constructed as evidence that socialism was failing to provide sufficient welfare for its citizens. Thus, policy discussions of abortion and contraception focused on providing additional material support for women, and it was difficult to acknowledge that women would avoid motherhood for any other reason.

After World War I, revolution, and the flu pandemic, population fell everywhere in Europe. The Soviet Union's population also shrank, but Russian fertility was still among the highest in Europe, so birth rate was not a primary concern. Because of socialist commitment to women's welfare, the Bolshevik government introduced key policies to enhance women's position in the family. The 1918 Family Law made marriage secular and allowed women as well as men to initiate divorce. All children became equal before the law regardless of their mothers' marital status, eliminating the distinction between children of married and unmarried mothers. In 1920, abortion became legal, and subsequently the development of contraceptive devices began. As legal specialists considered unwanted marriage exploitative for women and unnecessary, the 1926 Family Law enabled either husband or wife to send a divorce notification to the registration office. It also recognized common-law marriages, so marriage registration increasingly lost significance, and many people formed families without taking the steps to officially register.[46]

Revolutionary approaches to reproductive policies ended in the mid-1930s. After Stalin began rapid industrialization and collectivization of agriculture in the late 1920s, the birth rate fell. Further economic development made greater female participation in the labor force crucial. At the same time, to secure the future workforce, increasing the birth rate was also essential. Stalin also considered that the power of the state was in proportion to population size, so falling birth rate was a threat to building military strength. The 1936 Family Law was Stalin's answer to the question of what to do when the birth rate falls.[47] The law justified criminalization, arguing that progress and welfare in the Soviet Union had made legal abortion unnecessary. The state also repressed contraceptive development and distribution.[48] In exchange for introducing repressive measures, the law promised to expand medical facilities for mothers and children, as well as childcare, and provided new aid to mothers with more than seven children.[49]

Falling birth rate was not the only demographic problem in the early 1930s. Social turmoil caused by revolution, collectivization, and repressions produced a growing number of delinquent children who lived on the streets.[50] The 1936 Family Law and other legislation on family made it clear that the family, not the socialist state, bore primary responsibility for raising children.[51] The law also attempted to make all fathers responsible for raising their children by making divorce difficult and by setting high child support payments. In hindsight, the 1936 policy can be called "two-parent pronatalism," as it tried to pressure fathers back into family childrearing.[52]

By contrast, the 1944 Family Law enshrined one-parent pronatalism. Reversing the prewar policy, it would increase women's burden as caretakers of the family, as the law released men from responsibility for the birth and upbringing of out-of-wedlock children. The state designated the mother as the primary parent with the responsibility to care for children, physically, emotionally, and financially. This postwar pronatalism's highly gendered approach charged only mothers with full childrearing responsibility with some, but completely inadequate, state support. After the war, when the state demand for women's labor and birth rate growth was at its highest level, state policy further compromised women's welfare. One-parent pronatalism without sufficient state support essentially continued until the end of the Soviet Union, with long-term social and demographic consequences.[53]

The Great Patriotic War's Effects on Marriage

The 1936 Family Law aimed at making marriage more stable and binding by introducing measures such as a stricter procedure for divorce and high levels of child support payment. However, as long as the legal recognition of common-law marriage continued and the state was unable to enforce child support payment primarily from fathers, the state of marriage was never entirely clear, nor were child support responsibilities.[54] The Great Patriotic War multiplied ambiguities and complexities in marital relations because wartime society created high numbers of dislocated people and offered optimal conditions for new sexual unions among both the military and civilian populations in a variety of contexts.[55]

When the war and mobilization began, family members expressed their desire to meet again when the war was over. Departing soldiers had an almost existentially strong desire for their family members to wait for them to come back. They wrote letters to their parents, wives, lovers, and children to inform them that they were alive. "Wait for Me" was the strong sentiment shared by many mobilized soldiers, which crystallized in a very popular wartime poem with that title. Konstantin Simonov's poem created a powerful image as the very act of waiting became a lifeline to survival for soldiers.[56]

The realities of life during the war and into the postwar era proved very different from prewar expectations. The promise between lovers, married or not, to wait for each other would have been strong at separation, but wartime conditions made it difficult for many to keep. E. Sakharova, a doctor who remained in Moscow during the war, was waiting for the demobilization of her husband Sergo. While waiting, she confided to her diary that she feared that her husband might fall out of love with her when he saw her again, because she had changed so greatly during the war.[57] It was Ilia Erenburg, the most famous Soviet war correspondent, who cut closer to the truth in a poem he wrote on the very day of victory, May 8, 1945, or so he claimed. In it, a young man awaited reunion with his love, "as one waits only when one loves; I knew her as one knows only oneself; . . . The hour struck. The war ended. I made my way home. She came towards me, and we did not recognize each other."[58]

Civilian women who were separated from lovers and husbands sometimes united with men who were not drafted.[59] There were also sexual unions between military men and civilian women. Soviet military men visited women during business trips, leaves of absence, and re-deployments. When possible, they visited their families—but also women who lived nearby. Within the military, the most mobile personnel, such as drivers and those responsible for material procurement, tended to have excellent social opportunities.[60] Hospitalization provided another opportunity for civilian-military contact, as soldiers and officers sometimes checked themselves out to visit nearby towns or villages.[61]

Because the Soviet Army and Navy enlisted many young women in their late teens and early twenties, a significant number of military sexual unions, "cohabitations," and "marriages" were formed.[62] In the 1970s and 1980s, Svetlana Alexievich interviewed former female service women and heard many stories of love in the military.[63] When mutual, such attractions quickly turned into unions, often casually, but almost universally described as "marriage (brak)."[64] For example, Liubich knew a battalion commander and a nurse who fell in love with each other and "got married." The commander was severely wounded in battle and taken away to a hospital, leaving the pregnant nurse behind. The commander wrote to her to go to his parents' home and give birth to their child. Tamara S. Umniagina, a sanitary officer with the rank of junior sergeant, told Alexievich that she and her husband fought in the war together and vowed to get married if they survived, which they did.[65]

Other unions in the military were more hierarchical in nature and typically involved male officers with female soldiers or medical personnel.[66] The women in such relationships took care of the officers' sexual and other daily needs, such as washing and cleaning. Such relationships were understood to be a kind of "marriage," as these women were derogatorily called "mobile field wives (*polevaia peredvizhnaia zhena*, or PPZh)."[67] Not surprisingly, women became pregnant while in military service, and many attempted to abort.[68] However, whether they carried the pregnancy to term or an abortion attempt was discovered, these women were discharged.[69]

In Nazi-occupied areas, sexual violence and fraternization occurred. The German army set up military brothels, where local women were made available to satisfy soldiers' sexual needs on demand. In Gatchina, a Leningrad suburb, approximately 2,000 women were housed in an "isolation house" for sexual labor.[70] In Ukraine, younger women between ages thirteen and sixteen reportedly worked in officers' brothels.[71] In addition, a fair amount of fraternization took place between German men and Ukrainian women.[72] Erenburg quickly felt the complexities when the woman whose house he was billeted in briefly asked for his help in tracing her missing husband. He asked her how the Germans had behaved and she said that "No German ever set foot in here," only to be contradicted by her young son, "Mama, Uncle Otto used to come every day, he played with me, he played with you too."[73]

These wartime relationships and liaisons affected postwar formation of marriage and family in often fundamental ways. Many demobilized soldiers decided to stay with wartime partners; some demobilized soldiers demanded divorce when they learned that their wives had had other relationships; and many service women coming home felt that in order to be able to marry, they should be silent about their experiences.[74] Wartime complications in gender relations created many "common-law" marriages and resulted in many conceptions. The 1944 Family Law that redefined marriage would have great impact on many of these relationships and women's reproductive desires.

Women and Family in the Making of the Soviet Welfare State

Soviet state building was premised on the idea of creating a fair and just society, better than capitalism, that would provide all workers sufficient material conditions and social services to promote a healthy cultural life and provide care for all citizens in times of need.[75] This utopian vision was never fully realized. In the revolutionary period immediately after 1917, a new welfare system was introduced, but due to lack of resources, experts expected the family, not the state, to provide welfare.[76] On top of this, the government granted only workers social rights, excluding many disenfranchised people, such as formerly privileged classes of the prerevolutionary period and wealthy peasants.[77] But over time welfare measures expanded,[78] and by the 1970s the socialist welfare system provided a wide range of basic needs for all members of the population, including healthcare, education, pensions, childcare, family benefits, food, and housing.[79]

Theoretically, women's welfare was one of the key areas that differentiated socialist from capitalist welfare states, both because of the socialist theoretical commitment to women's equality with men and the socialist regime's expectation of women's participation in the labor force. As a step toward building socialist welfare for women, after the revolution, the new government introduced a new legal framework to enhance well-being, making women and men equal at law and abortion available on demand. In 1918, the Commissariat of Social Security was created with a department dedicated to the preservation of the welfare of mothers and children.[80] The Women's Department (*Zhenotdel*), created in 1919 within the Bolshevik Party, played a central role in women's welfare by teaching women literacy skills and social hygiene, providing political education, organizing institutions such as communal dining, milk kitchens, laundromats, and crèches, as well as maternity and pediatric care. Without sufficient financial and political support these institutions did not materialize in full, but the department produced visions of how to achieve women's economic independence and how to free women from traditional care work within the family by transforming daily life (*byt*).[81]

However, in 1930 the party closed the Women's Department on the grounds that activities aimed at improving women's well-being went against the unity among workers.[82] The government posited that women's equality with men had been achieved, and that the time had come to deliver welfare to all citizens. The 1936 Constitution guaranteed citizens' rights to rest, leisure, social insurance, free medical service, education, and maternity leave.[83] This promise was more real on paper than in reality. In the Stalinist 1930s, welfare provisions were not universal, but hierarchical and productionist. In this system, the state would provide various goods and services, such as housing, food, medical care, pension, and insurance, according to the type and level of jobs, or party ranking, of workers. "Stakhanovites" and shockworkers who outperformed production quotas received special recognition and rewards,[84] while the exclusion of large contingents of disenfranchised people continued.[85]

The hierarchical and productionist approach was extended to women's welfare. As demographic concerns emerged in the 1930s, the 1936 Family Law introduced the repressive reproductionist principle to women's welfare. Thereafter all pregnant women were required to give birth or otherwise suffer punishment. For those who met this requirement, the state would provide support. Like "shock workers" in factories, fertile mothers with seven and more children would receive special rewards from the state. In exchange for reproductive contribution, the government built a network of childcare facilities for working mothers. During the war this universalist reproductive principle was further expanded when penalties were introduced for insufficiently reproductive males as well.[86] The 1944 Family Law completed the universal reproductive hierarchy of citizens based on the number of offspring, where penalties and rewards were clearly defined.

Criticisms of this reproductive principle came almost as soon as the 1944 Family Law was promulgated and continued in the late 1940s. Soviet professionals and bureaucrats who observed women struggling with their reproductive lives proposed to reduce repression and support women's wishes. Some of their ideas were original and creative, such as painless birth without drugs.[87] Legal and medical specialists proposed amendments and accommodations to family laws and abortion surveillance. But as with other innovative ideas suggested in this period, few were implemented, and many of those who proposed them were disciplined.[88] In contrast to the Great Purge of the late 1930s, disciplining in the late 1940s generally did not involve physical repression, so those who proposed reform ideas generally survived. This laid the basis for some piecemeal reforms in the early 1950s.

The opportunity for transformation came after Stalin's death in 1953.[89] Professionals revived reform discussions, and in the field of reproduction this led to the 1954 cancellation of criminal responsibility of women for abortion and the re-legalization in 1955.[90] Women finally obtained universal access to clinical abortion, the only reliable method of fertility control available at that time. Re-legalization became the "symbol of women's reproductive freedom and the liberalization of sexual life."[91]

Yet this was a very limited reform. In its implementation, legalization was not fully liberating. The new access to abortion was not automatic, as women had to go through bureaucratic procedures to have the operation. The legal abortion system functioned as a new surveillance system, whereby the state could control the quality of the operation and learn about the women who sought this service.[92] The state made very limited investment in abortion facilities, so abortion was a painful and humiliating experience for women.[93] The new system was intrusive, rather than punitive, like many other systems developed under Khrushchev.[94] Despite the image of Khrushchev as a reform initiator, many reform initiatives made no headway during Khrushchev's reign, including key family law reforms.[95]

By 1970, the most repressive and reproductionist measures of the 1930s and 1940s were reversed or mitigated. However, family law reforms in the late 1960s were very limited in scope, and the principle of "one-parent pronatalism" was not reversed. As declining birth rate became a major political concern again in the late 1960s and 1970s, Soviet experts actively discussed women's welfare as workers and mothers. Sociologists and demographers, who had been silenced by Stalin's bludgeoning of these fields, returned from disgrace to join the discussion about how to achieve the right balance between women's roles in the workforce and at home in order to encourage a higher birth rate. While diverging policy visions developed based on distinct views regarding women,[96] Brezhnev's policies gradually moved toward considering women's inherent destiny as motherhood and homemaking.[97] Nonetheless, women were expected to stay in the workforce. Mikhail Gorbachev, upon becoming the Soviet Union's top leader in 1985, proved himself a reformer in many areas, but there would be no "New Thinking" on women.[98] A position among social scientists that called for a complete revamping of traditional gender roles as applied to family care never gained influence at the policymaking level. Instead, an essentialized view of women remained influential not only in the late Soviet Union but also beyond, feeding into post-Soviet nationalist discourse and anti-abortion movements.[99]

Women and the Socialist Reproductive Model beyond Russian Borders

The development of Soviet reproductive politics had important influence on women of different cultures and nationalities across the postwar Soviet Union and beyond. Legal abortion became available in European Russia, as well as in the Central Asian republics, where the population was primarily Muslim. Generally, Muslim women tended to have large families, but in the years following the 1955 re-legalization, abortion statistics grew rapidly.[100]

Beyond the Soviet Union, Soviet reproductive policy affected newly socialist regimes in Eastern Europe and China. After World War II, Central and East European nations under socialism adopted the Soviet-style system of centralized economy, women's full participation in the workforce, and secular families. China was not far behind. The Soviet origins of Chinese pronatalism are clear. After the founding of the People's Republic of China in 1949, China followed key features of the Soviet postwar system, adopted legislation similar to the 1944 Family Law, limited access to both abortion and contraception, and celebrated "Mother Heroines."[101]

After Stalin died and the USSR re-legalized, especially after the 20th Party Congress in February 1956 where Khrushchev attacked Stalin's cult of personality, most East European countries, under new communist leadership, also legalized or liberalized abortion.[102] In so doing, they came to share Soviet reproductive practice characterized by the multiple abortion culture without modern contraception, young marriage and birth, and low rates of childlessness.[103] This development set socialist women apart from women under capitalism in the latter half of the twentieth century, as the latter could use modern contraception and gained wider access to abortions. According to a 2007 collection of United Nations (UN) statistics, of the sixty-one countries that gather data on abortion rates, the top twelve were all former or current communist countries: Russian Federation, Vietnam, Kazakhstan, Estonia, Belarus, Romania, Ukraine, Latvia, Cuba, China, Hungary, and Mongolia.[104]

Recently, many countries in Europe, North America, and Asia have experienced problems of low birth rate and labor shortage, threatening the financial viability of the social security system. Increasing participation of women in the workforce can partially solve the present labor shortage, but to secure future workers, the birth rate also must rise.[105] The challenge is similar to what the Soviet Union faced many decades ago: how to realize a high rate of employment among women, while maintaining an adequate level of fertility. The Soviet Union succeeded in the former and struggled with the latter, making it an instructive historical case for comparatively analyzing welfare policies, women, and fertility.

Comparative studies of gender and welfare states have examined how different types of welfare policies affected men and women differently. Postwar European welfare states generally privileged income maintenance over social services for families because of the assumption of the male-breadwinner and housewife model.[106] However, this situation gradually changed as more women went into the workforce in the 1970s. Women's expanded access to birth control also supported this phenomenon. Initially, the common effect was declining fertility in all states. Facing this fertility trend, welfare state policies split into two main groups and within two decades demographic differences appeared. Those states that encouraged women to gainfully work outside the home and redirected substantial amounts of unpaid family care work from the hands of women to public institutions and/or the market saw recovery in the birth rate. In contrast to these success stories, welfare states that reinforced women's role as caretaker in the home, envisaged women's entry into the workforce as part time to supplement a main breadwinner's income, and provided limited social services for family care continue to experience declining or very low birth rates.[107] This result suggests that distribution of family care work away from women is a key factor that influences fertility when women's labor participation rises.[108]

Informed by this comparative perspective, this study pays close attention to policy changes that redistributed Soviet family care work to highlight the special place of the Soviet Union in the global study of gender and welfare states. Aside from the lack of the market, a salient feature of the Soviet welfare state that set it apart from capitalist welfare states was the common absence of a male breadwinner in the family and, in turn, the prevalence of women raising children officially or practically alone. In line with these developments, nearly all adult Soviet women by 1970 were in the workforce, and abortion was the only reliable method of fertility control. This made redistribution of women's role in family care work urgent, but the Soviet pronatalist measures of the 1970s and 1980s neither significantly reduced family care work nor delegated the task to someone else. Instead, they encouraged women to spend more time at home to take care of young children and household work without providing them full financial compensation. Combined with the Soviet Union's notorious shortage economy, lack of adequate housing, and absence of quality consumer goods and appliances to support household work, the socialist case undermined women's welfare and unwittingly produced the worst case conditions for fertility growth.

Russian demographers and demographers of Russia have not analyzed gender perspectives in existing studies of postwar Russian fertility decline. This work attempts to apply this approach to Soviet and post-Soviet pronatalist policies. Chapter 1 examines the policymaking process for the 1944 Family Law. As the victory over the Nazis came into sight and the demographic devastation became apparent, the Soviet leadership keenly felt the need to strengthen pronatalist policy. Several proposals submitted in 1943–1944 essentially expanded existing pronatalist measures without a fundamental change in the vision of population growth. However, Khrushchev submitted the most comprehensive overhaul from Ukraine based on a new vision for population and pronatalism. The government policy revealed a two-faced practice of Bolshevik language, claiming to "protect motherhood" when addressing the masses and non-Bolshevik discourse, population engineering language among the top leadership.[109] In the final law, policymakers prioritized giving men the incentive to father extramarital children over assuring the overall well-being of unmarried mothers and their children.

Chapter 2 introduces the work of Soviet obstetricians and gynecologists in the early postwar years up to 1949 and their fight against abortion. Gaining knowledge, practice, and self-sufficiency under extremely difficult wartime conditions, doctors had become used to expressing their own views and acting on them. Doctors of women's medicine understood that policymakers were interested in reinstituting the prewar abortion surveillance system, but doctors generally believed that most women needed safe abortion, not prosecution.

Yet a postwar purge in the medical field soon put an end to hopes for postwar alternatives in Soviet medicine, as contact with the West came under attack amid renewed calls for vigilance.[110] Soviet specialists in women's medicine were also attacked in the subsequent disciplining of professionals, because Mariia Kovrigina was one of the most active medical administrators to participate in the disciplining process. As Deputy Minister of Health in charge of women's and children's medicine, she also conducted a political purge of the main research institute under her control. The main outcome was the removal of many Jews from the institute, a common trend of workplace purges in the late 1940s and early 1950s. Under threat, medicine gave up on the idea of helping women individually through expert judgment and private consultation.

Chapter 3 describes how the 1944 Family Law affected marriage, divorce, and other family relations between men and women. Given the sex ratio, the new law created a situation where marriage had practical disadvantages for men and advantages for women. Men might try to divorce prewar "wives" in order to formalize new "marriages" made during the war, but many would try to avoid marriage because of the increased cost of divorce. Women, in contrast, wanted legal marriage for a variety of reasons.[111] Those who were pregnant wanted to register quickly, so that the child would not be born out of wedlock.

Because of the strict divorce law and men's unwillingness to legalize marriage, women's wishes often went unrealized. Often women and men would live together in unofficial marriages or separately, but without an official divorce, which was financially and psychologically disadvantageous for women and children. Not only did the "new class" of unmarried mothers with fatherless children voice their sense of injustice, but wives in legal marriage also complained bitterly about husbands' affairs with younger women and unpaid child support. Legal specialists and women party activists asked for amendments to the 1944 Family Law, emphasizing the harmful effects of the law on the physical and psychological health of out-of-wedlock children, but no signs of change appeared until 1948.

Chapter 4 analyzes the 1948/1949 interministerial abortion study and the beginnings of the abortion reform movement. The falling birth rate in 1948 became a political problem, and all demographic data were made secret in 1948. V. N. Starovskii, head of the Central Statistical Administration (TsSU), suggested that the rising number of abortions was the primary cause of the declining birthrate. The medical and legal professions undertook comprehensive study of both legal and illegal abortion, including a survey of illegal abortion, compiled through interviews with hundreds of women hospitalized after botched abortions. The results led to a shift in reformist focus from prosecution to prevention.

Chapter 5 discusses the final steps toward legalization. In the early 1950s, the Ministry of Health (MZ), Ministry of Justice (MIu), All Union Central Council of Trade Unions (VTsSPS), and state prosecutor collectively developed ideas to improve women's reproductive environment.[112] While a major political campaign targeting doctors derailed the process, after Stalin's death in March 1953, reform movements resumed. In 1954, journalist Elena Serebrovskaia began a public movement demanding reform of the 1944 Family Law, and many citizens joined her call. Medical and legal experts believed that the time was ripe for family law reform, but nothing came out of the public movement. Instead, medical experts advanced abortion law reforms in the early 1950s. Doctors also strived to improve contraceptive devices to prevent abortions. Despite these developments, the key elements of the 1944 Family Law remained untouched.

Chapter 6 traces the development of contraception policy, family law reform, and demographic policy from the legalization of abortion until the end of the Soviet Union. After 1955, the number of clinical abortions steadily rose. Soviet doctors of women's medicine began developing contraception to stop the prevalent practice of multiple abortions. However, their vision of preventing abortion as a way of improving the reproductive health of Soviet women increasingly contradicted the emerging pronatalism of the 1970s. As the introduction of contraception remained blocked, doctors again made it easier for women to get clinical abortions in the early stages of pregnancy. Key postwar practices would be reinforced into the post-Soviet era. Meanwhile, the reformed family law of 1968 brought only superficial improvement to the legal status of out-of-wedlock children. The one-parent pronatalism that allocated unequal parental responsibilities between the mother and father was largely unchanged from 1944 until 1991.

The epilogue analyzes the legacy of Soviet pronatalism in post-socialist Russia. In the 1990s, liberal policies supported by Western organizations introduced sex education and family planning to Russia, based on the idea that women have the right to contraception. However, this period ended quickly with the ascendancy of Vladimir Putin, who took an interest in history, learned from postwar pronatalism, and introduced rules that restricted women's access to abortion.[113]

In addition to an empirical base of archival documents on public health, legal cases, statistics, and internal party activities, as well as published professional journals, interviews, literary works and films are used to uncover hidden stories behind the primary and statistical sources. Similarities and differences drawn from the histories of different countries place Russia and the Soviet Union into global contexts as well. In so doing, this study shows how policies and practices developed after unparalleled wartime demographic devastation had long-lasting, unintended impacts on gender relations, reproduction, and population in Russia.

1

The Patronymic of Her Choice

Nikita S. Khrushchev and Postwar Pronatalist Policy

> The Great Patriotic War demanded of the peoples of the USSR an unprecedented exertion to secure victory over the Nazi-German invaders. Naturally, this led to significant population loss and the consequent important task of replacing as quickly as possible the lost population to assure future demographic acceleration.
>
> N. S. Khrushchev to V. M. Molotov (April 13, 1944)

At the end of the war, the Soviet Union was still a rural country, and the Soviet village was predominantly female. Svetlana Alexievich, the 2015 Nobel Prize Laureate in Literature, was born and lived in a Ukrainian village in the postwar period. Later, her family would move to Belorussia, the motherland of Alexievich's father. In her Nobel speech, Alexievich recalled the postwar village as a "world of women." As a child, every evening she listened to village women share their memories about their husbands who never returned.[1] Statistics supported this impression. In rural areas of the Soviet Union that were not occupied by Nazi Germany during the war, the number of men per 100 women between ages 16 and 54 stood at 94 in 1939; it had fallen drastically to 36 by January 1944. The Western part of the Soviet Union, including Ukraine and Belorussia, fared even worse. By 1944, only 28 men remained for every 100 women in this age group.

The implications of this world of women alarmed Soviet leaders for two reasons. The State Planning Committee (Gosplan) reported to the Soviet leadership that there was an "acute labor shortage" in the postwar Soviet village.[2] They worried too, about the future labor shortage, since the imbalance in the sex ratio would clearly prevent women from finding male marriage partners, and it undercut the birth rate of future workers. There might be

Replacing the Dead. Mie Nakachi, Oxford University Press (2021). © Oxford University Press.
DOI: 10.1093/oso/9780190635138.003.0002

little to be done to improve the immediate labor shortage, but the future was another matter. Nikita S. Khrushchev, head of the Ukrainian Communist Party at the end of the war, observed the women's world in the Ukrainian villages and developed a comprehensive postwar pronatalist policy to raise the number of Soviet workers in the future. His draft proposal became the basis for the All-Union Soviet 1944 Family Law.[3] Khrushchev thought it expedient that the Soviet Union make special efforts not only to "recover the lost population" but also to accelerate the birth rate.[4]

While participating countries in World War II lost population, most did not need pronatalist policies to recover from the demographic loss. The United States experienced a "baby boom."[5] Europe and Japan saw a modest but unmistakable rise, what could be called a "baby boomlet,"[6] as families started having children after demobilization brought back prewar and postwar husbands. In the case of post-imperial Japan, the loss of 40 percent of the empire's territory and the resultant repatriation from former colonies focused the leadership on overcrowding as the major postwar demographic problem, not population loss.[7]

The Soviet Union could not expect quick demographic recovery, primarily because 20 million men had perished during the war.[8] In addition, many people had been dislocated during the conflict, many prewar families and marriages disintegrated, and new forms of unions developed. Compared to the collapsed wartime birth rate, the Soviet Union's birth rate would also briefly rise in the postwar period, but the spike was very brief and would never reach the prewar level.[9] Soviet leaders, however, believed in social engineering and would not be deterred from trying to achieve higher birth rate targets.

Khrushchev already had expertise in the area of demographic policy-making, as in 1941 he had successfully convinced Stalin to tax singles in order to fund the increasing number of children held in state orphanages.[10] In 1944, Khrushchev developed a pronatalist approach well beyond the existing measures, such as criminalizing abortion, giving state aid to mothers with many children, and making divorce difficult. Khrushchev argued that all adult citizens must participate in population "growth," on average reproducing more than two children, and that those who did not raise two children should pay "bachelor" taxes.

Khrushchev's proposal considered the well-being of postwar mothers, particularly those who would raise children alone, but the policy goal was the acceleration of the birth rate. This priority was crucial in justifying the legal changes that reversed two key developments of Soviet prewar family policy: the state had mandated equality of all children, regardless of the marital status of their parents since the 1918 Family Law; and, the state had enforced paternal responsibility for childrearing since the 1936 Family Law. Previously, these changes were interpreted as a part of Stalin's going back to a more traditional family model, or a "Great Retreat" or "Revolution Betrayed."[11] In fact, the family model presented in the finalized 1944 Family Law moved away from the prewar family model, introducing "optional fatherhood" and thereby promoting unmarried motherhood.[12] One might say that, this development moved in the direction of the revolutionary vision of the family supported by Alexandra Kollontai, which advocated procreation as the result of sexual union based on love and considered the state as the responsible institution for childrearing rather than the family. However, a key difference was that this postwar development was not based on revolutionary ideology but on pronatalism, and it designated women to take primary responsibility for raising children.

Optional fatherhood and official promotion of unmarried motherhood would become central characteristics of the postwar Soviet family policy. Over time, this would lead to normalizing mother-centric families, where the mother took on most of the practical and financial responsibilities of raising children, with little or no involvement of the father in childrearing.[13]

This chapter analyzes the making of the 1944 Family Law by examining Khrushchev's draft proposal and attached explanatory documentation.[14] It reveals the development of an irresolvable tension between effective population management and protection of or support for women's well-being. The internal debate shifted the policy focus from women to men. While earlier proposals aimed at increasing support for women in the postwar period, Khrushchev's pronatalist idea encouraged men to father children outside of their official marriages and introduced greater punishments for women who underwent illegal abortions.

The tensions were represented by two groups of Soviet professionals. One group, consisting of statisticians and financial experts, primarily pushed for population management goals and tended to view women and children as nameless, faceless statistics. The other group, consisting of lawyers and doctors, were primarily concerned about the well-being of individual women and children. These differences of emphasis and empathy developed further after the promulgation of the law.

Khrushchev's original proposal aimed at incentivizing men to father children in non-conjugal relationships without undermining postwar single mothers' financial well-being. This would be possible by requiring the state to fully "replace" the father's obligation for child support for out-of-wedlock children by providing the full amount of state support for single mothers. However, the final law significantly reduced the level of state support for single mothers. This financial compromise kept all the professionals on board but compromised the policy goal of getting unmarried women to reproduce.

The World of Women and Children: The Ukrainian Origin of the 1944 Family Law

When the Soviet army recaptured the German occupied areas, they found complete devastation. While preparing his memoirs, Ilya Erenburg, a wartime Soviet correspondent, leafed through his notes from the summer of 1943. He had a long list of villages burned to the ground by the Nazis, whether for contact with the partisans or as part of scorched-earth tactics in retreat.[15] Erenburg described the "world of women" in these German-occupied areas. "There were hardly any young men, all were away fighting in the ranks of our armed forces. Those who [remained and] refused to submit [to the Germans] were murdered or deported to work in Germany."[16] These villages would not recover quickly. A count of kolkhoz residents in January 1948 revealed more than twice as many women than men between the ages of 16 and 60.[17]

N. S. Khrushchev also arrived in Western Ukraine with the Soviet troops in the spring of 1944 and found Ukrainian demography completely altered.[18] The Ukrainian population had risen and then fallen during the war. In 1939 the population of Ukraine was 30.96 million and in 1940 it had increased to 40.2 million due to the territorial gain and refugee influx that resulted from the Soviet occupation of Eastern Poland.[19] However, great losses followed. According to the 1947 report of the United Nations Relief and Rehabilitation Administration (UNRRA) that assessed the amount of aid needed in postwar Ukraine, during the three and a half years of German occupation "more than four million Soviet citizens had been murdered by the German invaders in Ukraine, and more than two million had been abducted to slavery in Germany. Of these so deported, a considerable number perished in captivity."[20] Many surviving citizens from Ukrainian villages, towns, and cities reported to the party detailed stories of how Germans shot civilians of various ages and genders, burned villagers alive, and took teenagers to Germany as forced labor.[21] In addition, Nazis almost completely exterminated Ukrainian Jews, mostly by shooting them at close quarters during 1941–1942. According to archival data, residents of Ukraine accounted for 48.2 percent of all victims in the occupied areas.[22] Many children became orphans after Nazi soldiers killed or took their parents to Germany, and some of them were sent to orphanages outside the republic.[23] Because of shifting postwar borders as the Soviet Union reclaimed western Ukraine and beyond, it is difficult to compare prewar and postwar figures, but basically the lost population was not replaced until 1960.[24]

Although the Germans were primarily to blame for the reduction of population in Ukraine, Soviet and Ukrainian nationalist fighting during and after the war further diminished the population. After the Soviet Union occupied western Ukraine in 1939, the Organization of Ukrainian Nationalists (OUN) began a new battle for independence with the Soviet forces. Their guerrilla attacks killed thousands of Soviets, and Khrushchev responded with arrests and deportations. The People's Commissariat of Internal Affairs (NKVD) also used extreme violence against the Ukrainian nationalists, even after the Soviet Union regained western Ukraine in 1944.[25]

The significant reduction of the Ukrainian population obviously threatened the labor force. The postwar Soviet government dealt with the immediate shortage by recruiting demobilized soldiers and young people (often by force), and using convicts.[26] The long-term labor supply, however, depended on the birth rate. Khrushchev likely to have pondered these issues from early 1944 on, as he began to mobilize workers to send to the front as it moved west, while screening for former Nazi accomplices.[27]

Like Alexievich and Erenburg, he would also have noticed that rural Ukraine was overwhelmingly female. How could future peasants be born, especially if women were also the only source of physical labor? During the occupation, the Germans had used women as agricultural labor, in particular, since Ukraine had been designated a grain exporter to Germany.[28] Unlike the Nazis, who wanted only labor, not children, from women and therefore legalized abortion in the occupied areas, Khrushchev wanted both production and reproduction.

The sex ratio, deteriorated reproductive health, and the breakup of family ties would all be obstacles to increasing the birth rate. These problems were worst in occupied areas because the Germans systematically killed civilians and took young people to Germany. Later, the Ukrainian nationalists, a significant percentage of the remaining males of reproductive age, went into the forests to hide. The extremely difficult living conditions would certainly discourage childbearing. Ten million people, nearly a quarter of the population, were homeless in Ukraine at the end of the war and lived in huts, dugouts, cellars, and rubble shacks.[29]

Already showing his awareness of the impact of demography on future economic development, Khrushchev had suggested to Stalin taxing the childless as part of the Soviet Union's pronatalism. The November 21, 1941, decree, "On taxing bachelors, single and childless citizens of the USSR," stipulated that the childless taxes would be subtracted from monthly salaries for practically all citizens who fit into these groups, with only rare exemptions, and the amount would be linked to class.[30] The funds raised would be used to support housing children in state orphanages.[31] Khrushchev had proved to Stalin his acumen in demographic issues and earned the leader's appreciation for his efforts.

Khrushchev's intimate exposure to Ukraine's utter destruction would have made clear that only comprehensive policies could effectively improve birth rate prospects in Ukraine. The Ukrainian leader understood that the Soviet Union as a whole faced similar problems with labor, demography, and the reproductive health of the population and, therefore, addressed his reproductive policies to the Soviet leaders in Moscow.

Ukraine's distinguished demographers and statisticians were available to help Khrushchev formulate postwar population policy. Kiev was the home of the first Institute of Demography in revolutionary Russia and the Soviet Union (1919–1938), which was headed by internationally prominent demographer and statistician Mikhail V. Ptukha. In the 1920s, Ptukha extensively researched and published on marriage and fertility in Ukraine and produced a long-term projection of population growth in Ukraine, which was discredited in the early 1930s when population and birth rate "suddenly" dropped due to collectivization and famine. He needed to explain the cause, but discussing famine and negative impacts of collectivization on population development was taboo. Ptukha most likely switched his research topic to the seventeenth- and eighteenth-century history of statistics in 1933 because of political pressure. Many of the Soviet Union's prominent demographers were purged after the 1937 Census; but Ptukha was spared, probably due to the shift in the direction of his research. Khrushchev most likely met him in the 1920s and later asked his advice in drafting postwar population policy; and Ptukha, who cared deeply about the postwar development of Ukrainian demography, agreed.[32]

The limited evidence suggests this. On September 28, 1944, M. D. Burova, head of maternity care of the People's Commissariat of Health in Ukraine, revealed that she, with Ptukha and others, had studied Kiev's future population, especially birth rate, the kind of work Ptukha had conducted earlier. The results, noted Burova, were discussed with "all of our leaders who are interested in these questions."[33] Most likely Khrushchev had gathered these obstetricians, gynecologists, demographers, and legal specialists in order to produce postwar pronatalist policy. Sometime in 1944, Ptukha also became the director of the Social Sciences Division at the Ukrainian Academy of Sciences, the perfect position from which to mobilize expertise for crafting the 1944 Family Law. Ukraine's demographic catastrophe and its scientific study by the Soviet Union's most eminent demographer, a Ukrainian, served as the basis for Khrushchev's all-Union pronatalist plan.

Discussions of Birth Rate and Family Law in Moscow

A wide range of data arriving at Molotov's office in the Kremlin alerted leaders in Moscow to the demographic catastrophe triggered by war and the extremely unbalanced ratios between men and women around the Soviet Union.[34] Moreover, in late 1943 and early 1944, several Soviet leaders foresaw postwar problems with the low birth rate and drafted new decrees for improving government support for mothers. Two factors determined the timing of these projects. After the Soviet Union's victories over the Nazis at Stalingrad and Kursk in 1943, Soviet leaders were able to consider allocating resources to priorities not directly for military use or postwar reconstruction. In 1943 the wartime collapse of the birth rate also became clear. As N. A. Voznesenskii, head of the State Planning Commission, reported to Stalin and other top leaders on March 15, 1942, the "inevitable reduction of the level of the birth rate during wartime" that he felt would "probably become manifest in the spring-summer of 1942."[35] As predicted, in 1942 and 1943 the number of births per thousand citizens was falling dramatically from 35.3 (1940) to 31.6 (1941), to 20.5 (1942) and 11.2 (1943).[36]

Vyacheslav Molotov, the first deputy chairman of the USSR Council of People's Commissars, considered two types of policy recommendations in 1943. One simply proposed to expand the government subsidies set by the 1936 law, or lower the number of children a mother needed to receive a bonus, or to increase the amount of bonus.[37] The People's Commissariat of Finance (Narkomfin) and the Central Statistical Administration (TsSU) assessed these options for the most cost-effective way of increasing births.

The second type of proposal introduced new ideas from the medical point of view. On October 12, 1943, the day on which Molotov received the second revision of the above ukase, Georgii Miterev, People's Commissar of Health, submitted to him a draft of a decree called "on measures for improving working and living conditions of pregnant women and nursing mothers."[38] Miterev argued that government support for mothers should be expanded to include all pregnant and nursing women regardless of the number of their children. This marked a shift in the pronatalist approach— from supporting women with many children to supporting all mothers, even those who had not yet given birth. Faced with a tripling since 1940 of the percentage of premature births, which reached 15 percent of total births in 1943, Miterev argued that the government needed to "carry out urgent measures for establishing maximally favorable conditions for pregnant and nursing women."[39] The new postwar issue was whether a woman could give birth to healthy offspring. Because premature birth was believed to relate to the state of pregnancy, Miterev proposed to shift the focus of support from women in childbirth as in the 1936 law to the inclusion of pregnant women and also to improve working conditions and diet for pregnant women, nursing mothers, and newborns.

Mariia D. Kovrigina, the new Deputy Minister for public health issues involving women and children at the People's Commissariat of Health (Narkomzdrav, hereafter, NKZ), was responsible for drafting Miterev's proposal for increasing support for all mothers and small children, rather than just mothers of large families.[40] The NKZ's proposal did not interrupt the ongoing discussion of state aid to mothers with many children, but the more comprehensive program of support aimed at qualitative, as well as quantitative, improvements. Yet, before either of these proposals could be finalized, events took an unexpected turn.

Khrushchev's Proposal and Informational Note

On April 13, 1944, Khrushchev, at the time the First Secretary of the Communist Party of the liberated Ukraine, submitted his draft ukase "on increasing government support to women in childbirth and mothers with many children, and the reinforcement of protection of motherhood and childhood" to Molotov. The draft was introduced by a cover letter and had an informational note (*spravka*) attached, which made clear the Ukrainian origins of the draft. After the preliminary drafting, Khrushchev had organized a conference of women in which forty people, including working women at Kiev enterprises, housewives, female students, peasant women, gynecologists, lawyers, and judges of the People's Court participated and discussed the draft ukase. In general, the cover letter argued, the women participants of the conference greeted the preliminary draft "with complete approbation."[41] The informational note, entitled "On Measures for Increasing the Population of the USSR," presented the policymaker's logic.[42]

Khrushchev's proposal was remarkable not only for presenting entirely new approaches to the question of increasing the birth rate, but also the draft ukase and *spravka* represented two ways of writing about his new policies for different types of readers. The draft ukase was written for the wider public, as if the state's main interest was the protection of mothers. The *spravka* was prepared for top echelon Soviet leaders and highlighted the acute problems of the declining birth rate in the Soviet Union and the need to take decisive action to increase fertility. For this reason the *spravka* more clearly articulated the pragmatic logic of postwar reproductive policies and detailed the policy's rationale at length. The existence of two versions clearly suggests that the leadership had consciously avoided open discussion of state-sponsored pronatalism, which introduced optional fatherhood and encouraged out-of-wedlock births. The legitimizing language they opted for was written in the paternalistic language of state care for women and children.[43]

Khrushchev's draft ukase was intended to become the law and so was written for public presentation. Its preamble reveals its goal without mentioning pronatalist thinking:

For the goal of increasing material support for women in childbirth and mothers with many children, of expanding the network of institutions for the protection of motherhood and childhood, of reinforcing criminal responsibility for crimes against the lives, health, and personal dignity of mothers and children, and also in relation to this, the introduction of some changes to the law on marriage and divorce, the Presidium of the Supreme Soviet USSR decrees . . .[44]

The draft consisted of thirty-nine articles, many of which were clearly labeled as government measures for increased protection of mothers. Other articles were included without explanation. The draft described new privileges such as increased state aid to mothers, particularly single women and mothers with many children. Single women would receive new types of government aid such as monthly subsidies for the maintenance of children, pegged to the number of dependent children.[45] In addition to the subsidies, they could send their children to free childcare facilities while maintaining the right to reclaim the child as desired. Not only single mothers but also some mothers with many children could qualify to send their children to kindergartens and crèches free, depending on their income bracket.[46] Other new privileges gave mothers with three and more children the right to transfer to the workplace most convenient for child-rearing, provision of double rations to pregnant (after six months of pregnancy) and nursing mothers, and the guarantee of rations to non-working mothers with many children.[47] Childcare and maternity institutions such as special rest homes for single mothers and weakened nursing mothers would be expanded.[48]

A comparison of Khrushchev's draft family law and the very different version already circulating in Molotov's secretariat before Khrushchev's appeared indicates that the two projects targeted different groups of mothers to increase the birth rate. Whereas the earlier draft aimed to give an extra incentive to mothers with four children considering one more, Khrushchev's proposal incentivized mothers with only two. Even more radical, Khrushchev's subsidies stated that all citizens should have more than two children or pay for those who did.

Alongside the new privileges, single mothers' loss of legal rights, more difficult divorce procedures, increased taxation for small families, and increased punishment for abortion were quietly included. Mothers would no longer be able to appeal to the court to establish fatherhood and levy child support from unregistered marriages.[49] The birth of a child outside of registered marriage would be recorded under the family name of the mother and her choice of patronymic.[50] The new law would recognize only registered marriage, require inclusion of information on marital status and spouse in the passport, and institute a complex public divorce procedure, which required the payment of 100 rubles to file a divorce case in the court, investigations, witnesses, publication of divorce announcement, and the payment of 300–1000 rubles for registering a divorce.[51]

The tax increase, from the 1941 taxation on childless citizens, was called an "amendment," included the new provision for the taxes on "parents who have only one child," and demanded one-third of the amount of taxes for the childless.[52] Only soldiers, pensioners, and students in middle schools and higher educational institutions would be exempt from tax payment.[53] Those with reproductive health problems and their spouses, who were exempted in the 1941 tax for the childless, did not qualify for an exemption in the draft ukase.[54] Most important, in the draft, punishment for women who underwent underground abortions increased from public censure or fines to three- to five-year prison terms.[55]

The draft ukase never explained why not only the childless but also citizens with one child should be taxed, why divorce should become harder, and why abortion should be punished more severely than in the prewar period. By excluding such information and emphasizing the "protection of mothers," the policymakers would be able to present the new project as a "gift" from the caring state to mothers.[56]

Unlike the draft ukase, the *spravka* stated explicitly that the new policies toward reproducing the population were necessary because the Soviet population had been significantly reduced during the war with Nazi Germany and the country needed to recover this loss. As a part of this general goal, the project proposed to make population increase a responsibility of all adult Soviet citizens and to penalize those who neglected this duty. The project separately targeted those who reproduced and those who were not reproducing. It was designed to provide privileges only to women who reproduced and to punish or penalize those who prevented conception or birth for themselves or others.

Reproduction as Civic Responsibility

The Soviet government first adopted the policy of increasing government subsidies for mothers with many children as a way to increase the birth rate in the mid-1930s. Khrushchev's proposal went beyond this prewar strategy by adding important, qualitatively different initiatives. First, he redefined a mother with many children not from the perspective of promoting large families, specifically those with seven or more children, which was deemed insufficiently effective, but from the perspective of rewarding those who participate in reproducing the population. Khrushchev and those who studied reproductive politics thought that promotion of the large family was not "sufficiently effective" for the goal of "stimulating" population increase.[57] Instead of encouraging a small group of fertile women to procreate more, the new project proposed to provide aid to all mothers of small families who would participate in the state project of increasing population: "In order to encourage procreation, it is necessary to establish payment of governmental subsidies to those mothers as well, who having two children, give birth to a third, thus entering on the path to reproducing the population."[58] For the third child, one-time government subsidies would be provided at birth. In addition, monthly subsidies for the child would be provided for five years, beginning from age two.[59] The new definition of mothers with many children as mothers who contribute to population growth by having the third child or more directly reflected the new demographic thinking of the policymakers considering regeneration of the Soviet population.

Rethinking the category of "mothers with many children" became especially necessary given the slowed birth rate in the villages, which had historically had large families.[60] This trend had begun already in the prewar period, but worsened significantly in the postwar period due to material difficulties and the lopsided sex ratio in rural areas, as many demobilized soldiers left for cities after initially coming home to the villages.[61] Policymakers in postwar Ukraine realized that it was unrealistic to hope for rapid growth of large families in villages. What seemed more realistic was to expect each adult citizen to have two or more children.

Similar to the system of giving privileges to women according to the number of children they bore, a system of punishment and penalties was necessary to incentivize citizens to bear at least two children and to help finance the increased government expenses to support childrearing. The policy anticipated crimes against reproduction, such as contraception, termination of pregnancies, or the killing of new-borns.[62] Khrushchev considered it important to increase punishment for abortion, contraception, and infanticide, and he wanted increased taxes on small families in this context.

The postwar reproductive policy recommended by Khrushchev defined crimes against population increase in terms of the three reproductive stages—conception, pregnancy, and birth—at which young life could be prevented or terminated without official permission.[63] The new project proposed severe punishment for all crimes against reproduction, with the type of punishment and intensity of prosecution varying significantly depending on the reproductive stage at which life was terminated. Regarding conception, the *spravka* strongly condemned the use of contraceptives and proposed to criminalize the production, sale, and diffusion of contraceptives, both methods and paraphernalia.[64] However, no further details were provided about prosecution.

In contrast, policies toward abortion (termination of pregnancy) and infanticide (termination of the newborn) were more detailed because they were of "particular social danger at the present time."[65] Both practices seem to have been particularly prevalent in post-occupation Ukraine. According to the head of the department of maternity care in Ukraine, this was because "the Germans had propagandized [for] abortion, because they could not take pregnant women to Germany for hard labor. Therefore, they permitted all doctors to perform abortions" despite the strict anti-abortion policy in Germany. When the period of occupation ended, Ukrainian women in both urban and rural areas felt entitled to clinical abortions under Soviet rule as well. Sympathizing with the difficulties of giving birth in destroyed Ukraine, doctors met women's expectations and continued to perform clinical abortions. This was probably because many Ukrainian women who had conceived with Germans toward the end of the war would want to terminate their pregnancies.[66]

The new proposal for fighting abortion intensified the old punitive method. It increased punishment for both abortionists and women who sought abortion, while intensifying medical surveillance over suspected abortion and hemorrhage cases in order to improve reporting to investigative authorities.[67] Under the 1936 law, the punishment for women undergoing abortion was limited to public censure for the first offense and a fine of up to 300 rubles for the second offense. Only abortionists would get prison sentences, and the length of the sentence depended on whether the abortionists had medical training or not.[68] The *spravka* particularly emphasized the importance of increasing punishment for women who had abortions and proposed prison sentences for all women involved.[69]

In addition to underground abortion, infanticide slowed population growth.[70] There were no accurate statistics on infanticide, which commonly occurred in the period between birth and birth registration. However, it is not hard to imagine that lack of contraception and difficult material conditions pushed some women to choose this path.[71] The new draft tried to reduce infanticide in two ways. First, it proposed to punish both mothers and fathers for infanticide, suggesting that there were significant cases of infanticide by fathers in postwar Ukraine. Under the existing Criminal Code of Ukraine, mothers who committed infanticide were imprisoned for up to three years. Second, it proposed to change the definition of the crime from "killing of newborn by the mother" to "killing of newborn by parents or one of them." The prison sentence for this crime would also increase to ten years.[72]

The other type of harmful practice identified in Khrushchev's draft was active avoidance of reproductive marriage: "Along with this, there should also be some measures of a compulsory character in relation to those who avoid married life, or those who despite being married and with full capability, refuse to produce offspring."[73] Bachelorhood and limiting family size were for the first time perceived to be offenses against the state that required a severe response. Given the imbalanced sex ratio, it is likely that this measure against remaining single was directed at men. Remarkably, the important policy considerations became how many times each man would impregnate a woman or multiple women and which children he would raise. In order to maximize the birth rate, the pronatalist government considered it most effective if men would produce offspring both inside and outside their conjugal relationships so that unmarried women could also reproduce.

Penalization of childless citizens had first appeared in the 1941 decree on taxes for childless citizens suggested by Khrushchev to Stalin.[74] It was the first manifestation of the idea that all adult Soviet citizens of reproductive ages were responsible for procreation and childrearing, and that the childless should subsidize state expenses for orphanages.[75] Whether or not Stalin and the tax collectors felt strongly about the reproductive obligation of citizens during the war is not clear, but certainly practical state financial interests in finding new revenue for running orphanages aligned with Khrushchev's proposal to create a new taxation system for the childless.[76] Penalization of childlessness was also directly tied to the government's need to pay a substantial increase in subsidies to mothers.

The *spravka* noted that in view of the significant expansion of government subsidies for mothers with three or more children, the rate of taxes to be collected from childless adults under the 1941 Law was insufficient.[77] The levy for a childless taxpayer was set at a quarter of the official per head childcare cost in the state orphanage in Ukraine. Calculations in line with this formula suggested that postwar taxes for the childless would double for workers, white-collar workers, and peasants.[78]

This financial projection was based on conditions specific to Ukraine. The new taxes would allow the government to cover the full costs of childcare in an orphanage for 135,000 children, 15 percent of the children born in Ukraine in 1940. Since, in most cases, the government paid part of the cost of childcare for single mothers, the project would be able to support more children and all single mothers.[79]

Khrushchev's project envisioned a radical shift from the principles of the 1941 decree. Then, people who could not have children for health reasons, military personnel, and students were exempt from the "childless tax," whereas the new project would significantly reduce exemptions:

> There is no need to exempt those who can not have children because of their health condition from these taxes because these taxes are also a form of participation of childless citizens in the national expenditure on the upbringing of the young generation. There is no need to exempt military personnel from these taxes. Exemption should remain for those military personnel who are on emergency service and who are in the ranks of front-line forces. In relation to pensioners, the first and second groups of pensioners are exempt, if the pension is their only source of income.[80]

In short, postwar reproductive politics made reproduction a civic responsibility.

Khrushchev's draft projected that those who had only one child would also be taxed one-third of the burden imposed on the childless.[81] Taxing one-child families was not only a financial measure but also a reflection of the new demographic thinking whereby population reproduction and growth were possible only when each woman had two or more children. Low birth rate was not limited to the barren; it also included women who could bear children but used reproductive practices that limited the number of children in the family to one, which harmed the stability of population and population growth. The *spravka* stated that "such practices as limiting the number of children are not compatible with government interests, especially at war and in the immediate postwar years." The new focus on one-child families materially disadvantaged the insufficiently reproductive, while stressing the negative views "of the government and society toward conscious limiting to a one-child-family."[82]

Together with state aid and penalties, the third way Khrushchev's project tried to motivate citizens for procreation was to make them aware of their moral obligation to provide children for the state through education:

> It is necessary to conduct a series of measures with the goal of inculcating into the consciousness of the wider masses the understanding of the state

and societal importance of population growth in the Soviet Union, especially in postwar conditions.[83]

Such education would have also undermined the obvious state effort to conceal the primary pronatalist goal of the new law. Probably due to this tension, educational measures did not appear in later drafts or the final law.

Khrushchev's plan for the postwar family law was single-mindedly pronatal, as the *spravka* revealed. Men would be targeted, if they remained single. Women would be watched carefully to avoid abortion or infanticide. Penalties and punishments would be liberally bestowed. For the first time, all Soviet citizens were caught up in a "reverse-birth-tax," where those who contributed to population growth received magnificent bonuses and all others paid. Although this was new, it was along the lines of the 1941 tax on bachelors. The major exception to the universal scheme were those fighting at the front for whom the war had not yet ended.

Encouragement of Out-of-Wedlock Births

One of the novelties of Khrushchev's pronatalist project was to encourage and support out-of-wedlock births.

> The question of stimulation of procreation among women who are not married for one reason or another (widows of those who died in the war and unmarried girls) has special significance at the present moment and in the approaching postwar period.[84]

With the seemingly inevitable rise of unmarried motherhood in the postwar period, the government anticipated an increased number of women demanding child support from their male sexual partners. In the prewar period, the Soviet government had already experienced the limitations of a child support system that could not ensure the welfare of children when too many fathers refused child support.[85] The system's failure resulted in masses of neglected and abandoned children. From the perspective of raising rates of childbirth, it also made mothers lacking child support unlikely to bear additional children. Moreover, in cases where fathers provided child support for children they had left, they were likely to limit the number of children in their new families, since they would have limited means for them. Thus, the existing system was doubly problematic for motivating citizens to procreate, both among those receiving child support unreliably and those paying child support who often became reluctant to reproduce in the new household.

Khrushchev's project instead proposed a system where both unmarried women and prospective fathers would not be discouraged from procreation in their relationships and where the welfare of their existing and future children could be assured. This was done by providing government support to single mothers, reintroducing out-of-wedlock births, and giving the unmarried mothers the "right" to leave their children in state orphanages. Because of the state's full involvement in raising out-of-wedlock children, women would not have to be afraid of getting pregnant, and male partners would not have to be afraid of impregnating their sexual partners. Khrushchev's proposal was designed to encourage both men and women to have non-conjugal sexual relationships that would result in procreation.

The project's description about the end of paternal support for out-of-wedlock children was written in the paternalistic language to show that the primary intention of the Soviet government was the protection of mothers, not an increase in out-of-wedlock births. For example, it described the governmental aid to single mothers as a policy that would "free women from claiming child support from the child's father."[86]

Another example is found in the way the project characterized the new system of supporting single mothers after the end of child support. Once these mothers could no longer expect to receive support from their male partners, the Soviet state was to give them the option of either receiving government aid for childrearing or of sending the child to an orphanage for free. The goal of this measure was described as "alleviating the single woman's burden in bringing up a child" and thus "cannot be applied to women still seeking child support from their husbands."[87] That a single mother might have other reasons to want to receive child support from her partner rather than receive government support was never considered in this policy statement.

The government was prepared to provide subsidies for childrearing, regardless of the number of children the single mother had. Here Khrushchev's project was based on the notion that "in order to increase the population of the USSR, [we] should carry out a series of measures directed . . . toward establishing the most favorable conditions for the upbringing of children who are born to unmarried mothers."[88]

The monthly subsidies would range between 150 and 300 rubles depending on the number of children in order to match the amount a single mother would have received under the prewar family law from a father who earned 600 rubles monthly, the estimated average wage of Ukrainian workers at the time.[89] Thus, Khrushchev's proposal justified promotion of single motherhood based on the assumption that the government support replaced prewar child support, a point that would be lost as the draft was revised in Moscow.

To release men completely from child support responsibilities required preventing unmarried mothers from making legal claims against biological fathers. This was to be achieved by recognizing only registered marriage as legally binding and by changing the birth registration system and allowing only legal wives to register their children under the patronymic and family name of the father. Under this arrangement, child support for the children of single mothers would become the responsibility of the state. In the case of two-parent families, the married couple should shoulder full responsibility for childcare, even in the case of divorce.

The idea of determining childcare responsibilities depending on whether the family is single or two-parent seems simple in theory but could not be easily implemented under the existing marriage and divorce laws. In the prewar period, common-law marriage was legally recognized, and the registration of newborns required the mother to report a father's name, so there were no legally fatherless children in the Soviet Union. Unless a mother decided to call herself "unmarried" publicly, she could identify herself as "separated" or "divorced" rather than "unmarried." Although this was sometimes legally contested in child support cases, as long as no official document was necessary to demonstrate marital status and as long as the mother had full control over identifying the father of her child through birth registration, a self-identification of unmarried status, instead of common-law, was a matter of maternal choice, and all children could have officially recognized fathers in the prewar Soviet Union. Moreover, the mother always had the right to demand child support from the official father. If she won the case, her partner would have to pay for child support, even if he had another family and other children. These financial and legal ties between two families blurred the distinction between single-mother and two-parent families in the prewar era.

The idea of the 1944 Family Law was to provide government aid to single mothers and fatherless children, but not to two-parent families, so the state needed to create a clear boundary between the two types of family. Once the family was formed, it was important that the legal status of the two-parent family, in particular, was stable. Any shifts in legal status of the two-parent family would result in reallocating childcare responsibilities. The prewar period had already demonstrated that fathers often did not fulfill childcare responsibilities. If this became common after the war, the new system of childcare would collapse, and the mothers without child support would limit the number of children they had. Moreover, if the state provided support to divorced mothers without child support, its expenditures would increase. In addition, if the divorced father provided child support, he would be less inclined to have additional children in later marriages.

The establishment of a clear distinction between single-mother and two-parent families affected the birth registration system, marriage, and divorce. The first was simple: only mothers in legal marriages would be allowed to register children under the actual father's name. "Only registered marriages were recognized as legal and generated rights and obligations between spouses."[90] With this definition of marriage, the government could easily identify single mothers and provide childcare support, while their male partners would assume no responsibility for childrearing. Similarly, the government could easily identify two-parent families, made fully responsible for their own childcare. To make marital status easily identifiable, the project proposed to include information about the place and time of marriage registration, as well as the name, patronymic, and family name of the spouse in all internal passports.[91]

Changes in divorce procedure aimed to stabilize marriage as a social, legal, and economic institution for raising children. The *spravka* condemned those who wished to divorce as being "frivolous toward family and family relationships."[92] Since the stability of marriage was the primary consideration, the new law also made divorce procedures more complicated and expensive. Similar steps had been taken in the 1936 Family Law, but to a lesser degree. While the 1936 law had raised divorce registration fees and increased the percentage of salary to be paid for child support, the postwar project would establish "increased material expenditures for the breakup of conjugal relations and increased procedures for dissolving marriages legally."[93] Divorce would become significantly more time-consuming and costly, involving many steps including publishing an announcement for filing a divorce case and paying fees for submitting a petition to the court and for registering divorce at the office of marriages, births, and deaths (known as ZAGS).[94]

These new policies marked a radical shift from the revolutionary family policies of the late 1920s, which legally recognized common-law marriages and ended out-of-wedlock births. The 1926 Family Law changed the 1918 one which recognized only registered marriage as legally binding, because lawmakers realized that the institution of de facto marriage without registration prevented many women from getting child support from their male partners. Thus, the historical reason for this redefinition of legal marriage in 1926 was to ensure child support, but it had the significant and enduring side effect of making marriage into an institution to be defined by subjective experience.

The 1936 Family Law placed limits on this notion of marriage as the product of individual will by creating a more complex procedure for divorce registration. It further disciplined fathers who failed to stay in either common-law or registered marriages and refused support to their children, especially after separating from the mother. This ended "postcard divorce" but recognized common-law marriage as the legal basis for the attribution of inheritance rights. The 1936 law left childcare responsibilities for couples in both registered and common-law marriages unchanged. Legal recognition of common-law marriages again became an important topic of discussion in 1939 when the Civil Code of the USSR was being amended. Some demanded an end to the legal recognition of common-law marriages, but countering arguments prevailed.[95]

Khrushchev described his proposed change as going back to the "legal norm" as defined in the 1918 law.[96] However, his attack on common-law marriage can also be seen as the introduction of Ukrainian family policy, which did not fully recognize common-law marriage, as the basis of All-Union legislation. The Ukrainian Law stipulated that only "registration with the public Registrar is indisputable evidence of the existence of marriage unless it is rejected in court," but it allowed marriage registration even when a member of the couple was in a common-law marriage with a different partner, suggesting that common-law marriage was not legally recognized.[97]

The *spravka* characterized the goal of the new marital policy as "further strengthening the family."[98] This concept of "strong family" was not about strengthening emotional ties among married couples and family members.[99] On the contrary, it could contradict the state's key goal, since, statistically, maximization of birth rate required that adult males impregnate more than one female partner. What the project tried to enforce was the social, legal, and economic form of marriage as a distinct and stable unit where various rights and obligations are clearly defined. The *spravka* proposed to give three-year prison sentences to those who entered a new marriage while already registered with another partner, and five-year sentences to those who neglected their childcare responsibilities, suggesting the primacy of childcare responsibilities over marriage.

These three administrative changes designed for population increase would result in the creation of the legal category of out-of-wedlock children, or fatherless children, for the first time in Soviet history. Despite the resulting financial, legal, and psychological disadvantages for millions of single mothers and their children, the language of the *spravka* rationalized the scheme as the natural outcome of a state policy aimed at improving single mothers' well-being:

> Unmarried mothers are freed from the necessity of claiming child support for the maintenance of a child, and therefore are not in need of formal identification of who indeed is the father of the child. Thus, the child would be registered at ZAGS under the mother's family name with the patronymic of her choice.[100]

In the postwar period, this linguistic technique to establish the image of the paternal Soviet state helped to legitimize the state policy of encouraging non-conjugal reproduction and creating the category of out-of-wedlock births. The legitimating paternalistic language helped to present the new policy as the provision of welfare measures by the caring state rather than as measures to increase births under any circumstances. The Soviet leaders recognized the need to use the power of language carefully. In the *spravka* which was prepared for the top Soviet leaders, the legitimating language was repeatedly deployed to emphasize the correctness of the policy proposal for solving demographic problems by creating illegitimacy. Such legitimizing language for the creation of out-of-wedlock births never appeared in the draft ukase. Instead, the project's focus on single mothers was intentionally obscured by not discussing them and not clarifying the distinction between unmarried mothers and war widows. In the *spravka*, such descriptive expressions as "mothers not in marriage," "women who are not in marriage for one reason or another (widows of those who perished in the war, girls who have never been married)," "single mothers not in marriage," or "mothers who have a child outside of conjugal relations" appeared.[101] In contrast, the draft ukase used "single mothers (*odinokie materi*)" to refer to all of the above except for one instance.[102] This word choice suggests that the Soviet policymakers wished to be less clear about their focus on out-of-wedlock births in the legal document for public use than in the internal document, because they were aware that governmental promotion of births among unmarried mothers was questionable and that the reintroduction of out-of-wedlock births was a black mark on the Soviet propaganda claim that all children were created equal. But the pronatalist imperative forced the Soviet leaders to set aside their ideological qualms.

Protection as Surveillance of Mothers

In order to promote demographic growth, Khrushchev's project proposed to significantly increase maternal privileges both for working mothers and housewives. That the postwar policy was prepared to treat women's reproductive work on a par with productive work was expressed in two ways. First, all pregnant women would receive double rations after the sixth month of their pregnancy and breast-feeding mothers for the entire period of lactation. Second, non-working mothers with more than four children, who in the past were not eligible for rations, were to be given a ration card equivalent to the normal portion of bread and other foodstuffs for a worker.[103] These proposals suggest a significant shift in the conceptualization of legitimate Soviet citizenship in that housewives' (non-workers') fertility was valued as the productive work of female workers.

The legal arrangement in the late 1940s that released mothers with young children from prisons also reflected the importance of women's reproductive and childrearing role.[104] Women's role in population increase and maintenance of children's welfare was considered so important that some petty crimes that women committed could be dismissed. Such privileges were not available to men, even if they had many children. This suggests that female fertility became an object of reward as much as obligation, but male fertility was a requirement in the postwar pronatalist state.

The 1936 law decreed that the government would build an extensive network of childcare facilities to help working mothers in cities and villages. The NKZ later put forth plans to expand this system. These plans were rarely fulfilled, but the number of kindergartens, crèches, and maternity homes increased in both urban and rural areas. During the war, some were destroyed or abandoned, and many others were taken over by other institutions, but postwar efforts to expand the network were renewed.[105]

All work places were to open kindergartens, crèches, rooms for nursing mothers, and milk kitchens.[106] At least two directions of institutional development were considered for the postwar expansion of maternity homes and childcare institutions. One proposed to establish new institutions for mothers who were active participants in the war. This idea of honoring veterans, which became common for men, was not adopted for postwar mothers.[107]

The other focused on accommodating unmarried mothers and their children. It proposed special rest homes for single mothers and weakened nursing mothers. Such a measure was considered necessary, particularly because it was believed that single women were often unable to give birth in their place of residence because of their unfavorable family relations or bad living conditions and that they should temporarily leave for a different place during pregnancy, childbirth, and post-partum recovery. Leaving single mothers alone in questionable conditions led them to often "place their children with relatives and abandon them, and sometime even kill them."[108]

It is clear that the major function of the home for single mothers was not only protection of single motherhood but also to "remove such phenomena" as abortion, infanticide, and/or abandonment by single mothers. If the TsSU's estimate was correct, that approximately a quarter of the total births per year would be out of wedlock, infanticide by single mothers could pose a significant danger to the whole project of population increase.[109] Moreover, single mothers were targeted not only because the policymakers believed they considered abortion or infanticide reproductive decisions but also as a way to protect single mothers from the "harmful vestige in the conscious-ness of backward elements about the fact that such a mother had 'committed' something 'illegal' and 'unnatural,' and considering her harmful morals, she can be subjected to public reproach and feel 'remorse.'"[110]

In this way, the rest homes for single mothers in the *spravka*'s conception shared some key elements with the Irish homes for mother and child, although the contexts were vastly different. In 1920s and 1930s Ireland, unmarried pregnant women, single mothers, and illegitimate children were forced into mother and child homes run by the Catholic Church to isolate them from a society where illegitimacy and abortion were considered religious and legal violations. Their key functions were to ensure that the unmarried woman did not resort to abortion, to "protect" her honor by hiding her from public eyes, and to raise illegitimate children.[111] In the Soviet Union, even though out-of-wedlock births were to be implicitly encouraged by postwar pronatalist policy, the project also envisioned accommodating single women to be monitored by the medical control commission that would determine who should stay in these facilities and for how long.[112]

Khrushchev's *spravka* outlined new family policies aimed at increasing the birth rate by defining participation in the reproduction of population as a civic responsibility for all Soviet citizens. The "quota" for each adult citizen was set at two children, which was the minimum for stabilizing population size. For women who had exceeded this quota, the government would provide privileges. Those who failed to meet it would pay taxes. Those who actively escaped from reproduction would be punished more severely than before. In this system, almost no adult person was allowed to get away from reproductive responsibilities, except those still killing the enemy.

The new pronatalist policy was developed according to the particular vision of gender relations that Ukrainian policymakers anticipated. The most acute issue was the excess number of adult women compared to adult men. The government leaders projected that there would be many women who would have non-conjugal relationships and, as a result, one-quarter of the total childbirths in the postwar Soviet Union would be out of wedlock. Policymakers assumed that most male citizens would marry and have children, while some of them would also father out-of-wedlock children. Projecting the rise of non-conjugal sex between men and women, the *spravka* neatly divided postwar society into single-mother families and two-parent families. Changes in marriage and divorce law, as well as state support, would make both of them into functional fertile family units. The 1944 Family Law, and even more so Khrushchev's draft, envisioned the creation of special new privileges, including exclusive spaces for the use of single mothers, but these would also enable the state to oversee women and their role in the demographic process.

Experts' Reactions: NKZ, TsSU, and Narkomfin

During the three-month process of preparing Khrushchev's proposals to become the final family law, various experts provided recommendations and suggestions. Some evaluated the proposal's effects on the well-being of women, at whom the new law aimed, encouraging them to give birth to a larger number of children than they would have in the absence of the law, and at children, whose status the new law would determine. Others treated women and children mostly as numbers and evaluated the feasibility and effectiveness of the proposal for the goal of accelerating the birth rate. Medical and legal experts recommended a number of qualitative changes, expressing concern over out-of-wedlock children not being allowed to register the name of the father under any circumstance.

On May 3, 1944, Miterev, the People's Commissar of Health, reported to Molotov about the NKZ's examination of Khrushchev's draft.[113] He expressed strong support for the proposed ukase's goal of "stimulating" the growth of the birth rate, calling it "timely" and "appropriate."[114] In order to show that Khrushchev's concerns based on Ukraine were relevant to the USSR, Miterev attached the analysis of the natural population movement for 1943 conducted by A. M. Merkov.[115] Merkov reported that between 1940 and 1943 the birth rate of the Soviet Union decreased by 68 percent and that already by 1942 the number of civilian deaths alone (2,403,818 persons) exceeded the number of births (2,030,160 persons), thus leading to depopulation.[116] He assessed the losses of World War II as "much graver than the demographic consequences of the war of 1914," where the reduction of the birth rate was only 22 percent. There was almost no increase in infant mortality in 1915, unlike the rapid rise in 1942.[117]

Referring to Merkov's demographic information, the NKZ harmonized with Khrushchev's basic message, arguing that the Soviet Union needed to take measures toward increasing the birth rate. But with a special professional interest in the public health of mothers and children, the NKZ considered it necessary to make various changes and additions to Khrushchev's draft ukase on issues such as the ukase's title, the period of provision for single mothers, the preservation of single mothers' rights to receive child support for cases predating the new law, the terms for the extra rations for pregnant and nursing mothers, the number of years that housewives would receive rations, and the degree of punishment for abortion.

The NKZ's particularly revealing suggestion was that the de facto father maintain the right to register children under his family name, if the mother, even unmarried, agreed to it. This demonstrates the NKZ's emphasis on the well-being of out-of-wedlock children, who would otherwise officially have no father. This suggestion, undoubtedly made and/or approved by Kovrigina, was never incorporated into any of the later drafts or the final ukase of 1944. She made the same suggestion again in 1948 and was again ignored.[118] However, this omission would haunt the 1944 Family Law until its ultimate revision in 1968, serving several times as a rallying call for would-be reformers both inside and outside the state bureaucracy.

The NKZ's suggestions for food allocations, maternity leave, and working conditions for pregnant women and nursing mothers were incorporated into the revised versions of Khrushchev's draft and the final ukase. The reduction in punitive measures against women and medical professionals in case of abortion or infanticide was also adopted. However, the suggestion to give de facto fathers the possibility of registering an out-of-wedlock child under their last names was rejected, because it concerned the very core of postwar reproductive politics initiated by Khrushchev. Between the late 1940s and late 1960s, several attempts were made to reform the family law, the birth registration procedures, and divorce requirements, but all failed, at least in part because legal experts were afraid that the identification of the de facto father with a child could create a basis for the child's mother to demand child support. Key amendments to the 1944 ukase had to wait until the 1965 law easing divorce and the 1968 law on the basic legislation of the USSR and Soviet Republics on marriage and family.[119]

Meanwhile, statisticians and economists made quantitative evaluations of the proposal's effectiveness. The TsSU collected and analyzed demographic statistics of the Soviet Union, and the data it produced were used for all spheres of Soviet economic, social, and cultural planning. Postwar reproductive policy-making also required financial assessments based on demographic data, such as the projected number of children, single mothers, and mothers with many children. On May 31, V. N. Starovskii, the head of the TsSU under Gosplan, reported to Molotov his analysis of recent birth rate figures and the projection for 1944–1950 as well as the breakdown of the families by the number of children. He discussed the sharp drop in the number of births from 4.63 million in 1941 to 2.09 million in 1942 and identified the primary cause as the "drawing of a significant part of the male population into the army."[120]

Starovskii projected that the birth rate would grow after the end of 1945 because of the demobilization of soldiers, partially compensating for the wartime loss of male population and many civilian deaths in the occupied regions. According to his optimistic projection, prewar levels of approximately 6 million annual births would resume by the beginning of the 1950s.[121]

Starovskii's report concluded that, based on his calculation from the census, "the number of children born to unmarried mothers will consist of about one-fourth of all births."[122] It is not clear exactly how the percentage of out-of-wedlock children was drawn from the data; however, Starovskii apparently expected the rate of out-of-wedlock births to rise slightly in the postwar period and assumed that prewar marriage trends would resume once conditions were normalized.

Finally, Starovskii presented an estimate of adult women of childbearing age broken down by the number of their children at the beginning of 1944, which showed that, of approximately 37.5 million women, 12 million were childless, 10 million had one child, and 8 million had two.[123] The data provided by the TsSU on birth rate trends and the number of children born in common-law marriage was transmitted to Narkomfin, which used it to estimate the costs of promulgating a revised version of Khrushchev's draft ukase.

After the NKZ's submission of its comments on Khrushchev's draft ukase, sometime in mid-May of 1944, a revised version of the draft ukase was prepared and submitted to Stalin. Based on the TsSU's projection, Narkomfin was able to calculate the cost of the increased government support for mothers. For example, the number of out-of-wedlock children for 1945 was estimated to be 500,000.[124] Narkomfin simply multiplied the estimated numbers of single mothers and mothers with many children by the proposed level of one-time and monthly governmental subsidies to calculate the approximate budget.[125] The total cost of the project for 1945–1950 was estimated at 58.8 billion rubles. Lacking data on the number of single mothers who would qualify as mothers with many children (three or more), these projected costs did not include government subsidies for single mothers with many children, suggesting that the actual costs would be higher.[126]

Narkomfin also actively proposed ideas to reduce costs. Considering the estimated 58.8 billion rubles too high, Commissar Zverev recommended the reduction of subsidies to rural mothers, who were set to receive the same as urban women. "It is expedient to reduce the amount of subsidies for single mothers and mothers with the third, fourth, fifth, and sixth children in the village to half of the amount set in the project." Zverev projected a savings of 17.4 billion rubles, if such village women received half of what their urban counterparts did.[127] Whose subsidies to reduce became key issues as the draft entered its final preparatory stage.

The "Birth" of the Mother-Heroine and the Maternal Status Hierarchy

The May draft was entitled "on the increased governmental support for pregnant women, mothers with many children and single mothers, the reinforcement of protection of motherhood and childhood, as well as on the establishment of the honorary title 'Mother-Heroine' and of the foundation of the order and medal 'Motherhood Glory,'" and included new awards of medals and other honors for meritorious mothers. These "medal" drafts when compared with Khrushchev's draft ukase highlight how the discussion of postwar reproductive policies developed after Moscow leaders accepted it as the basis for Union-wide reproductive policies.[128]

The medal drafts introduced several new themes to Khrushchev's draft ukase and modified Khrushchev's propositions to make them financially and legally practicable under All-Union conditions based on the evaluations made by legal, financial, and public health specialists. In general, the new changes were made to systematically categorize all adult citizens by the number of their children and to allocate privileges and punishments according to family size. Another characteristic of the medal drafts was the attempt to tone down the level of penalty for those who did not sufficiently contribute to population growth and to seek a balance between reward and punishment. In addition, single mothers became a permanent part of the document title, and financial considerations received renewed attention.

Some of the changes made between Khrushchev's draft ukase and the medal drafts reflect significant developments in thinking about reproductive policies. First and foremost, they introduced status "honors" in addition to cash subsidies for mothers with many children. The introduction of the medal system contributed to further categorization and differentiation of female citizens by the number of children they had. The introduction of this status hierarchy would be especially effective in developing renewed incentives for mothers with seven or more children, who had already been receiving grants before the war. Under the new system, mothers with four or more children would receive either the medal or order of "Motherhood Glory," or the honorary title of "Mother-Heroine." "Motherhood Glory" had a total of seven ranks for mothers with many children, while Mother Heroines occupied a special niche at the top of the hierarchy.[129]

The medal drafts clarified several important issues in Khrushchev's draft ukase. It stated that children who died or were missing in the war would be counted. This principle was applied to governmental subsidies to mothers with many children as well as to honorary titles.[130] In addition, the mothers of dead or missing children were exempted from the taxes for citizens with few children.[131]

The medal drafts dictated the timing for granting new aid to mothers with three to six children, specifically for children born following the publication of the ukase.[132] Likewise, single mothers would receive subsidies only for their children "born after the publication of this ukase."[133] This decision was consistent with Khrushchev's general position of disregarding citizens' prewar or wartime contributions to the state. Mothers with seven or more children, already eligible to receive governmental subsidies under the 1936 Family Law, would continue to receive the prewar subsidies. Only the delivery of postwar children would trigger the increased aid mandated in 1944.[134]

The medal drafts introduced the policy of differentiating between the rural and urban populations, proposing lower levels of subsidy to village mothers with many children, Narkomfin's idea originally aimed at reducing projected costs.[135] Three different versions, with the associated projected costs, were presented to Stalin.[136] These numbers were measured against a projected five-year revenue of 17.8 billion rubles from the new taxes on single people and citizens with few children, but the increased taxes would not cover new costs.[137] In the end, the 1944 ukase made no distinction between rural and urban on this issue, which suggests Stalin decided against it. In contrast, single mothers suffered a blow from the budgetary ax with projected monthly payments dropping from 125 to 100 rubles for the first child, from 225 to 150 for the second, and from 325 to 200 for the third and additional children.[138]

The medal drafts also incorporated expert legal opinion to establish more detailed, complex, and costly procedures for legal divorce. Instead of one, divorce would now involve two courts. Submission of a petition to the People's Court with a payment of 100 rubles would lead to an investigation and "reconciliation between the spouses." Only when reconciliation efforts failed there would the plaintiff gain the right to appeal to a higher court. To further discourage the estranged, the range of fees for registering a divorce at the local ZAGS jumped from the 300–1,000 rubles in Khrushchev's draft ukase to 500–2,000 rubles.[139]

The medal drafts made substantial changes to the new tax structure as well. Khrushchev's draft ukase proposed new taxes on single citizens and citizens who had only one child. Khrushchev proclaimed that all citizens of reproductive ages were responsible for participating in the process of reproducing the population, regardless of their physical condition. Some refinements were added to these basic premises.

Citizens with two children would be taxed 0.5 percent of their salaries, single-child families would pay 1 percent, and the childless 6 percent.[140] The tax on citizens with two children was significant because it suggested that only a contribution to growth rather than to stability was sufficient to fulfill one's responsibility to the state and society. Moreover, the new tax scheme significantly reduced the proposed tax rates for the childless and citizens with one child in comparison with Khrushchev's draft ukase, which originally proposed 10 percent and 3.33 percent.[141] The medal drafts expanded the pool of taxpayers, but charged lower tax rates.

The medal drafts further defined the age range for reproductive responsibilities. For men, the tax was levied on those between 20 and 50 years of age, and for women between 20 and 45 years of age. These ranges signaled the state's desire for citizens to begin reproductive life early. For a female citizen to have three children by age 20, she would have to begin childbearing at the age of 16 or 17, procreating regularly every year. Otherwise, penalties were unavoidable.

With this new scheme, the object of taxation shifted to citizens with two or fewer children. Accordingly, the terminology to describe the category of citizens subject to taxation changed from the childless, as in the 1941 Law, to the childless and "citizens with few children" or "one-child family" in Khrushchev's draft ukase, and to the childless and "small families" in the medal drafts.[142] This new tax scheme defined the ideal family size for state demographic politics in the postwar Soviet Union.

While widening the group of taxpayers, the medal drafts took greater account of postwar conditions by creating more exemption categories. Khrushchev's *spravka* proclaimed that "there is no need whatsoever to free from the tax payment those who cannot have children for health conditions . . . [or] soldiers."[143] Only soldiers and officers on active duty, students up to 23 years old (for women) or 25 years old (for men), and those who had pensions as the sole source of income were exempt in Khrushchev's draft ukase.[144] The medal drafts made concessions to bereaved families and invalids. They also exempted wives of soldiers and officers, women who received pensions and subsidies for single mothers, citizens whose children died or were missing in the war, and invalids of the first and second groups. Moreover, both female and male students up to 25 years of age would be exempt from the taxes.[145]

The input from relevant experts further developed Khrushchev's universal hierarchy of citizenship based on the number of children and the graduated system of rewards, penalties, and punishments. Those with two children were now integrated into the system as taxpayers. Only parents who replaced themselves and then had a third child to help replace the wartime dead would be moved from the category of taxpayers to that of the subsidized. Other novelties were consideration of reduced payments to rural mothers, concessions to war participants and their wives, and an expensive, two-tier divorce procedure.

In June, one more draft appeared, revising the scenario offering rural mothers half the subsidy of their urban counterparts and including several significantly new insertions. Interestingly, the June draft reintroduced explicit calls for population increase, language present in only Khrushchev's *spravka*. The introduction to the June draft clearly stated that "during the war and after the war, as a result of the need for an even greater increase of the birth rate, further expansion of these measures of governmental support are necessary."[146] Who proposed this insertion is unclear, but Molotov added: "During the war and after the war, when many families have more significant material difficulties, further expansion of governmental subsidies is necessary."[147] Molotov's version with the language of the caring state became definitive in the actual ukase. The reappearance of the direct articulation of the project's aim and its subsequent replacement with the idea of expansion of governmental aid to mothers confirms that Soviet leaders considered it inappropriate to publicly cite the demographic basis for postwar family policy.

The June draft also eliminated the harsher punishments "for crimes against health, life, and dignity of women and children" in Khrushchev's draft. Instead, a new article instructed the state prosecutor to "prosecute offenders for illegal abortion, forced abortion, insult or humiliation to the dignity of women-mothers, and persistent nonpayment of child support in accordance with the existing criminal code."[148] Reflecting the NKZ's recommendation, articles regarding infanticide were also eliminated. In this way, the key revisions made to Khrushchev's draft between April and June 1944 reflected considerations of financial costs, the definition of the number of children an adult citizen should have, and provision of incentives for women to have one more child.

The Final Ukase and Its Gendered Consequences

The final pronouncement, "On increasing government support for pregnant women, mothers with many children, single mothers, and strengthening preservation of motherhood and childhood; on the establishment of the honorary title 'Mother Heroine,' the foundation of the order 'Motherhood Glory,' and the medal 'Motherhood Medal,'" was published on July 8, 1944. The text involved only slight revision from the June draft, while aiming to reduce project costs. The amounts of government subsidies for mothers with many children and single mothers as well as the definitions of honorary titles were determined based on Soviet leaders' ideas about which mothers deserved state aid and how much incentive they needed for additional reproduction.

Notably, the 1944 Family Law made no distinction between subsidies for urban and rural mothers. Instead, it reduced subsidies to mothers with three, four, five, and six children in both areas.[149] At this stage, there was no further reduction proposed in the amount of subsidies for single mothers.

The final version of the 1944 Family Law modified the medal system in order to provide a graduated scale of reward so that all mothers would have sufficient and varied incentive to carry one more child to term. It replaced the medal of "Motherhood Glory" with a "Motherhood Medal" to be given to mothers with five or six children. Women considering a third, fourth, or fifth child were offered qualitatively as well as quantitatively different rewards for additional births. Thus, a third child would bring a one-time payment, a fourth guaranteed monthly subsidies, and a fifth came with status honors. This change might have been made to partially compensate for the reduction in subsidies for this category of mothers. In the course of a few months, Soviet leaders, bureaucrats, and experts had elaborated a system of reproductive rewards and penalties that would affect every female citizen. (See Table 1.1)

There is no evidence that the draft was widely publicized for public debate, as was the case with the 1926 and 1936 family laws.[150] While the pronatalist aim of the law seemed to have been obvious to contemporaries and later historians alike, the "true" aim of the law aroused various speculations. For example, some contemporaries speculated that the law tried to protect soldiers' wives from wartime girlfriends. But this argument was not made in the *spravka*, where the logic of postwar pronatalism under Stalin and Khrushchev was most clearly articulated.[151] It would be a decade before Khrushchev would make his pronatalism public.

Under the extraordinary scale of demographic damage done to the country by the war, Soviet leaders could have publicized their pronatalist intentions and promised full moral and material support for postwar single mothers and their children. Khrushchev's draft pointed toward this path, by

Table 1.1 The 1944 Family Law's System of Rewards and Penalties

Number of Children	One-time Payment	Monthly Subsidies	Honorary Title	Taxes for Small Families
0	–	–	–	6% of income
1	–	–	–	1% of income
2	–	–	–	0.5% of income
3	400 rubles	–	–	–
4	1,300	80	–	–
5	1,700	120	Medal of Motherhood II Degree	–
6	2,000	140	Medal of Motherhood I Degree	–
7	2,500	200	Order of Motherhood Glory III Degree	–
8	2,500	200	Order of Motherhood Glory II Degree	–
9	3,500	250	Order of Motherhood Glory I Degree	–
10	3,500	250	Mother-Heroine	–
11 and more	5,000	300	Mother-Heroine	–

Source: *Vedomosti verkhovnogo soveta soiuza sovetskikh sotsialisticheskikh respublik* 37 (1944): 1.

proposing to educate citizens about their reproductive responsibilities, to provide single mothers with government support at the same level as child support, and to increase punishment for insulting or humiliating unmarried pregnant women or unmarried mothers. However, the final law veered away from this path. One advantage of this choice was to avoid articulating men's role in the new pronatalist policy, which incentivized them to engage in non-conjugal sex by liberating them from the legal and financial responsibilities of fathering out-of-wedlock children.

Not only did the final law extensively employ the language of the caring state to conceal pronatalist intentions, but it also significantly reduced the amount of government support for single mothers from the level proposed by Khrushchev's draft, ostensibly for financial reasons, but in fact based on political and demographic calculations. Measures to protect single mothers from negative opinions were erased from the final ukase, which was consistent with efforts not to highlight the single mother in the law. In the end, the initial idea in Khrushchev's draft of replacing the biological fathers' child support fully with state aid was not realized. Postwar, unmarried mothers would receive less financial help from the state than they would have received from biological fathers under the prewar law. The state aid for single mothers, as well as mothers with many children, was cut in half in 1947, because, the law stated, at a time when the Soviet economy was expanding and the ruble was strengthening, "it would be unjust to preserve the high level of aid set up during the war."[152]

One of the concepts added in Moscow was a new status hierarchy for fertile mothers. The new definition of "mothers with many children" created millions of qualified women, making the concept of "mothers with many children" less special than in prewar years. The introduction of titles such as "Motherhood Medal," "Motherhood Glory," and "Mother-Heroine" solved this problem by creating numerous differentiated categories. Through award ceremonies, Mother Heroines became publicly recognizable. Given the rapid fall in fertility among Ukrainian and Russian village mothers in the postwar period, the majority of these glorified mothers came from Central Asia.[153]

Beyond the Soviet Union, this provision would have an unexpected impact on Communist China. After the 1949 Revolution, China would adopt Soviet policy on family and marriage and attack contraception, sterilization, and abortion as a cultural invasion by the capitalist West.[154] Chinese mothers with many children were awarded similar honorary titles and were also celebrated in the press.[155] In this way, glorification of especially fertile mothers became postwar socialist practice beyond the Soviet Union.

Unlike other pronatalist policies of modern states in the early twentieth century, the newly promulgated Soviet family law treated women equally without differentiating on the basis of ethnicity, class, and/or health. Instead, a new social divide between married and unmarried mothers opened. Not only would the latter find themselves without rights in their intimate dealings with men, but their children would also face prejudice as "fatherless" or "out-of-wedlock," a category the Soviet Union had proudly eliminated in 1918.

After the promulgation of the law, how postwar unmarried mothers chose patronymics for their children got to the heart of the matter. There were likely two main variations. Some would have wanted to include the biological father's name, like Galina, who used the biological father's first name for her son's patronymic.[156] Others would have wanted to bury the memory of the person who had abandoned them.

Cultural representations offer examples of both. In the 1973 movie *Stepmother*, Natalia, the former lover of Pavel, used the biological father's first name for the patronymic of her out-of-wedlock daughter Svetlana. Natalia raised Svetlana alone without ever telling Pavel about his daughter. Pavel only learned about Svetlana when he received the news of Natalia's death. By then Pavel was married to Aleksandra and had two children. The couple decided to adopt Svetlana, then eight years old. They simply changed her family name from Natalia's to Pavel's, as she already had Pavlovna as her patronymic.[157]

In contrast stands the famous 1979 movie *Moscow Does not Believe in Tears*, set in the late 1950s. Factory worker Katerina, the main character, falls in love with Rodion and spends the night with him after a romantic dinner. As a result, Katerina becomes pregnant. She fails to get an abortion, and Rodion refuses to help her, calling it a "woman's business." Katerina gives birth to a baby girl while living in a factory dorm. She names the baby Aleksandra, after her own father, Aleksandr. At a party celebrating the birth of the baby, Katia's friend's husband pauses while delivering the first congratulatory toast to ask what the baby's patronymic will be. Katia answers, Aleksandrovna, again referencing her own father. No hint of the traitorous biological father is allowed.[158]

The reintroduction of out-of-wedlock status can be understood as a partial, gendered adaptation of Alexandra Kollontai's revolutionary idea of "free love," widely considered a euphemism for responsibility-free sex.[159] Most Bolshevik leaders in the 1920s frowned on this idea, and there is no reason to think that Khrushchev was a supporter. Ironically, however, postwar leaders promoted responsibility-free sex in the name of population increase. In the absence of socialized childrearing and reliable contraception, responsibility-free sex was never real for women.

2

Abortion Surveillance and Women's Medicine

It is necessary to expand criteria for [clinical] interruption of pregnancy and introduce criteria about everyday-life conditions.

Academician B. A. Arkhangel'skii (1945)

We will act individually. When we consider that a woman who is a war victim has the right to an abortion from the medical point of view, we will give her permission.

Dr. A. L. Estrin,
Chairman of the Moscow Central Abortion Committee (1945)

Medical professionals succeeded in convincing postwar policymakers not to levy additional punishments on women for abortion.[1] After the promulgation of the 1944 Family Law, doctors would continue to view a growth in the birth rate as linked primarily to improved reproductive health and women's well-being rather than due to increased sexual encounters and reduced number of abortions. Doctors understood that long family separations, as well as Nazi occupation of the western part of the Soviet Union, led to many unwanted pregnancies. Many women were undergoing illegal abortions, but not everyone could find medically trained abortionists, and unfortunately women died from botched abortions. As their husbands and lovers were often absent, dead, or handicapped, many postwar women would have to singlehandedly earn a living and raise children. Under these harsh conditions, Soviet doctors wanted to make safe abortion available.

In the postwar years, doctors of women's medicine in various countries faced a rise in unwanted pregnancies and chose pragmatic, extralegal, or illegal solutions to meet the challenges of postwar problems. In Germany, the anti-abortion policy, spelled out unequivocally in paragraph 218 of the

Replacing the Dead. Mie Nakachi, Oxford University Press (2021). © Oxford University Press.
DOI: 10.1093/oso/9780190635138.003.0003

German Criminal Code, officially remained in effect in the postwar period. Nevertheless, when an estimated 2 million German women in Berlin were raped by Red Army soldiers in the spring of 1945, many women demanded safe abortions, and doctors helped them. Doctors' response soon led to the granting of legal abortion for victims of rape.[2]

Similar horrors befell Japanese women. After the Soviet Union declared war on Japan, the Red Army crossed the border into Manchuria, where Japanese colonist women were targeted for rape and many became pregnant before being repatriated back to Japan. Although abortion was a crime, the Japanese government secretly set up abortion clinics near the ports where pregnant women were landing.[3] In both cases, doctors performing abortions did not face prosecution; rather, their extralegal actions were supported or encouraged by the local or national government. Doctors and policymakers supported women's decisions and justified extralegal abortions not only out of sympathy for them but also in support of ideas about racial purity, eugenics, health, and the protection of postwar family.[4]

The postwar suspension of anti-abortion policy sometimes brought about long-term policy changes. This was not the case in Germany; both the Western and Soviet-occupied zones of Germany had restricted abortion by 1950.[5] In Japan, not only rape victims, but also women who wished to limit family size in difficult postwar socioeconomic conditions, demanded safe abortions. The confluence of women's demand for wider access to safe abortion, rampant underground abortions, and the eugenic concerns for racial purity and healthy race among medical professionals and policymakers, as well as concerns about overcrowding on the part of US occupation forces, pushed through a dramatic legal change.[6] As a part of the Eugenic Protection Law, abortion became widely available in 1949 in Japan and persists today.

Soviet doctors also wanted to provide postwar women with wider access to safe abortions. In the case of Russia, mass rape was not the central concern. Rather, massive postwar demobilization increased sexual encounters, many of which ended in unwanted pregnancies and venereal diseases.[7] Unlike in Germany and Japan, pronatalist Soviet top leaders demanded greater anti-abortion surveillance. Nonetheless, Soviet doctors wanted to give access to safe abortion to many women who would not qualify for legal abortion under the very restrictive prewar regulations. Thus, they were forced to take illegal actions to deal with the situation created after the war. Doctors asked among themselves how to make safe abortion available in such a way that it could be justified to an anti-abortion and pronatalist regime. Top specialists of women's medicine took two major positions, as represented in the epigraphs. The first position was to change the law, by expanding the existing list of criteria for clinical abortion; the other was to allow doctors to make judgments individually and provide abortion depending on the patient's conditions and needs.[8]

Soviet doctors wanted to help women terminate pregnancies less over racial or eugenic concerns than over issues of health and provision of effective prophylactic care. During the war, doctors had realized that the existing abortion surveillance system had frightened women away from seeing doctors. This problem would block doctors' efforts to improve postwar reproductive health and the birth rate. In this context, this chapter discusses the abortion surveillance system that developed after the 1936 criminalization of abortion. It covers wartime abortions and reproductive health problems that became common in the postwar period, ranging from infantilism and amenorrhea to infertility. The mounting problems with women's health became the basis for medical specialists to argue that abortion surveillance work was preventing them from improving women's health and undermining doctor-patient relations. To counter this doctors supported the "individual approach," where they attempted to provide clinical abortion through legal and almost illegal subterfuge. Here the Soviet practice of "*blat*," doing favors based on personal relations, was often at work. Mariia D. Kovrigina, Deputy Commissar of health in whose bailiwick women's medicine lay, did not criticize these ideas in the immediate postwar years.

However, a dramatically changed political climate from 1946 onward adversely impacted the ability of Soviet professionals and bureaucrats to decide the policy and practice of women's medicine. A 1947 show trial found two medical researchers, Nina G. Kliueva and Grigorii I. Roskin, guilty of disclosing their secret cancer cure (that did not work) to Americans and led to the disciplining of scientists and intellectuals. The field of women's medicine was also heavily affected by the so-called KR affair, leading to a purge of the Moscow Institute for Gynecology and Obstetrics.[9]

The Soviet Abortion Surveillance System

When the Soviet government criminalized abortion in 1936, it claimed that the achievements of socialism had made it unnecessary. Now that women were equal to men, capitalistic exploitation had ended, and the material well-being of women was growing, the earlier legalization could be reconsidered. Since 1920, Soviet women had practiced fertility control through legalized abortions, and so criminalization had a significant and enduring effect on women's reproductive health and practice. Women, especially in urban areas, who used to seek clinical abortion for fertility control, could no longer rely on this method legally. At the same time, education about contraception essentially stopped, and contraceptive devices became even scarcer.[10] Despite the law's claim, women did not find themselves receiving sufficient economic and social support for childbearing and childrearing. Instead, they began to seek the safest possible option for underground abortion.

In order to deter these crimes, a system of abortion surveillance was set up in 1936. It consisted of a system controlling clinical (legal) abortion, and another system for prosecuting non-clinical (illegal) abortion. The former system was operated by the centralized network of abortion committees established in local women's clinics. Each local committee consisted of a gynecologist, a therapist, and a local medical administrator. When gynecologists considered that their patients needed an abortion, these women presented their medical records to the local committee. The local committee reviewed the applications based on the criteria for clinical abortion defined in November 1936.[11] Questionable cases were forwarded to the central medical committees, located in regional centers, which granted permission on an individual basis. Only after approval by a committee could women get clinical abortions.

In contrast, the system of prosecution was coordinated by the NKZ, the People's Commissariat of Justice (NKIu), and the state prosecutor, involving doctors, legal experts, and prosecutors. At the central level, Narkomiust outlined the legal aspects of the surveillance system, and the NKZ determined the definition of non-clinical and criminal abortion. At the practical level, doctors reported to the prosecutor about non-clinical abortions and provided medical evidence of the abortion. Only when sufficient medical evidence was presented would the prosecutor investigate the case to establish criminality. Under the 1936 law, women were sentenced to public censure for the first offense or a fine of 300 rubles for repeat violations. The success of abortion prosecution greatly depended on the cooperation of doctors to report non-clinical abortions and provide medical evidence of criminality.

Soon after criminalization, doctors found various insufficiencies with the system of granting clinical abortion. Many considered it necessary to make clinical abortion free of charge because it was a medical necessity, and they demanded a legal change in the fee basis.[12] Lacking contraceptives, doctors asked how to protect women who had chronic conditions that required clinical abortion if they became pregnant. There were also problems with the way certain conditions included in the criteria for clinical abortion were diagnosed because not all of them were gynecological or obstetric. For example, the diagnosis of schizophrenia, which soon became one of the most common for women applying for clinical abortion, was apparently made not by psychiatrists but by obstetricians and gynecologists, suggesting that doctors quietly tried to provide women with clinical abortions whenever possible.[13]

Not only the system of granting clinical abortion but also the punitive abortion system faced several problems once put into practice. For example, doctors did not report all incomplete abortion cases to prosecutors. Sometimes, they did not provide prosecutors with necessary medical documents to prove criminality. Prosecutors also showed limited willingness to force compliance. Some did not always take up doctors' reports and others dropped cases where the accused woman had died.

Since women were trying to control their reproductive lives without contraceptives, and abortion surveillance was not enthusiastically and thoroughly monitored by legal and medical professionals, it is no surprise that the number of abortions began climbing after only a one-year dip in 1937.[14] These results and malfunctions of the surveillance system were attributed to insufficient instructions about prosecution of abortion in the 1936 law. To plug these holes, in November 1940 an order entitled "Instructions on the Battle against Criminal Abortions" was issued, providing a detailed definition of criminal abortion and the relevant tasks for both doctors and prosecutors. In this document, a criminal abortion was defined as "any intentional interruption of pregnancy, in the absence of appropriate paperwork." Within twenty-four hours of an examination, doctors or other medical personnel were required to send signed documentation to the local prosecutor regarding suspected cases of criminal abortion. The fact of criminal abortion would be legally established only by a woman's medical history and the evidence of artificially interrupted abortion provided by a doctor. In case of death, medical personnel were to report to the prosecutor, and an autopsy would be conducted.[15]

The 1940 instructions confirmed the primary role of medical specialists and the secondary role of prosecutors in abortion surveillance. One important new detail of the procedure outlined was that prosecutors were generally not allowed to interrogate medical personnel or to summon them as witnesses. This was included because of the consideration that a doctor's legal confrontation with patients would negatively affect doctors' relationships with female patients in general. Doctors were supposed to stay behind the scenes once the investigation had begun. Only when there was a "real necessity" were the investigators allowed to request a doctor's involvement.[16]

The prewar abortion surveillance system created space for doctors to autonomously influence the fate of women who wanted to get a criminal abortion. Doctors could ensure that a woman did not end up in the court by performing an abortion without reporting it to prosecutors or by not reporting to prosecutors incomplete abortions that ended up in a hospital or clinic. They could also report an incomplete abortion case to prosecutors without providing sufficient documentation for prosecution. Both doctors and female patients were aware of doctors' autonomous power and doctors used it to their own benefit. By becoming the state's first line of defense against abortion, medical professionals also became women's last hope in a struggle with Soviet pronatalism. The effectiveness of the 1940 instructions in prosecuting abortion cases could not be fully tested before the war began in 1941.

War and Abortion

Wartime sexual liaisons without condoms resulted in unwanted pregnancies, and the rate of abortions shot up from 31.2 per 100 births in 1940 to 52 per 100 births in 1943.[17] However, for the most part, the intention of the 1940 instructions to improve abortion surveillance lost steam after June 1941. After many doctors were mobilized to the Red Army, local medical committees were effectively dismantled. The Central Abortion Committee in Moscow never met with local abortion committees during the war. As the absolute number of abortions declined together with the fall in conception numbers, anti-abortion work seemed less urgent than before. Due to evacuation, women's mobility was very high, making it difficult for medical institutions to keep track of pregnant women. The only exception might have been the Red Army with 600,000 women volunteers sent to the front.[18] Many pregnancies happened in the military. As pregnant women in the army had to be discharged, many tried to abort. Others regarded it as their chance to leave military life, though they understood that their families would not welcome them back pregnant and discharged from the service.[19]

Besides wartime organizational difficulties, many doctors and prosecutors lost interest in prosecuting abortion. This problem was discussed by the representatives of the NKZ, the Narkomiust, and the State Prosecutor's Office at a meeting recorded as "On the Question of the Battle against Abortion" on December 25, 1943. N. Ia. Sosenkova, a representative of the USSR People's Commissariat of Health (NKZ SSSR), reported that abortion committees had ceased to function, and doctors were often granting clinical abortion for any reason they thought appropriate, including socioeconomic ones. Many physicians left insufficient medical records explaining the reasons for clinical abortion.[20]

Dr. E. K. Isaeva, a representative of the People's Commissariat of Health, Russian Soviet Federated Socialist Republic (NKZ RSFSR), discussed cooperation with prosecutors. In 1940, she had worked with a prosecutor specializing in abortion cases, but during the war, no prosecutor worked on abortion cases.[21] This was a common finding among doctors during the war. Dr. G. L. Vainshtein from Tashkent reported in 1944 at the First Joint Plenum of the Council of the NKZ SSSR and the NKZ RSFSR on Maternity Care that a local prosecutor had been indifferent when the physician "personally called the district prosecutor and told him to send someone quickly because a woman wanted to inform [him] about where she had received an abortion. The prosecutor answered, 'I have no time.'" For a whole month, no investigator came to interview the doctor, and the woman died.[22] Because prosecutors were generally not interested in pursuing abortion cases, they often terminated investigations when women died of botched abortions.[23] Prosecutors' lack of interest in pursuing abortion cases would remain an issue for as long as abortion remained illegal.

Some doctors appeared frustrated with uninterested prosecutors, but others did not want to be involved in helping to prosecute abortions.[24] No doubt, many doctors were sympathetic with women who decided to terminate pregnancies because their husbands were absent, it was hard to raise multiple children, or the pregnancy was the result of casual or forced sex. Doctors often believed that anti-abortion policy should be accompanied by measures to improve mothers' living conditions. During the war, Dr. Vainshtein suggested to the local Communist Party organs in Tashkent that state aid to mothers should be given not from the seventh child, but from the third or fourth to encourage women with two or three already not to get an abortion.[25]

But what became the most fundamental problem for doctors was that their involvement in prosecution caused distrust between doctor and patient. Dr. Isaeva complained that the prosecutor was an intruder in the maternity clinic. Doctors should avoid non-medical tasks, since "if doctors begin to fulfill investigative functions, prosecutors will have nothing to do. What will happen to maternity clinics then? But [if] we allow doctors to confront women, what good does that do?"[26] Another NKZ representative V. A. Iushkova also expressed the opinion that the doctor's role as an informant was chasing women away from maternity clinics. "If two-thirds of pregnant women avoid maternity clinics, it is because they are afraid that clinics report their pregnancies to [investigative organs]."[27]

Prosecutors complained about doctors' work. Urakov, a representative from the State Prosecutor's Office, accepted doctors' criticisms but pointed out that doctors were also to blame for the poor quality of documentation submitted to the prosecutor.[28] "Can we send cases with such [poor documentation] to the court? No, we cannot, if we do not have objective medical information which demonstrates that there was an abortion as a result of criminal intervention." He added that the prosecutor's work to investigate abortionists, which did not always require medical documentation, had improved, implying that a doctor's involvement could be an obstacle to prosecution.[29] Thus, neither prosecutors nor doctors had strong interest in prosecuting women for abortion during the war, and doctors were concerned that strict surveillance would chase women away from clinics.

Prosecution of underground abortions was simply neither practical nor a priority in the liberated areas. Ukraine was an important case. Ukrainian doctors reported that self-induced abortion was one of the most harmful social phenomena for the postwar effort to increase birth rate. Since the promulgation of the 1936 Anti-Abortion Law, the number of underground abortions and induced miscarriages was steadily increasing.[30] The growing phenomenon was particularly alarming "not only because the birth rate has significantly decreased, but also because we have lost many women who were physically healthy and capable of procreation."[31] Since the liberation, the reapplication of the Soviet anti-abortion law was also ignored because of Ukraine's loss of experienced personnel to investigate and prosecute abortion. Newly hired investigators and prosecutors in the postwar period needed to be trained to enforce the criminalized abortion policy of the Soviet Union.[32]

Instead of prosecution, doctors were seeking to help improve women's health. As Professor A. Iu. Lur'e, an obstetrician in Kiev, complained, because women in Ukraine took clinical abortion for granted, it was difficult to conduct anti-abortion work: "We sometimes cannot work or provide gynecological support, because abortions suffocate us. Due to this, there is an incorrect atmosphere among women, who consider that abortion can be conducted without punishment."[33] Because there were few maternity care institutions in postwar Ukraine, and since many women with hemorrhaging came for medical assistance, doctors often had to accommodate women with incomplete abortions together with pregnant women. Some doctors considered this practice harmful to the morale of the pregnant. Lur'e argued, "It is politically incorrect to have pregnant women lying next to women with [abortion-related] hemorrhage. We should establish the abortion-only hospital. Ukraine has entered this path. The NK[Z] (of Ukraine) has issued an order about the establishment of abortion-only hospitals in Kiev. It would be very important to have such a directive from Moscow."[34] Although Professor Lur'e criticized women feeling entitled to clinical abortions, his proposed measure was actually to satisfy women's demand, by providing them with an institution dedicated to terminating pregnancies to save their health and lives.

A central directive was never issued, but a similar development took place in Leningrad.[35] Following the examples of Leningrad and Ukraine, several local health administrations also organized special hospital wards for botched abortion cases to provide efficient and effective care, while separating these patients from other gynecological cases.[36] Practices that developed in some of the most devastated areas influenced other parts of the country.

Postwar Women's Reproductive Health Problems

During the war, much of the medical infrastructure was destroyed or occupied by other Soviet institutions. The dire shortage of instruments and drugs, common to all fields of medicine, was worse for maternity care, which was considered secondary to directly war-related specialties such as surgery and epidemiology. For the same reason, most obstetricians and gynecologists who were mobilized to the army worked outside their specialization.[37] The importance of gynecology and obstetrics also diminished because the number of births dramatically declined during the war, and many women stopped going to maternity clinics.[38] But the 1944 Family Law, which clearly stated the Soviet government's commitment to improving conditions for women, helped revive the fields of women's medicine, gynecology and obstetrics, within Soviet medicine, both materially and in terms of prestige. In November 1944, the government issued a decree requiring that all spaces formerly used as maternity homes, women's clinics, and childcare facilities be returned to their original functions in the service of motherhood.[39]

Gynecologists and obstetricians were tasked with responsibility for birth rate growth. This was challenging because, in addition to general postwar public health problems, such as untreated infections, malnutrition, and unsanitary living conditions that negatively affected the health of women and newborns, there were many indications that these conditions and even worse ones during the war were causing infertility, miscarriages, and premature births. Compounded by all negative health phenomena was the continuing increase in criminal abortion. Since the NKZ had recommended against increasing punishment for abortion in the discussion of the 1944 Family Law, the medical establishment would bear a special responsibility for reducing abortion by other means. Despite this expected role, postwar doctors actually believed in the comprehensive and prophylactic approach for enhancing reproductive health. At the newly founded Academy of Medical Science, Professor M. S. Malinovskii, a renowned obstetrician, clearly stated in August 1945 that population growth was possible through a comprehensive approach to multi-faceted postwar problems in women's health:

> The essential problem and today's task . . . is a fight for the health of the mother and her newborn. . . . In the postwar period, this task particularly supports the most important task of the postwar period—natural population growth. This is a colossal, greatest problem of Soviet industry. For us, it is above all a problem of all-round maintenance of the highest function of motherhood, the establishment of optimal conditions for its multi-sided maximal development.[40]

Abortion was a part of this comprehensive approach, and doctors expressed this position openly among themselves in the early postwar years. Then, the question was how to provide clinical abortions for women in need under the existing anti-abortion system.

Soviet gynecologists and obstetricians were responsible for improving women's reproductive health so that women were healthy enough to conceive and that this resulted in the maximum number of births for each woman. This task involved improvements in all facets of women's reproductive health, including the treatment of several acute and frequent gynecological and obstetric conditions. The discussions focused on various damages caused by wartime conditions that affected young women's ability to conceive and carry pregnancy to term, such as sexual infantilism and amenorrhea.

The rise in the infant mortality rate, a major indicator of the overall level of public health, was alarming for Soviet medicine as well.[41] In September 1945, USSR Commissar of Health G. A. Miterev, while chairing the conference on maternity care, reported that in Moscow maternity homes the infant mortality rate was 8 to 10 percent per year, sometimes rising to 16 percent per year. Such appalling conditions alarmed not only medical administrators but also the public. The results were complaints, rumors, and fear.

> I have received so many signals both from mothers and responsible organs that demonstrate that this issue is going beyond the medical profession. All these deaths generated the opinion that some kind of wrecking organization exists in Moscow which artificially infects the navels of newborns, especially of baby boys. With the war over, this group will be reactivated, strengthening its activities in order to prevent replenishment [of the population].[42]

Miterev went on to say that such ideas were groundless, but he still considered it an important reflection of mothers' distrust of maternity homes.

Since the field of maternity care was responsible for the health of newborns, gynecologists and obstetricians should have considered fighting infant mortality one of their most important tasks. In reality, they tended to consider their primary task helping women, not infants, and thought improvement in maternal reproductive health during pregnancy could help bring down infant mortality.[43] Soviet doctors of women's medicine believed that "mothers' interests are supreme" and "naturally, the mother always comes first."[44] Due to this general orientation, women's reproductive dysfunctions became the focus of postwar maternity care.[45]

During and immediately after the war, infertility was recognized as a widespread problem among Soviet citizens, female and male. For the pronatalist state this was a core concern. As Academician B. A. Arkhangel'skii pointed out, gynecologists understood little about mechanisms or treatments, recognizing a wide range of causes, including abortion and "wartime conditions." In order to provide useful information to women who wanted to get pregnant, he called for specialized research on infertility.[46]

Postwar infertility was discussed among women's temporary reproductive health conditions and within infertile marriages. For the former, the spread of venereal disease during the war—in particular, untreated gonorrhea—was identified as a major cause.[47] One common postwar cause of infertility as well as miscarriages and premature births was "infantilism" among young women, characterized by the disrupted physical development of sexual organs under wartime conditions. Malnutrition, poor housing, and unhealthy work places were blamed. Professor Malinovskii, the great authority in obstetrics, stated that doctors "must pay particular attention to those women who were on the verge of sexual maturity during the war years. We must take into account the possible negative impact of infantilism and a whole series of diseases related to infantilism, such as premature births, stillbirth, etc."[48]

Among infantilism's symptoms, Professor A. M. Agaronov from Odessa argued that underdevelopment of the uterus was particularly prevalent. His opinion was based on his 1935 study at a medical institute in Erevan of Armenian women who were repatriated from Turkey after the Armenian genocide in 1915. Those between 8 and 15 years old during that period suffered from underdeveloped uterus, infertility, and premature births later in life.[49]

If this turned out to be the case in the postwar Soviet Union, as a prophylactic measure against miscarriages and premature birth, women with infantilism had to be located and treated before they became pregnant. Professor A. P. Nikolaev articulated the importance of conducting prophylactic work during adolescent development,[50] which would require the universal examination of all young women.

Among adult women, a widespread postwar symptom was amenorrhea. Professor V. P. Mikhailov argued that the shock of experiencing bombardments, the departure of relatives to the front, and the stress of constant tension at home and work all contributed to widespread amenorrhea. For example, a 30-year-old female doctor suffered from amenorrhea right after her husband's conscription, but her periods resumed when her husband visited her in 1942. Similar cases were widely cited in support of this theory.[51] Importantly, they suggested that amenorrhea was not a result of infertility, but this could not be confirmed. Further research on amenorrhea was called for to secure the health of "the nation's [child] bearers."[52]

Lack of mass data on women's reproductive health was an obstacle to researching female infertility. Dr. Osenbaum of the Institute for Obstetrics and Gynecology of the Academy of Medical Science stated that in order to conduct successful academic studies of female infertility, it was essential to gather detailed materials, not only on infertile, but also on fertile women.[53] Special attention should be made to detect syphilis, tuberculosis, endocrine diseases, and anamnestic data. Abortion records would also be crucial. Such information would help in understanding the process of becoming infertile, the dynamics of the disease, and effective methods of treatment.[54] But mass data, particularly of those not suffering from infertility, would be extremely hard to collect without women's desire to share their information with doctors. Again, doctors needed women's participation in order to develop effective treatment.

In addition to female infertility, doctors discussed "fruitless marriages," a phenomenon that directly undermined the goals of the 1944 law. This topic was hotly debated at the Second Plenum of the Joint Council for Maternity Care of the NKZ SSSR and RSFSR at the end of 1945. The first problem was identifying the infertile party. Professor P. V. Manenkov argued that men could be held responsible in more than a third of the cases.[55] Professor I. L. Braude emphasized that, going beyond women's medicine, gynecologists should study male infertility by researching sperm.

This discussion revealed the Soviet Union's prewar efforts in artificial insemination. Dr. Ivanov of a Moscow maternity clinic shared his clinic's experience in artificial insemination since 1935. Out of 2,000 infertile couples, artificial insemination was tried thirty-two times, and eleven cases had positive results.[56] Although the rate of success was low, artificial insemination had technically been proven feasible. However, there were legal issues that posed difficulties for doctors interested in this technique. The key issue was whether the sperm donor should be a relative of the husband or remain anonymous. Professor M. N. Pobedinskii voted for the former to avoid congenitally undesirable traits. In the legal fog generated by new technologies, this seemed to be the safest route.[57] Others, such as Professor Braude, took up considerations of anonymous donors.

> I think that from the legal point of view, it would only be less dangerous if the donor was anonymous, for who would be considered the father of the child born of artificial insemination? The biological father would be the donor, but this would be very difficult to establish from the legal point of

view. Thus, it seems that limiting the donor to relatives *a priori* would be wrong.[58]

Dr. Ivanov agreed with Braude, particularly since sometimes husbands had no relatives. At his clinic, mutual anonymity prevailed. The two parties signed a contract with the doctor as mediator. Even the suggestion that an additional witness be present often provoked protests from the female recipients.[59] Because artificial insemination still had many legal and technical problems, as well as a low success rate, most gynecologists and obstetricians regarded the treatment of female infertility as primary.

Besides conducting infertility research, all doctors agreed that prophylactic measures were necessary to reduce infertility among women, especially young girls. Doctors considered it necessary to educate girls about "marital hygiene," involving discussion of venereal disease, abortion, and various reproductive disorders.[60] Some doctors argued that in such meetings the importance of a stable marriage needed to be emphasized as the core prophylactic practice. Professor A. G. Butyrin said that this was particularly important because "the war has brought some dissonance and will bring [further] dissonance to this foundation [of our family]."[61] Thus, doctors understood that successful research needed to go hand in hand with prophylactic and educational work. Increased fertility could only come from women's mass cooperation and participation. However, in reality Soviet women were avoiding medical professionals, fearing their role in abortion surveillance.

Doctors' Conflicted Roles

As the importance of increasing women's participation in medical care became apparent in the immediate postwar period, doctors roundly condemned the existing surveillance system and suggested new approaches. The first point of conflict concerned the doctor's role as investigator of illegal abortions, which prevented women from seeking medical aid. At a meeting with Mariia Kovrigina in May 1945, outspoken Academician B. A. Arkhangel'skii sharply criticized the existing abortion policy and called for a radical change in the surveillance system.

I consider that the [current] measures for fighting abortion are wrong. The doctor is made into an investigator. He collects evidence, for which he alienates women from himself and from the maternity clinic. It is necessary to expand criteria for [clinical] interruption of pregnancy and introduce criteria about everyday-life conditions. Also, instructions need to be given to maternity clinics regarding the application of contraceptives.[62]

Arkhangel'skii's demand to make contraception available to women was a point other doctors had also raised before the war so that doctors could help women who could qualify for clinical abortion not to conceive in the first place. Many doctors were interested in the possibility of reviving the prewar project of developing contraceptive devices.[63] In December 1946, at a Ministry of Health (MZ) maternity conference, Dr. N. M. Polinovskii criticized the lack of contraceptive devices for women who had conditions that qualified them for medical abortion. As a result, some had repeated pregnancies and medical abortions. At the conference, doctors identified types of contraceptive devices and chemicals for women and requested significantly increased production.[64] Repeated earlier requests had not led to any perceptible increase.

Since the surveillance system operated on women through fear, many would simply avoid official visits to doctors.[65] This undermined general prophylactic and educational measures, but even worse, it meant that many nonclinical abortion cases would only come under medical supervision after the damage was done. Ironically, by scaring women away, punitive surveillance produced its own victims. The rising casualties of the war on abortion could also serve as statistical proof of the surveillance system's necessity. The process was as circular as it was deadly.

Doctors found that, fearing prosecution, many women were avoiding the maternity clinic and its record-keeping. Moreover, after unsuccessful abortions women often waited until the last minute to seek medical intervention, hoping that their problems could be resolved without going to the doctor or fearing that the doctor might save the fetus.[66]

Realizing the unintended effects of abortion surveillance, Professor Nikolaev expressed his frustration:

Is it useful to turn doctors at maternity clinics and maternity institutions into investigators? Suspicions . . . are driving women away from the maternity clinics and forcing them to put off hospital visits until the last minute.

As a result, women often come to the hospital when they are already beyond medical assistance.[67]

Pre-pregnancy examinations were most desirable, everyone agreed. However, as long as there was a possibility of pregnancy, and therefore abortion, women feared the indelible ink of the medical chart.

Sharing the view that the doctor's role in surveillance work prevented improved medical care for women, Dr. Isaeva, head of the RSFSR maternity care, argued that the key issue was one of trust between doctor and patient: "I categorically protest that doctors in any way publicly participate in this [judicial-investigative] work. A woman should not know that her doctors report to prosecutors. Otherwise she will not trust the doctor and will not consult our medical institutions. Abortion will go underground."[68]

Dr. M. K. Gesberg, Director of the First Gynecological Hospital, warned that doctors' support for abortion surveillance work was cooling. "Doctors should not be required to conduct investigative confrontations with their patients or satisfy endless summons to judicial-investigative organs. Such conditions disturb the doctor in his immediate work and reduce his desire to conduct work in the present [anti-abortion] direction."[69] M. M. Kliachko, a counselor of the Moscow municipal medical administration, discussed how a confrontation between doctor and patient ruined their relationship and invited mutual mistrust. She complained that investigators often did not understand this:

Confrontation between doctor and patient should never be tolerated. This reduces the doctor's authority and puts him in a difficult position. What could a confrontation do? A woman told the doctor that she had an abortion, but told the prosecutor, subsequently, "No, I did not say that." However, unfortunately, judicial-investigative workers do not understand how much damage they would bring by organizing confrontations. They do not understand and do not want to understand. I will give you one example. A prosecutor of Rostokin raion called up a doctor and asked him to come over while the woman, about whom the doctor had provided relevant materials, was in the prosecutor's office. The doctor said: "I will come later. It is not necessary that the woman knows about this."[70]

Doctors also expressed frustration that prosecutors were not doing their job in abortion surveillance. Dr. A. L. Estrin said that prosecutors frequently did not respond quickly when doctors reported a case of abortion, and often no action was taken. Because some women understood this, they were not afraid of going to a maternity clinic with hemorrhage.[71] Kliachko thought that prosecutors did not consider abortion a crime and complained that they were not developing a method of investigation. Dr. Gesberg suggested that investigative organs establish a group to work exclusively on abortion cases. He said to the state prosecutor, "Even if these are uninteresting cases from your point of view, you still have to work on them." Isaeva agreed with Gesberg about the need for special investigators for abortion cases, a practice initially begun in 1940.[72]

Doctors depicted legal investigators as insensitive and unsympathetic, but the lawyers counterattacked, hinting broadly that doctors' unwillingness to establish a criminal case of abortion was also to blame for the failure of surveillance. After the doctors' speeches, Khlevnikov of the NKIu cautioned against criticizing only the prosecutors. He insisted that a major cause of poor surveillance work was a lack of efficient information exchange among the medical, investigative, and judicial administrations. In particular, many discrepancies often existed between medical and legal materials. As an example, Khlevnikov noted that even the clearest evidence of abortion, such as incomplete abortions, did not always result in a criminal case.[73] The fact that the prosecutor did not begin registering abortion cases until 1944 may be partially responsible for this malfunction. However, insufficient desire among doctors to get involved in prosecution of abortion cases was also responsible for the poor rate of prosecution. To prove this point, he argued that cases that got to the court with sufficient documents provided by the doctor generally got appropriate sentences.[74]

Comrade Braslavskii, state prosecutor of the USSR, admitted that prosecutors were not doing a very good job with abortion cases, but he also defended them by blaming doctors for producing inadequate materials for investigation. For prosecutors, abortion was especially difficult to investigate because it was a crime in which the victim had no interest in revealing the criminal and actively wished the investigation to fail. Under such conditions, prosecutors needed close contact with doctors, without making that cooperation public knowledge. Braslavskii agreed that investigators needed more experience with abortion cases and that some of them should specialize in this area. Practically, however, there were not enough investigators available for abortion cases. Without specific ideas for immediately improving surveillance, he proposed working-level discussions involving doctors, prosecutors, and legal specialists.[75] These exchanges show that many of those who were involved in abortion surveillance did not relish their roles but could not criticize the system in public, so instead they blamed others.

Instead of official visits to a trained doctor, many women preferred unofficial care. In the villages, they visited *babki*, women healers, midwives, and abortionists who were not trained in Western medicine. In cities, women tried to arrange unofficial visits to doctors or babki through networks of friends and acquaintances. There were always doctors willing to help women obtain illegal abortions, particularly since some doctors did not consider it a real crime.[76] Cash bribes might not have been the typical payment for such an arrangement, but since doctors' salaries were so meager, receiving food or rare items was appreciated.[77] But as Lena's example, in the Introduction, and other interviews and anecdotal evidence shows, paying a high fee was common in cities.

This kind of informal exchange of favors though a network of friends and acquaintances called *blat* was prevalent in the Soviet Union and important in obtaining good health care. "Good" health care meant expedited treatment based on personalized attention, which could not be obtained if one went as a patient without any relationship with the doctor. Sometimes such personalized medical service arranged through blat would be provided for free, and other times at the normal fee, but what was provided was access to personalized, attentive care without waiting in queues.[78]

Doctors considered treating botched abortions and miscarriage far more important than prosecuting abortion, but due to the legal issues, they were forced to act differently depending on whether the case was a miscarriage or self-induced incomplete abortion. When an abortion case was identified as non-clinical, doctors needed to focus on producing evidence of illegality and the method of pregnancy interruption rather than providing the woman with the most effective treatment. From the medical point of view, this was counterproductive since they needed to minimize damage to women's reproductive organs after abortions and miscarriages. Given how widespread these were in the postwar period, some doctors considered it harmful to prioritize legality over improved medical care. Dr. E. S. Popova, Deputy Commissar of Health of Turkmenistan, suggested that doctors focus on preserving the fetus in all forms of interrupted births, both miscarriage and abortion, in order to maximize the birth rate. Practically, this was an invitation to consider criminalized abortion policy secondary to prophylactic measures to prevent miscarriage.

Prophylactic measures for both miscarriage and abortion required women's participation. Popova particularly emphasized the importance of identifying women who were in danger of abortion and hospitalizing them for medical supervision. Citing prewar experience, Popova argued that a doctor's engagement with a woman at risk could greatly contribute to saving the pregnancy. In 1939, in Gynecological Hospital No. 5 in Moscow, 69.6 percent of miscarriages, under medical supervision, resulted in births. In 1940, that figure rose to 75 percent. This meant that the lives of 1,001 (in 1939) and 1,096 (in 1940) children were rescued in one hospital alone.[79] By emphasizing the medical logic rather than legal logic, Popova implicitly criticized the punitive abortion policy that prevented doctors from providing care. No one contested her views on that ground, probably because most doctors agreed with her.

This opinion seems to have been strong, particularly among doctors who worked in areas such as Leningrad where the abortion rate was particularly high. At the Second Plenum for the Council of Obstetrics and Gynecology in August 1945, Professor V. A. Polubinskii reported on the work of fourteen women's health consultation rooms in various Leningrad enterprises. In Leningrad, it appears, the number of abortions paralleled the recovering birth rate. The number of abortions there increased from 2,294 (1942) to 10,368 (1944), as the birth rate rose from 12,408 to 22,565.[80]

For Professor Polubinskii, the importance of prevention rather than punishment of abortion was obvious. In Leningrad, all forms of abortion and premature births increased during the years of blockade due to hunger, lack of vitamins, neuro-psychological shock from bombing, and the physically demanding work of defending the city, which was shouldered by women. For every hundred normal births, there were around forty-five premature births and seventy-five abortions. If the war caused socioeconomic and medical problems for women, women were not to be blamed. Instead, doctors should try to help them by providing the best possible care. In order to fight abortion, the government had taken primarily punitive measures, but was still "far from achieving the goal." [81] Polubinskii argued that abortion prevention was extremely important because abortion was believed to cause 25 percent of all gynecological problems and to raise the probability of death during labor by a factor of ten.[82]

When prophylactic work failed and women had abortions, Dr. L. I. Bublichenko, who spoke after Polubinskii, considered timely aftercare and hospitalization critical. In his view, immediate medical care was more important than prosecution:[83]

Despite all our efforts for the fight with abortion, undoubtedly, some abortions will remain, and we will have to deal with those complications that result from abortions. In this regard, we can also reduce the amount of these complications through a whole series of measures, and preserve the possibility of timely treatment and the possibility of future pregnancy and procreation for women.[84]

Bublichenko's study showed that whether failed abortion created further complications depended on how soon a woman was hospitalized. If the treatment was timely and effective, sometimes the fetus could be saved. In order to provide effective post-abortion care to save both mother and child, he suggested the organization of specialized abortion care within hospitals.[85] His idea resonated with Professor A. Iu. Lur'e's suggestion to expand special abortion clinics from Ukraine to the rest of the Soviet Union.

The immediate postwar issues of Soviet obstetrics and gynecology flowed directly from the wounds of war, as did the 1944 Family Law, which sought to address a part of these. Prophylactic measures involving not only the sick but also healthy women were considered necessary for a reduction of all infertility, miscarriages, and premature births. Improvement in women's reproductive health needed universal participation to achieve effective prevention and timely treatment of abortions and miscarriages alike.

Two Options

Despite these conflicts in the surveillance and treatment roles of doctors, these physicians were still expected to reduce abortion. Alarmed by the rapid increase in abortion as the war ended, Commissar of Health Miterev convened representatives of the NKZ, the NKIu, and the state prosecutor in August 1945 to discuss "measures for the battle against abortion." In her opening speech, Kovrigina stated that the existing measures for the fight with abortion were "apparently" insufficient and would not eliminate the problem. It was clearly she who was responsible for solving this crisis at the NKZ. In 1944, the number of abortions per 100 births in the Soviet Union, excluding Ukraine, the Baltic republics, and Belorussia, was 30.5 and that of the RSFSR was 46.2. The city of Moscow had 73 abortions per 100 births, a "simply dreadful figure." The NKZ felt powerless in the face of this situation and therefore invited help from the other two institutions involved in abortion surveillance.[86]

Various issues concerning the surveillance system were addressed at the meeting, with the most active discussants being the doctors who dealt directly with failed abortion on a daily basis. They pointed out problems with restoring the prewar surveillance system in the postwar context. The one thing that doctors agreed on was that the list of criteria for clinical abortion was outdated. Two potential solutions emerged from the discussion. First, as Professor Arkhangel'skii had argued, some doctors considered that, because the war produced many severe health conditions for women, the criteria should be expanded. Professor Nikolaev, Deputy Director of the Moscow Institute for Gynecology and Obstetrics (MIGO), expressed this view. "It is necessary to take into account that the [present] list of criteria does not include many of the diseases that we now often encounter.... We must think about whether it is possible or necessary to add the after-effects of war to the criteria for clinical abortion." Nikolaev's examples included cases of women with abdominal wounds and limb amputations. He also mentioned stress-related high-blood pressure among many girls who saw the face of battle, a previously rare syndrome whose effects on pregnancy were feared, but not well-studied.[87]

The key debate over expansion of criteria was whether or not non-medical criteria, such as poor material conditions or not being married, could be included. Professor Arkhangel'skii recommended that socioeconomic criteria be added to the list. But most Soviet doctors, including Professor Nikolaev, rejected the idea because such a broad expansion of eligible conditions would undermine efforts to increase the birth rate.[88]

The second position was not to make changes to existing abortion surveillance, but to delegate authority to individual doctors to give permission for clinical abortion to those who were suffering from wartime conditions. Dr. Estrin, chairman of the Moscow Central Abortion Committee, presented this possible solution to the tension between limited prewar criteria and deteriorated postwar reproductive health. As shown in the epigraph, his proposal was for doctors to deal with women's postwar problems on an individual basis and permit clinical abortion on the merits of each case without changing the law.[89] Given the authority to make decisions for individual women, concluded Estrin, doctors should minimize the number of clinical abortions granted outside the criteria.[90]

In order to provide the most effective care, Estrin considered it important that doctors study the patient carefully and cultivate an influential relationship.

I consider it indispensable to conduct individual treatment of each woman in the doctor's office. The doctor to whom the woman went to express her desire to get an abortion, should study her from "A" to "Z (Ia)" and do everything so that she does not get an abortion. This is the most effective method [for the battle against abortion].[91]

The key issue for this solution was for doctors to understand women's medical, social, and economic conditions fully so that they could make good judgments about either providing permission or dissuading women from seeking non-clinical abortion. To do so, doctors needed the chance to examine women during a private consultation in a closed office.[92]

This suggestion was an endorsement of the wartime practice. Due to extreme conditions, doctors sometimes acted on their individual sense of necessity and justice instead of Soviet laws and provided abortion— for example, to handicapped and raped women. As Estrin himself implied, he granted a clinical abortion to a woman who had lost parts of her body. Perhaps more commonly, doctors provided false diagnoses to permit clinical abortion.[93] At the end of the war, the highest ranking doctors outspokenly promoted this semi-legal practice as an immediate solution to urgent problems with women's health.

According to an authoritative 1945 pronouncement by N. A. Semashko, the first Soviet Commissar of Health, "the interest of the collective is above the interest of the individual patient."[94] In this official understanding, if the important collective interest was immediate growth in the birth rate and enforcement of criminalized abortion law, obstetricians and gynecologists should strictly follow the law even at the expense of trust in doctor-patient relations and of the development of prophylactic care through universal participation.

Clearly, the individual approach violated the spirit of the 1944 Family Law, but it would be easier to implement than expanding criteria, a proposal unlikely to be supported by the pronatalist postwar government. Even if the idea was approved, amending the policy would require a major time-consuming bureaucratic effort. Moreover, because women had experienced so many varieties of physical damages during the war that an expansion of criteria for clinical abortion might have no limit. It was also possible that in a few years, the kinds of health problems women had because of the war-time conditions might dissipate, making the list of criteria obsolete. In short, the individual approach was an extension of the status quo and, for the time being, many doctors wanted an immediate solution to the problems they encountered every day.

The special conference on abortion surveillance produced no real results. In her closing remarks, Kovrigina lamented that because there were no real ideas emerging from the conference, she had no choice but to organize a working-level discussion. Frustrated and desperate, she reminded the assembly that "this year we must achieve real results. Information exchange is not enough. Information exchange is good and necessary, but not the most important matter. What is most important is the reduction of the number of abortions, and consequently, an increase in the birth rate."[95]

Nonetheless, the conference produced no new measures for surveillance work, though the discussions among doctors, prosecutors, and legal specialists revealed some of the underlying reasons why the prosecution system was not working, while clarifying the medical profession's primary role in this "failure." Doctors considered that the prewar criteria for medical abortions were inadequate for the postwar reality of women's health, so they were making individual decisions during private consultations about granting clinical abortion, essentially violating the 1936 law. They were reluctant to participate in surveillance work because the role of policing was harmful for cultivating trust with patients, which, in turn, endangered effective clinical and prophylactic medical care. So they tried to stay out of sight in abortion investigations, often undermining the prosecutors' need to acquire legal and medical evidence and documentation of illegal abortion.

Kovrigina was not able to respond quickly to this overwhelming criticism of punitive abortion policy. An expansion of criteria would have been difficult for the government to accept, since it had just introduced the pronatalist policy. A formal acceptance of individual doctors' authority in providing permission for clinical abortion, a practice which she would have been aware of, was problematic too, because the basis of judgment could vary among individual doctors. Doctors increasingly expressed views that enhanced prophylactic work was more urgent than prosecution and that, for such work, doctors must attract women to maternity care, and the list of criteria should be expanded.

Not all doctors wanted to change the existing abortion surveillance system, believing that fuller implementation of the 1944 Family Law's welfare measures for mothers would suffice. For example, Dr. R. N. Umanskaia focused on a proposition to provide state aid to pregnant women without fail.[96] O. D. Matsepanova, head of the RSFSR administration of maternity homes and maternity clinics, also focused on the consultation work for pregnant women at an early stage of pregnancy so these women could be informed about government support for mothers. There were female activists among female factory workers who helped medical personnel discover pregnant women. Other workplaces even conducted clinical examinations of the workshop employees to discover pregnant women, presumably in order to support pregnancies, but also preventing them from terminating pregnancies.[97]

By mid-1946, Kovrigina had endorsed improved prophylactic care as something doctors could strive for. In her concluding remarks at a meeting of administrative leaders of Maternity Care USSR in June 1946, Kovrigina stated:

> The battle against non-clinical abortions must be closely coordinated with the prosecutor. The role of doctor-obstetrician and gynecologist is great in the protection of the health of women and newborns. We must strive for attracting the pregnant in the early stage to maternity clinics, closely coordinate material questions with consultants on socio-legal issues, improve everyday life conditions of the pregnant and conduct sanitary-educational work broadly.[98]

There is no evidence from any of the many meetings in 1944–1946 over which Kovrigina had presided to suggest that she was against the idea of expanding categories of women eligible for clinical abortion or against some doctors' suggestion to act individually to solve women's problems. This would soon change as she became heavily involved in emerging Cold War politics.

Cold War Politics and Kovrigina's Purge of Obgyn

The postwar attack on the intelligentsia began in August 1946, when the journals *Zvezda* and *Leningrad*, two Leningrad-based publications, were attacked for "serious ideological irregularities." This campaign aimed at cultural repression is commonly known as *zhdanovshchina* (Zhdanovism), after Politburo member Andrei A. Zhdanov, although recent archival studies have revealed that it was initiated by Stalin. The main political sin was alleged "servility before the West" and anti-patriotic attitudes among cultural figures, such as Mikhail Zoshchenko and Anna Akhmatova.[99] In 1947, the KR affair triggered a wave of Cold War–related attacks on Soviet medicine. In February, Stalin convened a Politburo meeting to discuss scientists Nina G. Kliueva and Grigorii I. Roskin, who were developing a "miracle cure" for cancer at a laboratory of the Mechnikov Institute for Epidemiology and Microbiology in Moscow. These scientists were believed to have sold their research on the anti-cancer drug "KR" to the United States.[100] Studies show that Kliueva and Roskin were merely following bureaucratic orders when they sent their manuscript to the United States, and the charges against them were essentially "staged" by Zhdanov. However, as the Soviet Union developed secret scientific research in many fields (especially atomic energy), sharing what was considered to be an important scientific breakthrough with the emerging "main" enemy could be interpreted as treason.[101] A few other associated scientists were arrested with Kliueva and Roskin including V. V. Parin, the first Academician-secretary of the Academy of Medical Sciences (AMS), the "most powerful man in the Presidium [of AMS]."[102] Miterev, Minister of Health, was fired for insufficient caution, despite his knowledge of the correspondence between the two Soviet doctors and American ambassador General Walter Bedell Smith.[103] Miterev was soon replaced by Efim I. Smirnov, head of military medicine within the Red Army.[104]

The Cold War anti-Western campaign hit Soviet medicine particularly hard, because during the war there was much direct communication between Soviet and Western doctors. Wartime cooperation made it clear to Soviet doctors that Soviet medicine was lagging behind the West in many areas, especially medical instruments and medical technology. They were eager to learn from Western medicine, with Commissar Miterev himself promoting information exchanges and asking permission to subscribe to key Western medical journals. The AMS, modeled on Western academies, was founded for the purpose of elevating the level of Soviet medicine.[105] Western allies were also eager to learn from Soviet achievements in science and therefore initiated collaboration and exchanges during the war, most notably over penicillin production.[106] When the anti-Western campaign began, it was inevitable that it would affect Soviet medical personnel and the AMS.

The trial of Kliueva and Roskin took the form of a "Court of Honor," organized within the Ministry of Health (MZ) in June 1947.[107] This political disciplining campaign condemned "servility before the West" and promoted patriotism among Soviet intellectuals, as was the case in *zhdanovshchina*. The MZ's court of honor was the first one and was a model for all the other courts.[108]

No gynecologists or obstetricians were purged in the KR Affair, but it resonated through their specialty. The Moscow Institute for Gynecology and Obstetrics (MIGO) represented these subfields in the AMS, which was under fire after Parin, the Academician-secretary, was arrested in the KR affair. After the KR Affair, the party intensified political education in the AMS and emphasized the importance of learning and developing on the sole basis of Russian and Soviet medical achievements.[109] Because the institute was a part of the AMS system, it automatically came under scrutiny. The termination in 1947 of publishing a table of contents in English for the most important academic journal in the field, *Akusherstvo i ginekologiia* (*Obstetrics and Gynecology*), is a reflection of the end of wartime collaboration with Western scientists.

Another reason the Moscow Institute was targeted for discipline was that Kovrigina, who served on the MZ Court of Honor, was in charge of supervising the field of maternity care in the Soviet Union. As a politically vigilant top medical administrator, she would have wanted to eliminate questionable individuals and practices before anyone else criticized them or her. Using the rhetoric of the anti-Western campaign, Kovrigina purged the MIGO where what she identified as "private practice" and "nepotism" were flourishing. She replaced them with the principles of need-based free medicine, professionalism, and patriotism among postwar doctors in her field of supervision.[110] Her role in this affair helped pave her path to the ministerial level and a place on the Communist Party's Central Committee.

That Kovrigina disciplined one of the most important institutes in women's medicine is not surprising, but what is interesting are several additional characteristics of this purge. Along with "servility before the West," "anti-patriotic behavior," and "careerism" used as charges in the KR affair, her purge attacked "private practice" and "nepotism." The overall result was a sharp reduction in the percentage of Jews working at the Moscow Institute. These results also affected the ongoing discussions about abortion surveillance work by making clear that henceforth doctors would not be allowed to pursue their own professional opinion wherever it might lead. The abandonment of private medical consultation as a pathway to abortion led both medical practitioners and desperate women throughout the USSR to look for alternatives.

On December 22, 1947, Minister of Health Smirnov issued a prikaz to form a commission, headed by Deputy Minister Kovrigina, to investigate the MIGO.[111] By January 10, 1948, the investigation was complete, and

Kovrigina wrote a report to Smirnov condemning servility before the West and capitalist remnants observed at the Institute.[112] In essence, the "problem" discovered revolved around the Director of the Moscow Institute, M. S. Malinovskii, one of the most prominent obstetricians in the Soviet Union.[113]

It became apparent that Malinovskii had had difficulty organizing a new scientific institute under wartime conditions when experienced doctors were all mobilized except for those who were old or inexperienced, young doctors. He therefore had to choose new cadres from the limited pool of specialists.[114] Allegedly, recruitments were often arranged through the personal network of Malinovskii and his wife, T. A. Komissarova, who was also his assistant at the First Medical Institute, and some members were placed in positions for which they had no expertise. Thus, the institute was condemned for its nepotism, which produced an "in-group" surrounding Komissarova, the Director's wife, and, money-making by doctors through their private practice. Komissarova's friends, many of them hired through personal networks, were able to distribute resources favorably among themselves.[115]

The report explained that the in-group also extended its favoritism to patients and was making profits through private practice. Patients were accepted only through their acquaintances or "even worse, for presents."[116] Those private medical practitioners who were taking patients only for profits were rude, but no one could criticize them because they were protected by Malinovskii's wife.[117]

Interviews provided the most shocking descriptions of private practice and the group of doctors who supported each other. Dr. V. I. Bodiazhina reported that Dr. A. B. Gillerson had "a large private practice and sent his patients from private reception to hospital beds." Because of the prevalence of this practice, the admission of new patients to the institute's clinic was done "illegally." Bodiazhina claimed that "an ordinary dying woman cannot get into the institute. To get in, she has to go to a private meeting with Professors Malinovskii, Gillerson, or Gittel'son." Kovrigina quoted this in her report to Smirnov to make the point that private practice was a "violation of the Soviet principle of universally available medicine."

Interviewees further suggested that private practice was also about questionable treatments and operations from which doctors made profits. Nurse Koter reported that in the surgical department, most patients came from the professors' offices, and many of their operations were not recorded.[118] Bodiazhina described incidents that happened when she was on duty. When patients arrived without sufficient symptoms of disease, she rejected them.

In such cases, Dr. E. D. Zhuravskaia went to the head doctor F. G. Klebanov, and the patient was unconditionally admitted. But favoritism was apparently practiced mutually. Later, Zhuravskaia reported to the commission that no action was taken when she complained to Dr. Bodiazhina, her superior, that "at our institute criminal abortions were conducted," suggesting that Bodiazhina was aware but did nothing.[119]

Free tickets to sanatoria were given to patients who came from private practice, rather than to those who needed special treatment. Moreover, Koter reported that in the department "a surprisingly large number of patients were Jewish women," implying that many of them came from private practice. Bodiazhina insinuated that patients coming from private practice were paying enormous sums to doctors. In 1946, a patient named Fillipova, for instance, paid a total of 16,000 rubles to Professors Gillerson and Aleksandrova.[120]

In her report to Smirnov, Kovrigina argued that "the Institute must synthesize and reflect this field of medicine in the spirit of pure Soviet patriotism from the standpoint of relentless criticism of the bourgeois school and demonstrate the development of pre-revolutionary Russian and our Soviet school of obstetrics and gynecology."[121] According to this principle, Soviet medicine would attain highest quality when doctors were patriotic and critical of the West. However, the institute failed in that task. Kovrigina exposed the institute's pro-capitalist orientation by condemning illegal profit-making operations among some doctors. Among other questionable actions, she reported that a 43-year-old citizen T. E. Shapiro, with permission from the No. 51 Moscow Oblast' Abortion Committee dated December 15, 1947, was granted a clinical abortion. The order for such an operation was based on a private note from the head doctor Klebanov, suggesting a special arrangement. M. E. Smurova, age 39, was registered with a private note from Professor Gillerson. Such private notes were found during the investigation.[122] Some of these were written by Malinovskii himself. It was assumed that doctors received compensation for private treatment. Kovrigina assessed private practice as "crudely trampling on the highest and loftiest principle of Soviet public health—provision of medical aid for free—the Institute's clinic was reduced to a patrimony of the Director and his close associates, into an additional source of their enrichment."[123] These kinds of arrangements were quite similar to "individual decision-making in the doctor's office" as promoted by Dr. Estrin. Most institutions at the time likely tolerated informal or semi-formal arrangements.

At the first conference at the institute to discuss the result of the investigation, Kovrigina cited Stalin insisting that Soviet scientists "not only catch up, but overtake in the near future the achievements of science outside our country" as Kupriianov, the public prosecutor at the KR trial, had done.[124] To achieve this, it was essential that Soviet doctors fight a "decisive battle against servility and cringing before foreigners and the battle against all remainders of capitalism in the consciousness of our people." Kovrigina especially attacked the spread of private practice among doctors, who enriched themselves at the expense of Soviet women. These doctors sent their private patients to be hospitalized at the institute and presumably received fees for this service, a practice Kovrigina called "a shameless trade in government hospital beds."

Results of the Purge

After the investigation, the Moscow Institute went through a complete streamlining based on Kovrigina's recommendations. Numerous individuals were fired or demoted, and the overall number of personnel was dramatically reduced.[125] Externally, the institute lost its position as the leading academic institute in the field. In the summer of 1948, the Moscow Institute was removed from the academy and integrated into the Ministry of Health. The Leningrad Institute for Gynecology and Obstetrics instead became the AMS Institute to represent gynecology and obstetrics.

The internal restructuring of the Moscow Institute involved lay-offs and demotions. Director Malinovskii was fired, and Deputy Director Nikolaev replaced him. A number of doctors who were considered incompetent were fired, whereas some doctors who were competent, but criticized during the purge, were demoted. Academic and clinical staff were reduced from 152 to 108.[126] Some new recruitments began, but often positions were left vacant.

The composition by nationality changed significantly, disproportionately affecting Jewish doctors. While the purge reduced Russian doctors by 15 percent, it removed 55 percent of Jewish doctors.[127] However, it would be inaccurate to interpret the purge as entirely motivated by anti-Semitic sentiments. After the reform, four Jewish doctors were assigned to head institute departments, including M. I. Olevskii. The primary reason they remained was that they were recognized as professionally competent in their fields and held academic titles.

It might be possible to interpret this purge as a campaign to reverse war-time developments in Soviet medicine, as was the parallel case in the Finance Ministry.[128] Among other chilling effects, this purge put an end to the open discussion of doctors' discretion as the solution for postwar abortion surveillance. The next solution would be an expansion of criteria for legal abortion, an institutional change. Some doctors suggested that such an expansion would help reduce some of the illegal abortions. At a 1949 meeting, having succeeded Dr. A. L. Estrin, Dr. A. I. Dmitrieva, the head of the Moscow Central Abortion Committee, mentioned that doctors had tried hard to provide legal abortion to women by diagnosing non-existent conditions, but she thought that the time had come to revise the legal criteria themselves:

> Is it possible to work in the course of many years under the threat of Article 140 [of the Criminal Code]? Why should we draw on myocardium-dystrophy in order to establish the myth of medical evidence? Why should we not present this question to the government? Comrades, the war happened, significantly impairing the health of some parts of the population, for whom living conditions have altered. However, the list of medical evidence for abortion has not changed since 1936. It is long [over]due to present the question of expanding the list of evidence [needed to receive legal] abortion to the government.[129]

Thus, Dr. Dmitrieva implied that many doctors had been certifying women with non-existent conditions to qualify for legal abortions, but she considered that that practice alone could not improve the situation. Formal expansion of legal abortion was necessary. She even suggested including socioeconomic reasons to help would-be single mothers.

In 1949, Japan took precisely this path of adding economic indications to qualify for legal abortion. However, unlike Japan, where overcrowding was a major concern, the Soviet Union was trying to increase the birth rate by encouraging extramarital births. In this context where socioeconomic reasons were often referred to as "without child support from the biological father," doctors' attempts to cite socioeconomic reasons for legal abortion would have been an attack on the policy itself. The makers of the pronatalist policy were not yet ready to recognize the harm they had done to the welfare of mothers and children by promoting single-mother families without providing sufficient financial and institutional support. Dmitrieva agreed that the postwar family law that created illegitimacy and irresponsible fathers was leading to a great number of abortions and that this should become the basis for including non-medical reasons in the criteria for legal abortion. However, understanding the political significance of this subject, she also cautioned that measures should be taken to prevent healthy, well-off women from getting permission for legal abortion. In her opinion, the standard of living was improving among Soviet people and for most of them it was possible to raise one or two children.[130]

The logic of expanding criteria to prevent underground abortion worked, because sympathetic doctors were basically cognizant of the emerging postwar problems that drove many women to terminate pregnancies. Already at the First Joint Plenum in September 1944, guidance counselors at maternity clinics had warned that the 1944 Family Law's creation of out-of-wedlock status was affecting women's reproductive environment and decisions. For example, Professor S. E. Kapelianskaia reported that when a mother in a common-law marriage found out that she could not register her newborn twins under the father's name, she asked her to take the babies to an orphanage. In another case, it was the pregnant woman's mother who made the same request. The reason given was that her daughter was unmarried and the newborn's grandfather was a sick invalid, so the baby would have been an additional burden. In both cases, pregnancies happened well before the legal change and were carried to term.[131] However, those who would become pregnant after July 8, 1944, in similar socioeconomic conditions would immediately opt for illegal abortion.

By 1949, doctors had become aware of women's attempts to avoid out-of-wedlock births, child support deficiencies, and men's irresponsibility as factors affecting women's reproductive decisions. According to O. V. Makeeva, 12 percent of all aborting women in Moscow were single mothers.[132] In Makeeva's opinion, in order to solve problems of underground abortion, men should be included in the upbringing of their children, by which she meant "child support." In short, she wanted the 1944 Family Law revised.

> Why is Papa responsible for nothing? I mean the unofficial father. After all, there is a mass number of those children [of unofficial fathers]. We present this question . . . because perhaps this question needs to be raised so that fathers become [real] fathers.[133]

Makeeva's implied criticism that the Family Law's creation, single mothers, were major contributors to abortion statistics was widely supported by medical professionals, especially among those who were involved in the work of the social and legal consultation office. Along similar lines, Comrade Kravets expressed the opinion that the issue of child support was essential to the question of reducing illegal abortion: "We cannot ignore the issue of child support. Indeed, there are women whose situation is so insecure that they would do anything to avoid having a child."[134]

Kovrigina's 1948 purge of Soviet obstetrics marked a turning point. No longer would doctors be allowed to develop individual practices to accommodate the contradictory roles they had been assigned in abortion surveillance and medical care. No longer could doctors openly argue that abortion surveillance was not the goal in itself, but a part of their effort to provide comprehensive and prophylactic care for women. Instead, medical views on abortion policy shifted toward amendment of the criteria for legal abortion, which would eventually lead to legal changes in the mid-1950s, after Stalin's death. Another emerging concern was that postwar marriage relations were affecting women's reproductive decisions. While the doctors and medical administrators debated their next step, individual women began to chart their path through the new postwar realities created by the 1944 Family Law.

3

Postwar Marriage and Divorce

The New Single Mother and Her "Fatherless" Children

At this time my wife is not in Osipenko and it is not clear where she is. Now I must divorce her, because I found for myself a different wife, who is a real Soviet woman.

A Demobilized Soviet Man (1944)

I still want to have a child, but I don't have a husband. There is no one to marry. Men of my age are either at the front or married. Until now I didn't particularly think about these questions, but now I must think. If I give birth to a child out of wedlock, I will not have the right to register him under the father's family name. I have to write down my own family name. It turns out that he will be "illegitimate." Is either the child or I guilty that the war robbed me of my husband? The child will grow up and ask, "Who is my father?" What should I tell him? Everyone will point their fingers at him and say, he is illegitimate. I can't agree with them. I consider that the right to receive child support can be curtailed, as long as the government has taken these responsibilities upon itself, but the right to carry a father's family name must be upheld. After all, this morally destroys a woman.

A Postwar Soviet Woman (1945)

With the 1944 Family Law, the USSR created the new category of *odinokaia mat'*, commonly translated as "single mother." Such women were denied the right to include the names of their children's fathers on their birth certificates or to demand child support. The choice of this term was probably intentional. In Russian, as in English, the term is demographically broad and includes all women raising children without fathers, such as widowed mothers. Legislators clearly avoided the more specific term for an unmarried

Replacing the Dead. Mie Nakachi, Oxford University Press (2021). © Oxford University Press.
DOI: 10.1093/oso/9780190635138.003.0004

mother (*mat'-odinochka*) because they did not wish to highlight their focus on unmarried women as the object of pronatalist policy. Only indirectly, in the description of the offspring, was the intended meaning of single mother revealed. Legally, such a son or daughter would be "a child from a mother not in registered marriage."

More informally, an out-of-wedlock child was called *nezakonnorozhdennyi* (illegitimate), *vnebrachnyi* (out of wedlock), or simply *bez ottsa* (fatherless). These Russian words and phrases had different nuances. "Out of wedlock" was the more technical phrase. In contrast, "illegitimate" and "fatherless" invoked a negative moral judgement of out-of-wedlock children emphasizing lack of normative status, either legal or biological. In the new context of the post-1944 Family Law which forced the name of the father to be left blank or marked with a dash in the birth certificate of an out-of-wedlock child, "fatherless" felt the worst of the three, denying the presence of the father in any form.[1] For example, in the woman's epigraph above, "out of wedlock" is simply the objective state of affairs that leads to labeling as "illegitimate," a word associated with "guilt" and moral degradation. In another lament, a woman complains that her child will be branded "fatherless," which she considers a "most dubious title."[2]

However, in the immediate postwar years differences among these terms seemed not so important, as unmarried mothers rejected all three. Before 1944, revolutionary family law recognized de facto marriages as legal and relationships that produced offspring as de facto marriages. The existence of offspring practically defined marriage. In that world a child was never out of wedlock, nor illegitimate, nor fatherless, all terms associated with the discredited, unjust traditions of the imperial era. Postwar women, particularly those affected by this legal change, found all three categories unacceptable, offensive, and illegitimate for socialist society.[3] Some resisted vocally and their voices are highlighted in this chapter. Like the Soviet Woman in the epigraph, single mothers hated these words for undermining the welfare and well-being of themselves and their children.[4]

In various ways, European women suffered from changing legal, social, and cultural contexts for reproduction between wartime and postwar periods. One of the tragic cases took place in France. While the country was under Nazi occupation, many French women had children with the Germans, which was socioeconomically advantageous and culturally tolerated. However, after the liberation, those women were called "collaborators" and had their heads shaven in public.[5] In the Soviet Union, during the war women thought conceiving a child would entitle them to have a husband and family, but after the 1944 Family Law, they would instead become unmarried mothers of "fatherless" children. In both cases, women and their children personally suffered for a long time from postwar reproductive practices.

During the decade following the war, a total of 8.7 million out-of-wedlock Soviet children were registered, and the number continued to rise. No doubt, this was a significant number, but it did not necessarily constitute proof of a successful pronatalist policy aimed at increasing extramarital births.[6] Even without the pronatalist measures, there would have been non-conjugal sex and many births by women not in registered marriages. Whether these relations would have yielded fewer than 8.7 million babies over this decade would depend on calculations that factor in prewar reproductive patterns, as well as the enormous wartime and postwar changes that affected women's and men's sexual and reproductive behaviors. Such comparative estimates would be both difficult and unreliable.

Assessing the effects of the pronatalist law by looking only at the number of women becoming unmarried mothers ignores how women experienced it. The new law impacted both the legal and material environment for single mothers and the stability of marriage. The creation of state support for single mothers was intended to provide material support to encourage unmarried women to become mothers. However, successive drafts of the law continuously diminished the amount of aid for single mothers. Then, on November 25, 1947, aid to single mothers, along with other state aid to mothers, was cut in half. Even before this cut, of course, state aid was, from the mothers' point of view, insufficient and a weak incentive. Some single mothers used their new right to leave their children in orphanages, but whether this could become an acceptable solution for increasing population depended on the state's ability to raise orphans. In terms of legal environment, the issue of visible illegitimacy could serve as a strong disincentive to having an out-of-wedlock child.

The 1944 Family Law claimed to strengthen the family by creating a legal distinction between single and two-parent families.[7] In two-parent families, both the mother and the father were responsible for the well-being of their children. Since the law had made divorce quite difficult, this type of family was now supposedly stable. If a divorce did occur, the departing parent, most likely the father, would continue his responsibilities through child support. In contrast, in single mother families, mothers were solely responsible for raising the children, with the help of the state. In this way, the framers of postwar pronatalism hoped that women who otherwise would not be able to marry and have children due to an imbalanced sex ratio could nevertheless reproduce.

Policymakers expected most single mothers to raise only one child. In contrast, they hoped that married women would raise multiple children. The assumption largely held true in the short term; however, over time the stability of legal marriage did not guarantee the stability of marital relations. In fact, increased extramarital births directly impacted the stability of marital relations and women's reproduction.

This chapter examines the gendered patterns of marriage and divorce practices that developed after the introduction of the pronatalist law.[8] It begins by looking at the state of marriage at the end of the war and how men and women expressed their feelings about marriage and divorce. It then shows how the new law shaped the efforts of legal experts to resolve discrepancies between the law and reality. The experts proposed amendments and supplementary instructions to the 1944 Family Law, some of which were adopted. Finally, it discusses how new practices of marriage and divorce negatively affected single mothers and their children. Not surprisingly, women were the chief critics of the law. So-called stable marriages suffered in this environment, and these new forms of marital malaise were reflected in the steadily growing number of abortions.

Gendered Life in the Postwar Era

Postwar society treated wartime sexuality of men and women differently. After the war women alone were condemned for non-conjugal sexual relationships. Women themselves were willing to tolerate their husbands' wartime infidelity. On the other hand, when husbands found out that their wives had engaged in wartime liaisons, especially with German soldiers, they often filed divorce petitions. Aside from this gendered understanding of sexual morality, the postwar sex imbalance also supported and rewarded men's infidelity.

Official propaganda celebrated demobilized women for their heroic role in achieving victory, but in their private lives they often faced particular difficulties.[9] In the case of the marriage between the battalion officer and nurse, mentioned in the Introduction, what happened to the nurse after the officer, her lover, was killed is unknown. At best, she could have gone to her husband's parents and given birth to a child. She might also have discovered that the officer already had a wife and family back home, or she might have found herself unwelcome because the officer's parents believed that girls from the front were promiscuous. Even if she and her child were accepted by his parents, the young woman would have had difficulty registering herself as a military widow since there was no official record of their marriage, and potential witnesses might have perished.

If the pregnant nurse had gone to her husband's parents, she could claim that she was the wife of their son and pregnant with his child. However, when the so-called field campaign wives were discharged upon becoming pregnant, they had no place to go to be safe from stigma, especially those from rural areas. After the war, some demobilized women felt compelled to hide the fact that they had served in the army. Some even refrained from wearing their medals because female soldiers' reputations were tainted.[10] Although military men commonly had sexual liaisons with women, this point was not much discussed, nor did it ruin the reputations of demobilized men. In the 1980s Nina V. Il'inskaia, who served in the war as a nurse, lamented:

A man returns and he's a hero. A [potential] bridegroom! But if a girl returns, then she is immediately looked upon askance as if to say, "We know what you did there." . . . And the whole family wonders, "Why marry her?" To be honest, we covered it up and didn't want to say that we had been at the front. We wanted to become normal girls again. [Potential] brides.[11]

The extent to which demobilized women were stigmatized can be seen in the case of Tamara Umniagina, who married a man with whom she fought in the war. They had vowed to unite, if they survived, and on June 7, 1945, they did. Complications ensued. When her new husband took her to his home town, they found that his family was deeply unhappy. Her mother-in-law cried bitter tears and rebuked her son, "To whom did you get married? To a girl from the front. . . . You have two younger sisters. Now who will marry them?" The family tried to hide Umniagina's past and destroyed Umniagina's photographs from the front.[12]

Many demobilized men preferred to find a bride who had not served in the army. Nikolai Borisovich, interviewed by Svetlana Alexievich, explained that this was not because they considered women from the front "dirty" but because after going through the hell of war, soldiers wanted "something beautiful, beautiful women" to help them leave their wartime experiences behind. One of his friends in the army, for this reason, did not get married to a comrade whom he fell in love with at the front. Instead, he found a pretty girl back home and got married. He soon regretted this choice, but at the end of the war, he could not even consider marrying someone whom he had seen only in military attire. The urge to forget was too strong.[13] Nikolai also married a woman who had not served in the army and who despised women from the front. She considered demobilized women aggressive sluts. Nikolai did not agree with his wife's views, but, in the interest of family harmony, he was also ready to forget the war.[14]

The spontaneous, temporary, and ambiguous nature of wartime "marriages" as well as the tragic postwar fate of military women who became pregnant is shown in an extreme form by the marriage of Tatiana N. and Andrei R. Tatiana joined the army medical corps at age 18. In 1943, when she was assigned to a reserve regiment in Petropavlovsk, she met Andrei, a 25-year-old company commander. They began living in one room as husband and wife. This was general knowledge among the officers. Tatiana became pregnant in 1944 and gave birth to a son in June 1945. The son was registered under Andrei's family name and patronymic.[15] When Tatiana became pregnant Andrei had begun treating her badly and started meeting with other women. When friends and associates reminded him that he was married, he said, referring to his relationship with Tatiana, "It is only temporary." In fact, Andrei frequently came home drunk and beat Tatiana, shouting "You are not my wife!"

When Andrei was transferred, Tatiana briefly went back to her rural parents, but soon came back to the regiment, because it was shameful to return to village society with a child, but no husband. Later, Tatiana's parents regretted that they had let her leave the village. Sometime in the spring of 1946, they lost contact with their daughter. When they requested an official investigation concerning the whereabouts of Tatiana and their grandchild, they discovered that in 1947 Andrei had gone to Iuzhno-Sakhalinsk and married another woman. When Andrei was questioned about Tatiana and her son, he admitted that he had lived with her for a while but denied that they were married and insisted that the child was not his.

The investigation revealed that Andrei's and Tatiana's marriage was not registered, although their child was registered as Andrei's son. Witnesses noted that Tatiana was a "shy girl, stainless in her behavior, never met with any officers, and never went out, because she was embarrassed by her very noticeable limping." One of Tatiana's friends thought that Andrei and Tatiana had definitely registered their marriage, because Tatiana had expressed a strong negative view of common-law marriage. In August 1958, Andrei finally admitted that he had murdered Tatiana and her son before going to Iuzhno-Sakhalinsk. He was imprisoned for ten years in Minsk.[16]

The murder of a wartime wife is certainly an exceptional case, but Tatiana and Andrei's history had common characteristics with many wartime unions and postwar separations. They lived in the army as "husband" and "wife," without official marriage registration. The "husband" considered the "marriage" temporary, and as soon as he discovered that his "wife" was pregnant, he began seeing other women. The "wife" could not force the husband to register the marriage, even after the 1944 law made it clear that rights would be forfeited without registration, and despite her belief that marriage should be official. The "wife" could not return to her home village because she was stigmatized for having a fatherless child. The "husband" later denied that the "marriage" was real and that the child was his. He moved on to a subsequent relationship without any consequences.

This was a real parting of the gendered ways. In the prewar period, a man and a woman in a sexual relationship could easily refer to each other as "husband" and "wife." Shared military and conjugal experiences continued this practice in the Soviet Army right up until the war's end. Women often considered themselves to be in common-law marriages, even after the 1944 Family Law created the distinction between legal marriage and other sexual relationships. But the "husbands" contested this practice because they believed the new law was on their side. From 1945 onward, massive demobilizations again created the potential for separations and conjugal recombinations on a mass scale last seen during the mobilizations and evacuations four years earlier. Terrible family dramas became a common postwar Soviet experience, as the battle of the sexes accelerated.

Divorce in the Wake of War: Men's and Women's Motivations

When the law was promulgated on July 8, 1944, many prewar family members were still missing, and most wives in the rear were still waiting for their husbands to return. On the other hand, many demobilizing male soldiers, who were married in the prewar period and had wartime "marriages" as well, were contemplating which "family" to return to. Such a moment was depicted in Vera Ketlinskaia's wartime story "Nastia," in which the hero Pavel tried to decide whether to go back to his wife and children or stay with his wartime lover, Nastia.[17] Irina (born in 1929) talked about another woman whose husband did not want to be with his wife after being demobilized from the war. "They had three children. She chased him in town, at work, in the metro, but that didn't do anything. He went to another woman, got married, and had two children. He just didn't want to live with her."[18] Some without prewar commitments were conflicted about whether to continue a wartime relationship or seek new postwar partners.

Although any demobilization might well create the opportunity or necessity for life-changing choices, the 1944 law shaped conditions under which men could avoid legal marriage, while women desired it. Legal cases sharply reflected this gendered chasm, particularly regarding the three most common areas of legal action: divorce, child support, and proof of married status.

Soon after the 1944 Family Law was introduced, legal experts noted that men filed the large majority of divorce cases.[19] In 1944, of 470 divorce cases in the city of Moscow, 386 were filed by men and 84 by women. In Moscow oblast, of 50 divorce cases, 38 were filed by men and 12 by women. The majority of those who filed for divorce were between 30 and 40 years old and had been married for five to ten years.[20] In Ukraine of 32 divorce cases, 25 were filed by men and 7 by women. In the city of Leningrad, of 59 cases examined from September to December 1944, 51 were filed by men and 8 by women.[21]

According to the NKIu's study of 1944 divorce cases, the three most common causes for divorce in RFSFR and Ukraine were existence of another common-law family, infidelity of the spouse, and "dissimilarity of characters."[22] In Moscow and Leningrad, the presence of another marriage was the most common reason for divorce.[23] For example, Comrade Shiriaev of Khar'kov was typical, filing for divorce in December 1944, because his new "wife" would soon give birth. He wanted to make the new marriage legal and register the child under his family name.[24]

Some men initiated divorce because their wives were unfaithful during the war. The wife of N. Shepel' of Moscow, a demobilized soldier, for example, "married" a man from Omsk when she was evacuated to that city. At the time of writing, Shepel' did not know whether his wife had left her current "husband," but Shepel' himself wanted a divorce.[25] Repulsion toward wartime infidelity was also expressed by V. I. Stepanov, another veteran. After he entered the army in 1941, Germany occupied Leningrad oblast where his wife, daughter, father, and mother lived. Not hearing any news from

Stepanov and believing her husband might be dead, the wife "got married" to a Russian "collaborator" with the enemy, but this "husband" was soon killed by partisans. For his part, Stepanov wanted a separation from this woman so that she would not carry his family name or collect funds meant for his parents and daughter. Stationed 7,000 km away from Leningrad oblast, he wanted the divorce processed in his absence.[26]

As in postwar France, women were attacked for wartime sexual intimacy, real or suspected, with German men during the occupation. In the context of divorce petitions, condemnation was strongest when the woman's new sexual partner was German or from another enemy population, a relationship most likely to develop in occupied areas. When infidelity was the reason for divorce, the husband often condemned his wife's wartime sexual behavior, such as fraternization with Germans. Captain I. M. Sukach wrote, "During the German occupation of Ukraine, my wife got married to a German militia man in order to avoid labor deportation to Germany. She lived with him for a while, that is, until the arrival of the Red Army. Then he was killed, and she was left alone. I learned about this directly from her in the letters she wrote to me. She asks me to accept her again. But because I was at the front for the whole time, and she got married to a German lackey, I decided to break off all ties with her. . . . Please explain to me what I need to do so that my official documents do not include my wife, who got married to a German lackey."[27]

As in Sukach's letter, when demobilized soldiers wanted a divorce, they often based their entitlement to divorce on their military service, a sentiment strongly expressed by I. T. Avdeev, an invalid veteran, who in the epigraph to this chapter invoked patriotism in petitioning the court for a legal separation.[28] Avdeev wanted a divorce because when he went back to Osipenko in Zaporozhskii oblast, which was under German occupation during the war, he found out that his wife had lived with a "German fascist invader" until the German retreat. Avdeev emphasized that he should be given a divorce because he had defended his country, and his former wife was a blemish on his record that needed to be removed. Demobilized soldiers also asked the government to grant them an automatic or free divorce without a court procedure.[29] Some even asked for punishment of wives for infidelity.[30]

Other demobilizing soldiers were indignant at the possibility that single women who conceived children by Germans could be entitled to state aid. The 1944 Family Law, however, did not respond to patriotic sentiments. Legal experts insisted that there be no exceptions to the 1944 law's divorce clauses. Furthermore, Soviet law had no provision for punishing adultery, whether with allies, enemies, or countrymen. Children forcibly conceived with individuals from enemy countries were equally protected and entitled.[31] Despite demobilized soldiers' expectations, legal experts did not allow exceptions based on their wartime service.[32]

Avdeev's indignation regarding his wife in part masked his own desire to legalize his own wartime relationship—also adulterous. Avdeev had found a "true" Soviet woman to marry. Strictly speaking, the fact that he had already found this woman before legalizing his divorce could also be considered infidelity, but as the epigraph shows, Avdeev self-righteously presented his position as that of a hero entitled to special consideration.[33]

Like Avdeev's case, husband-initiated divorce cases based on the wife's infidelity or sexual dysfunction were often motivated by the presence of a new postwar family, a direct outcome of the war's corrosive impact on the social fabric. The existence of second families was probably much more prevalent than statistics indicated, as many men were able to disguise them.[34] NKIu Ukraine reported that according to the analysis of cases between February and March 1945, military men often blamed the breakup of their families and the formation of new ones on their long absences from home. However, many of them initially covered up the presence of the new family or intimate relations with other women and made up "irrelevant motives" instead.[35]

Men used reasons other than a wife's infidelity to hide their own motivation for divorce. One interesting case shows a combination of the logic of reproduction and the Soviet discourse of culture as justification for divorce. In Moscow, one Sychkov filed a divorce case against his wife Sychkova. They had been married in 1930 and had two children. He reported his motives as age difference (his wife was eight years older) and "cultural level." He said, "I was always ashamed of her because I have higher education and she only has secondary education." At the court hearing, it became clear that "the true reason for divorce was the presence of a second family, with a younger woman, formed during Sychkova's evacuation."[36] Sychkov was implying that more reproduction was likely if he married the younger woman.

A second notable motive for postwar divorce was venereal disease and consequent infertility. In Ukraine, a number of husbands filed for divorce because their wives had been infected with sexually transmitted diseases while their men folk were serving in the army. The implication of "sleeping with the enemy" hovers just below the surface. Venereal disease was commonly presented as evidence of promiscuous behavior, even in areas that had not been occupied by the German army. In Tashkent, one Matsokin filed a divorce case, claiming that "during his service in the Red Army on the front-line of the Great Patriotic War, his wife Matsokina was leading a dissolute way of life." The result for both of them, he claimed, was venereal disease. Wives also filed divorce cases based on venereal disease and presumed infidelity of husbands.[37]

Infertility and sexual dysfunction also served as grounds for divorce. In Uzbekistan, infertility was one of the most common motives, justifiable on the grounds that the government was committed to increasing the birth rate. In 1945, Khurmatov Muitdin, after thirty years of childless marriage, filed a divorce case. He reported that he and his wife, Khashimova, had adopted children and that she, but not he, had undergone infertility treatments. Muitdin did not explain his sudden desire for divorce from his 45-year-old wife, but without further ado, the Tashkent court ordered a divorce under the banner of patriotism.

Although the majority of divorce cases motivated by infertility were filed by husbands, wives also demanded divorce based on male sexual dysfunction. M. O. Beliaeva filed a divorce case in Tashkent oblast court, claiming that her husband suffered from "impotence." As a result, she claimed she had developed neurasthenia, leading to premature births, when she finally conceived. It is not clear if contemporary doctors recognized any scientific basis for this claim, but the court ordered divorce based on reproductive incapacity.[38] Similarly, in Ukraine, a woman, Bezpal'ko, asked for a divorce due to spousal infertility.[39] In the Russian Soviet Federated Socialist Republic (RSFSR), divorce was sometimes granted for "lack of children."[40]

Moreover, some evidence suggests that women sometimes considered themselves inadequate wives and invoked their own lack of sexual capacity when seeking a divorce. Z. P. Gubareva of Kiev, for example, claimed that she was "physically much weaker than her husband" and "unable to satisfy his physical demands." Moreover, this mismatch had become a bone of contention in the family. Remarkably, the court granted them a divorce.[41]

The fact that infertility and sexual dysfunction became common motives for legal divorce makes sense under the pronatalist policy; men and women alike quickly learned to speak the language of the reproductive imperative. Moreover, in this era when gynecological problems and venereal disease had reached epidemic proportions, such claims were readily accepted by the courts, even though they often masked other motivations, such as the desire to marry another person. Sometimes these intentions and the pressure from the "other woman" were revealed inadvertently or because the parties were unaware of judicial practice. For example, A. S. Mel'nikov, born in 1895 and married in 1914, was conscripted in 1943 and by 1945 was living "unregistered" with another woman. Apparently he was hoping that his first marriage which took place in the church would not be recognized in the Soviet Union; under that condition, he could divorce his wife and remarry, but the NKIu soon dashed his hopes. A second request for divorce was based on his wife's gynecological diseases and the most common cause for divorce proceedings, the de facto presence of a second family.[42]

Significantly fewer cases of divorce were filed by women than men, in part because women, especially the middle-aged, had little chance to find a new husband. Also, prewar wives and their children enjoyed financial advantages such as inheritance, state aid, and pension, but only if they did not divorce or remarry, even after husbands had died or gone missing in the war. As with men, new partners figured prominently in divorce proceedings initiated by women, but women presented their motives quite differently, emphasizing the interests of their children rather than their own. Women typically emphasized their desire to avoid out-of-wedlock births and to unify the family, including stepchildren and themselves, under one *familiia* (last name). In fact, so central was the arrival of a new child to most divorce cases filed by women that few bothered to hide the existence of a second marriage. Generally, concern about their children's interests eclipsed most women's accusations regarding a husband's wartime infidelity, even when such behavior was well known.[43]

Women also demanded that divorce be granted by simplified procedures on the grounds that the marriage had already ended in the prewar period. Z. M. Petrova was married in 1924 to a significantly older man. They lived together for thirteen years, despite "his sharp temper," which filled married life with "unpleasant events." After a "family scandal," in 1937, her husband left home and never returned. She eventually "remarried." When Petrova learned about the 1944 Family Law, she tried to get a divorce from her former husband, but the judge did not accept her petition, telling her to publish a divorce announcement in a newspaper and wait for five years. Petrova considered this approach overlong and "crudely formalistic."[44]

Other cases were complicated by the fact that husbands had gone to the army and not yet been demobilized. L. P. Kumukova (Stavropol') had married in 1937 in Karachai Autonomous Oblast where she was assigned to teach. According to her, this marriage was unhappy because her husband, a Karachai, forced her to observe Karachai rules and customs. She left him in

1940 and returned to live with her sister in Stavropol'. She attempted divorce, but her husband prevented it and then left for the front in 1941. She "remarried" in 1941 and had a child. However, without an official divorce, she could not register either her second marriage or first child.[45] Kumukova's case was further complicated by the fact that the Karachai husband was missing in action. For this reason, her divorce case could not move forward until his fate was officially determined.

Being left in limbo, with their children's legal status endangered, was unacceptable to some women. A. A. Safonova (Vladivostok) was one of them. She made two inquiries with the NKIu regarding divorce and remarriage. Her first letter was not filed in the archive, but from the legal expert's reply, it is clear that she believed that her registered husband was missing or dead in the war. The NKIu assured her that without a document confirming her husband's fate, the court would not process her divorce case. She would have to wait until the war was over. If her husband returned, she could file for divorce. Only a death certificate would allow her to register her second marriage without court proceedings.[46]

Safonova did not consider this advice useful and without fearing to appear unpatriotic, complained that she was being asked to wait "for an indefinite period of time," when she had to deal with urgent real-life problems. The raw emotion that she expressed stood out among a couple of hundred letters on marital problems archived together. In an indignant rebuttal to legal advice, she clearly demonstrated her sense of entitlement to a happy postwar family life after the war had destroyed her prewar family.

> Your admonishments mean nothing to me personally nor to anyone else. Such an answer does not do anything for me. You know I am a living person, however small I am. Nevertheless, I am but a small screw in the grandiose government machine. I carry out complicated work, but at the same time since the beginning of the war I am deprived of the right . . . to a family, like millions of citizens of our vast fatherland.
>
> My first husband went missing, and his child died. My family was destroyed. However, I patiently waited, thinking that perhaps there had been a mistake. I contacted all administrations that might give me some information about him and wrote to his military unit. However, my search was not successful. No one gave me an answer. . . .
>
> I got married again, to a person whom I consider my legal husband in all respects. I have lived with him already for half a year and I will soon have a

child. The child will have a real father, but will not be permitted to bear the family name and patronymic of the father. In official documents the child will have the status of "fatherless," which is what I, the mother, consider a most dubious title.[47]

The second reply to Safonova repeated the first. Her case would be reviewed only after her husband's return or confirmed death. Only after getting an official divorce could she get married to her second husband. Until then, the child could only be registered under the mother's family name.[48] Like so many women, Safonova plead for her child's regularized legal status and postwar family happiness, but the law would not accommodate her desire. Although she had created family stability, her absent husband condemned her child to be born fatherless.

Gendered Consequences of the 1944 Law

In many divorce proceedings, women had a strong concern about obtaining child support from their prewar common-law husbands. This was heightened by confusing language in the 1944 Family Law. The law did not discuss who would be responsible for child support for children born to unregistered, common-law marriage partners before July 8, 1944. It stipulated that mothers whose children were born after the introduction of the law would receive state aid, but there was no clause stipulating whether the state or their biological fathers would provide for those born earlier. In addition, there were many such children because common-law marriage had the same legal significance as registered marriage prior to the 1944 law. Finally, the issuance of the law precipitated deeply gendered conflicts of interest as mothers rushed to register their marriages, and fathers, convinced that child support was now the state's burden, refused to make this commitment. The presence of another family, spousal alienation after a long wartime absence, sheer selfishness, and various combinations of these factors prevented ready resolution of the great divide, driven by the 1944 Family Law. The victims were usually the children.

Suddenly, in late 1944, many women in prewar common-law marriages lost their marital status and child support. Seeking help, one such mother, E. Nazimova (Arzamas, Gor'kov oblast), wrote to the local paper, *Arzamasskaia Pravda*. She reported having entered a common-law marriage in 1939 in Leningrad and bearing a child in 1940. When her husband was mobilized into the army, she and her child were evacuated to Arzamas. From the spring of 1943 her husband sent her money monthly for child-rearing. However, in September 1944 he wrote to say that under the 1944 law, common-law marriage was not recognized, and he had no intention of registering. Furthermore, he considered himself "free" and would not feel responsible for future child support. Nazimova wanted to know if she had the right to demand child support from him.[49] The legal expert who responded to her could only say that the NKIu was currently discussing the issue. G. M. Prianichnikova was in a similar situation. After passage of the 1944 law, her common-law husband declared that he no longer wanted to live with the family. She wondered if he would provide child support and felt that the new law was justifying "disreputable paternal behaviors."[50]

Regardless of what the law said, mothers felt that fathers should take part in childrearing, at least financially. P. M. Nikitichna wrote to the editor of the journal *Working Woman* (*Rabotnitsa*) after receiving no help from the court:

> Dear Comrades! Please put yourself in my shoes and advise me. I am in a very difficult family situation. My husband, Razuvaev Ivan Leont'evich, with whom I lived eleven years together in one room, has now left me for another woman, leaving me with two children. . . . The father categorically refuses to help his children and said "You are not my legal wife. Our marriage was not registered. The new law abolished child support, so I will not pay it. Go ahead. Sue me." I contacted people's court in Pervomaiskii raion. My case was not accepted.[51]

This was forwarded to the NKIu, which examined the case and determined that the people's court handled the case correctly.[52] Nikitichna received neither solace, nor support. Her case was part of the groundswell of maternal discontent provoked by the 1944 law.

Fathers also inquired about their child support obligations under the new law, but these questions were often inspired by diametrically opposed conceptions of personal interest. Men wanted to know the limits of their new "freedom." For example, I. I. Garban' (Ivanovo oblast) asked if he should be paying support for the three children of his prewar common-law marriage. Already before he was mobilized into the army, he had separated from his wife and began paying 25 percent of his salary as child support.[53] After demobilization, even before locating his family, he wanted to know the personal implications of the new law.[54] The legal expert had a very clear answer to this question: those who were already paying child support in the prewar period were responsible for child support until their children turned 18.[55]

Similarly M. S. Pestov raised questions regarding the child support he had been paying since the prewar period. Pestov's common-law marriage had ended in the prewar period. His former wife then lived with another man for two years, without children or pregnancies. Although the details remain unclear, Pestov and his former wife reunited for a short, but consequential, week. Eight months later, a child was born. With the "infertile" husband as witness, his wife brought suit against Pestov for child support. The court agreed, but Pestov demurred. He appealed to a higher court, where a blood test revealed that he, his former wife, and the child had the same blood type, while the new husband had a different one. Based on this "evidence," the court ordered Pestov to pay child support. He wanted to appeal again, but the war intervened. He now hoped that, according to the 1944 law his child support obligation would end.[56] The answer from the NKIu legal expert was that prior court decisions remained in effect, although Pestov was free to pursue his appeal while continuing to pay his child support.[57]

Although the finding emphasized continuity, this case is a striking demonstration of the changes wrought by the 1944 law. In the prewar period, Pestov's wife could lawfully demand child support for her child born of a brief sexual liaison, despite her de facto marriage with another partner. In the postwar period, women in common-law marriages had lost all rights to child support from the biological father, no matter how clearly established. Legal marriage became the sole basis on which to make a claim. Thereafter, children who did not receive paternal support would be "fatherless" and their mothers "single."

Child support aside, the establishment of the very fact of marriage was an option no longer available to women whose common-law husbands returned to the new realities of the 1944 law. Ironically, in the cases where husbands were missing or deceased, women in prewar common-law marriage could successfully establish their dead marriages at law. Obtaining such legal marital status was important because they could receive various forms of state aid and pension as long as they did not remarry. Already on April 28, 1943, Sovnarkom SSSR issued a decree providing lump sum payments to the wives of general and high-ranking officers of the Red Army who were missing or dead in the war. The amount of the aid was substantial: up to 100,000 rubles.[58] Around the same time, the government also provided lump sums or pensions for wives and families of rank-and-file service men and lower-ranking officers.[59] To be eligible for such aid, wives had to provide marriage certificates and proof that they had not subsequently remarried.

Providing proof of marriage was not always easy for postwar wives. Many had lost official documents during the general evacuation. Offices from which replacement marriage certificates might be obtained had themselves been evacuated. Many wives in common-law marriages had also never recorded their marriages officially. To accommodate these two cases, on November 10, 1944, it was decided that those who were in either situation could establish the fact of marriage through the court.[60] Once procedures had been clarified, war widows rushed to the court to become eligible for state aid and pension, or sometimes property inheritance, in the postwar period. These wives were generally required to call witnesses who could state that they had lived with the soldier as wife and husband until the war had begun.[61] With the 1944 Family Law, legal recognition of prewar marriage without the presence of both spouses became technically more complex. However, it appears that the courts adapted slowly to the new circumstances and generally established the fact of marriage without careful cross-examination of witnesses.[62] For example, the court "married" Anna, although witnesses testified that they knew about the couple's engagement, but not about the marriage, thus enabling Anna to inherit a house.[63]

Women could have a difficult time providing proof of marriage if their common-law marriage with a now-missing soldier had taken place before they had divorced a previous husband. One woman's claim for state aid was challenged on these grounds, but three witnesses who testified that "she was indeed the wife . . . and lived with him until the time of his mobilization in 1941" convinced the court to recognize her marriage and claim.[64]

The generally easy-going attitude toward the establishment of the fact of marriage based on witnesses' testimony occasionally created problems when more than one wife asked for legal recognition of marriage with one missing or dead soldier. In February 1944, M. G. Il'ina submitted a petition at a Moscow court asking for recognition of her common-law marriage with K. G. Feoktistov, a battalion commissar who died in 1941, and recognition of their two children. The court agreed, and the woman received a lump-sum payment.

In 1948, however, the USSR Supreme Court began reinvestigation of this case because a 1943 case in Chkalov oblast had already recognized A. N. Zekhova as the wife of Feoktistov and had awarded her payment, too. Since Soviet law did not recognize polygamy, only one of these women could be considered Feoktistov's wife at the time of his mobilization. An investigation established that although Zekhova was in a common-law marriage with Feoktistov between 1931 and 1941, his acquaintance with Il'ina had resulted in twins in 1937. Feoktistov had recognized them and was paying child support. Il'ina insisted that their relationship dated to 1933 and that only in 1937 had she learned of his previous marriage and children. But this was already a recognition of Zekhova as Feoktistov's first wife. The court resolved this conflict in Zekhova's favor.[65]

Thus, the legal recognition of marriage allowed the widows of prewar common-law marriages to receive postwar benefits for bereaved wives. At the same time, they were given financial incentive not to remarry, at least legally. Ironically, wives whose prewar common-law husbands came home from the front were penalized. Neither legal recognition nor financial benefits became available as many demobilized husbands made full use of their "rights" under the new family law in refusing to register marriages or provide child support. Wives whose children were born before the 1944 law could wish their husbands dead, but it was too late.

The NKIu "Successfully" Implements the 1944 Law

As soon as the 1944 law was promulgated, citizens' reactions and questions revealed basic inadequacies in dealing with postwar realities of marriage and divorce. Legal experts quickly focused on issues such as child support, the recognition of paternity for "fatherless" children, and the confused division of labor between people's courts and oblast/city courts in handling divorce cases. An analysis of how legal experts discussed key problems with the 1944 law shows the tension between their desire to resolve family legal problems and their official responsibility to implement postwar pronatalist policy. In interpreting and implementing the law, such experts generally strove for practical solutions that would allow the true state of marriage and divorce to be reflected in the legal record. Because so many prewar families were broken up during the war, jurists wanted legal recognition for de facto divorce. At the same time, they wanted to allow the legal establishment of paternity for fatherless children when the biological father voluntarily recognized paternity. However, these measures contradicted the pronatalist goals of the state in Khrushchev's conception, which limited access to legal divorce and separated out-of-wedlock children (single-mother families) from legitimate children (two-parent families) in order to stabilize family life at high rates of reproduction.

Caught between the two tasks, legal experts at different levels tried to do both. The result was a series of painful compromises on the part of the experts and the citizens. Unable to process divorce cases promptly, legal experts failed to create a system where legal records of divorce reflected the true state of marriage. Frustrated with the legal system, citizens began to disregard the law, left their spouses, and formed common-law marriages without registering divorces. Because the practice of separation developed outside the legal realm, divorce statistics remained low, inaccurately reflecting levels of family stability within Soviet society. If fathers had been able to recognize their out-of-wedlock children, this might have been a psychological boon to the children. But legal experts could not pursue this solution, because pronatalist policy considered recognition a brake on birth rate. As early as July 1944, legal experts discussed three specific sets of issues in preparation for supplementary instructions to the 1944 law: child support for children who were born before the 1944 law; rights of out-of-wedlock children (born after July 1944) and their birth registration; and registration of common-law marriages and of de facto termination of marital relations.

The 1944 law had not clarified who would provide support for mothers who had children in prewar common-law marriages in cases where their prewar partners refused to legalize the marriage. Sometimes common-law marriages had been dissolved before the war began, but the mothers could not make legal arrangements to receive child support, because the father was mobilized into the army. This situation was complicated further if either parent was in occupied territory. In some cases, a plaintiff (the mother) had already filed the child support case at the court in the prewar period or during wartime, but the case was postponed because of the husband's absence at the front. This predictable postponement discouraged many women from going to court, as they knew they might appear unpatriotic for suing a soldier as he was risking his life for the fatherland. Another complication was that some prewar child support was arranged voluntarily without court involvement. After the war, some fathers stopped paying child support, believing that mothers had lost the right of appeal.

Regarding the issue of child support for children born before the 1944 law, NKIu legal experts decided to apply prewar standards to make biological fathers responsible for child support, even if the father had not legalized the marriage with the mother of the child. In cases where a plaintiff could not appeal to the court for child support during the war because her common-law husband was mobilized or either parent was located in occupied territory, the case would also be examined under the prewar law. If the prewar child support arrangement was made voluntarily, and the father stopped paying child support after the war, the mother could appeal to the court. Moreover, children who were born into prewar common-law marriages would have the same legal rights, that is, for inheritance, as children in registered marriages.

The status quo ante approach limited the number of children that fathers could support in a postwar new family, undermining the pronatalist goal of the 1944 law. Fathers who carried child support responsibilities and had children in a new family could easily fall into difficult financial conditions. Some of them asked for reduction of their child support responsibilities at the court. For example, on December 30, 1947, one Petr from Engels (Saratov oblast) petitioned for a reduction of child support. He paid 50 percent of his salary for child support, while supporting a second family of four. He demanded a reduction from 50 to 25 percent of salary on the grounds that he had another family to support, he was a war invalid, and his former wife was not particularly needy. The court rejected this claim, even after Petr's second appeal. Eventually, however, the plea of fathers who were experiencing difficulties in supporting too many families did not fall on altogether deaf ears. Fixed rates of child support could not provide an even distribution of resources for all offspring and still encourage further reproduction. This issue would be revisited during the 1960s reform movement.

The question of out-of-wedlock children was even harder to resolve. The new law provoked problems and complaints, and significantly, legal experts would soon argue that out-of-wedlock children should have equal rights with legitimate children regarding inheritance, pension, and state aid for families of service men, just as before the war. In this version, the only right that postwar out-of-wedlock children would lose was child support from their biological fathers. The opinions of legal experts were divided regarding the birth registration of out-of-wedlock children. The initial consensus when the discussion for supplementary instructions to the 1944 Family Law began was that the children should be allowed to register under the biological father's name, if the father wished and the mother agreed.[66] Apparently, this was a sensitive issue, because the editor of this draft, most likely the head of the NKIu SSSR N. M. Rychkov,[67] crossed out this statement and instead added one paragraph at the end of the letter stating that, during the discussion of the instructions, the issue of registering out-of-wedlock children under the father's name had been raised. However, because this proposal was a "significant" amendment to Article 21 of the 1944 law, it would not be included in the draft supplementary instructions. "I think this matter should be discussed separately," added the postscript. Clearly, the Commissar and his advisors were at odds on this issue and required consultation with cadres higher up in the Soviet leadership.[68]

The postwar registration of de facto marriages and de facto divorces was the other area of concern for the NKIu. It proposed to modify the 1944 law in order to expedite the registration of marriage and divorce. Regarding the registration of marriage, two situations were considered. The first was when the spouses were living far away from each other and, therefore, unable to appear together at ZAGS, the office of marriages, births, and deaths, which the law had required for marriage registration. However, especially among those who were in common-law marriages during the prewar period and who wished to legalize their status, there were many whose spouses were still not demobilized or had not returned from evacuation. In such cases, the NKIu proposed to allow registration with a letter from one of the spouses.

The second situation in which the NKIu considered it necessary to expedite the registration of marriage concerned women who were in common-law marriage in the prewar period and lost their spouses during the war. If these women had lost their marriage certificates, they could appeal to the court to establish the fact of prewar marriage. Considering that this question would have a tremendous positive impact on the bereaved's right to pension, state aid, and inheritance, the NKIu proposed to extend the same procedure to cover prewar common-law marriages, definitively ending this debate.

The proposal that the NKIu made regarding registration of de facto divorce was also a practical measure to allow simplified divorce procedures in limited situations. One such situation was marriages that had ended long before the 1944 law was issued but had not been officially voided at ZAGS. For such cases, the NKIu offered automatic divorce if either party requested this in court.[69] This proposal clearly showed that legal experts sought practical solutions so that the postwar record could reflect the true state of marriage and divorce, and fewer children could be unjustly identified as "fatherless."

The vast geographic territory of the Soviet Union became relevant to establishing criteria for expedited divorce procedure. Akin to the process of marriage registration where the physical separation of spouses prevented simultaneous appearances in court, the NKIu proposed to make a minor amendment so that divorce petitioners with small children would not have to travel. Moreover, if one of the spouses did not appear at a scheduled court hearing, the case could be postponed twice, and then the judge would proceed. This was a measure to prevent intentional avoidance of reconciliation efforts in people's court. If child support was involved, the court could subpoena either party. Clearly, the NKIu wanted these messy cases settled and removed from the docket. Clarification and expeditiousness took precedence over pronatal considerations. In other situations, the NKIu considered simplified divorce procedures as satisfying both criteria. Thus, they allowed hundreds of thousands of those missing in the war, disabled physically or mentally, or convicted of crimes to be removed from marriages at spousal request, so that these spouses could have a chance to form a new, legal, fertile family. Here the NKIu skipped the reconciliation process in people's court in favor of an immediate decision in city/oblast court. Moreover, the divorce fee of 500–2,000 rubles was waived.[70]

Some of these NKIu proposals were approved by Molotov, while others were not. In general, the government adopted proposals concerning child support and marriage that essentially were about prewar legal responsibilities and rejected those concerning out-of-wedlock children and divorce provisions that postwar Soviet leadership had introduced as new pronatalist measures. The November 27, 1944, and January 20, 1945, NKIu instructions decreed that biological fathers of children born prior to the 1944 law be held responsible for child support even if they were not in registered marriages with the mothers.[71] None of the measures that tried to improve the legal rights of postwar out-of-wedlock children was mentioned. Regarding divorce cases, simplified procedures were applied to the case of spouses missing in the war, the mentally or physically disabled, or those convicted of crimes. However, other cases were not considered. Despite the NKIu's proposal, easy divorces for marriages that had ended de facto before the 1944 law were disallowed. In sum, some of the legal experts' proposals that tried to simplify divorce procedures and all of those recognizing paternity for out-of-wedlock children were denied.

Although the top leadership of the NKIu decided to follow the party's pronatalist policy, local-level legal practitioners did not always find it so easy to ignore real life exigencies. Many documents show that local authorities violated central instructions in order to expedite divorce procedures. One of the reasons was that courts often received the instructions late. For example, in Ukraine, the November instruction first arrived in December.[72] Due to the limited number of copies, some courts never received them, so not every judge could study the instructions. Slow communication and lack of paper in the postwar period meant that sometimes courts did not receive instructions or did not have time to study them, but it is also likely that some local judges intentionally ignored the rules, considering the new instructions not useful for dealing with real divorce cases.

Judges in the people's court were especially likely to violate central instructions. The 1944 law stated that the first stage of a divorce case in people's court should consist an attempt at reconciliation. Only if reconciliation efforts failed would the case be examined at the city/oblast court. However, the NKIu found many violations of this two-stage procedure. It immediately concluded that violations were due to the inadequate definition of the division of labor described in the law. Detailed definitions followed making it clear that people's court would conduct the initial collection and examination of case materials and then oversee the attempt to reconcile the spouses. Most important, the NKIu emphasized that people's courts were not to make any decisions concerning divorce, child support, or division of property.[73]

However, there is abundant evidence that courts continued to violate the instructions on divorce. The NKIu's general court department, which studied divorce cases, generally determined that common motives for postwar divorce, such as long separation, the presence of a second family, a missing spouse, and even certain types of diseases and health conditions, were all caused by the war.[74] Just as the effects of war were irreversible, prewar families could not be mended. Probably, the court tended not to make special efforts at reconciliation or to cross-examine cases carefully. One of the common "mistakes" of the people's court with regard to postwar divorce cases was that it had hearings with both spouses but did not make efforts to understand the relationship, rendering reconciliation unlikely. Another kind of "mistake" was that people's courts made decisions about divorce, child support, and the division of property.[75] The city and oblast courts also tended to grant divorce more easily than the lawmakers had intended, leading the NKIu to complain that judges were allowing legal divorce too easily. The reluctance of many judges to strictly follow the instructions that were aimed at preventing divorce suggests that, unlike lawmakers, they understood that it was often a waste of time to attempt to repair broken bonds.

Occasionally there were cases where couples wanted to restore a prewar family even after a de facto breakup, but it usually happened when one side initially thought, mistakenly, that the other spouse had died in the war. For example, in Moscow a wife filed a divorce petition against her second husband. She had a five-year-old child from an unregistered prewar marriage. Her first husband was mobilized into the army and never contacted her again. Considering him dead, she "remarried." However, her first husband returned in 1944. "In order to restore the family," she wished to return to him. During the hearing, she, her first husband, and her second husband agreed that her return to the first husband would be the most "correct" decision. In another case, a husband who was demobilized looked for his wife and child in Moscow and Smolensk oblasts, to which they had been evacuated during the war. After the search failed, he considered them dead and got married. However, a few months later he found his former wife and child. He filed a divorce case with the second wife, wishing to return to the first wife, although by then the second wife was pregnant. Such cases were few. In the city of Moscow and Moscow oblast, "restoration of the prewar family" did not rank in the top five motives for divorce.[76] In the RSFSR, it ranked seventh (2.9 percent) as compared to "the presence of a different marriage," which ranked first (28.1 percent).[77]

The leaders of the NKIu, eager to show the party and government some evidence that the anti-divorce measures were strengthening the Soviet family, ignored the work of those who studied postwar divorce cases. In November 1944, NKIu SSSR Rychkov reported to A. S. Shcherbakov about divorce cases in the city of Moscow and Moscow oblast. He emphasized that the number of divorces had significantly declined since July. In contrast with the pre-1944 law period when the monthly divorce cases increased from 455 (January 1944) to 708 (June 1944), the average between July and November 1944 had decreased to 120. Based on this, he concluded that "the basic goal of requiring a court order to dissolve a marriage, namely, a decisive reduction in the number of divorces, can be considered achieved."[78]

This misrepresented the situation. The 1944 law certainly reduced the number of divorces, but this was an administratively created result rather than an actual reduction in marital collapse. There were many reasons that the number of broken marriages was much higher than the number of official divorces in 1944. Between July and November 1944, many courts simply stopped reviewing divorce cases because the 1944 law lacked detailed instructions about how to handle divorce.[79] Only after the issuance of supplementary instructions in November did courts resume taking divorce cases. Divorce filings were also delayed because, typically, newspapers delayed the required publication of a divorce announcement. A local newspaper could only publish a limited number in each issue, so plaintiffs often had to wait a few months. Courts understood that without publication, the case could not proceed and tried to solve this problem. In Moscow, courts asked the *Evening Moscow* (*Vechernaia Moskva*) to publish the backlog within two to three months and to publish forthcoming announcements within one month of their receipt.[80]

Probably the most important reason that the official divorce statistics were a poor reflection of reality was that failed prewar common-law marriages were not counted, the category of relationships most threatened by the 1944 law. The actual number of such breakups cannot be known, but the significance of this phenomenon can be seen in the prevalence of postwar child support cases, which involved mothers of prewar common-law offspring.[81] When their common-law husbands left them in the postwar period, no registration of divorce was necessary, but these women were entitled to ask for child support. One was Elena (Engels, Saratov oblast), who was in a common-law marriage between 1933 and 1944 and had a daughter born in 1934. Her husband left her and said that he would not pay for child support because he was no longer responsible under the 1944 law. The court ordered the husband to pay one-fourth of his salary for child support.[82]

A woman in the city of Saratov "married" in 1937, and then had one daughter and two sons. Without having been registered, the marriage ended in "de facto divorce" in 1945. The court ordered the husband to pay 50 percent of his salary for child support.[83] Another woman, Zinaida (Engels, Saratov oblast), was in a common-law marriage between 1942 and 1944 and had a daughter in August 1943. Her husband left Engels for work in Khar'kov in November 1943. For a while he sent letters, but then he disappeared. Later she found out his current address through the address bureau in Kiev. The court ordered him to pay a quarter of his salary for child support.[84] Zinaida's marriage was shorter than Elena's, but before the 1944 law both would have been considered as legally binding as registered marriages. However, the breakup of prewar common-law marriages was not counted as a postwar divorce. The authorities would not allow the harrowing personal experiences of millions of women to demonstrate instability of marriage in the official statistics.

Despite the difficulties of the procedure, divorce numbers began to climb. As Rychkov reported it, the number of divorces dropped after the 1944 Family Law in urban areas of the RSFSR from 205 in 1943 to 107 in 1944 per 1,000 registered marriages.[85] Yet the number of divorces in all regions of the RSFSR rapidly increased between 1946 and 1955 from 7.9 (1946) to 68.3 (1955) per 1,000 registered marriages. [86] Analyzing various statistics on marriage and divorce, demographer V. B. Zhiromskaia explained the postwar increase in divorce statistics by describing two scenarios: legalization of registered prewar marriages that had ended in de facto divorces before 1944, and remarriage of men with women much younger than themselves, leading to divorce from prewar wives.[87] This demonstrates that despite all the bureaucratic obstacles, couples made great efforts to straighten out their legal status so that their children could have the father's name and/or they could marry their postwar partners.

The Movement to Protect Out-of-Wedlock Children

The NKIu was thus responsible for providing a rosy, yet inaccurate, picture to the party and government in November 1944, claiming that the 1944 law's pronatalist measures were already a great success. In reality, the NKIu's reluctance to resolve contradictions between the law and real practices, and the single-minded focus on cutting the divorce rate, had detrimental consequences for the well-being of Soviet family and marriage. Many children who lived with their biological fathers were officially designated as out-of-wedlock children because either or both of their parents could not get an official divorce. Most important, the new divorce law encouraged men to disregard their legal responsibility to register marriage and divorce. Because divorce was too difficult to obtain, men who found another partner simply walked away from the marriage, without going through the legal divorce and taking up a non-registered "marriage." Given the postwar demographic sex imbalance and the cost of divorce, women were often willing to accept unofficial marriage. This created many serial marriages where official and unofficial marriages overlapped with each other. Moreover, the disregard of legal procedure regarding marriage and divorce created many spontaneous marriages and divorces that were not reflected in the legal record.[88]

Communist Party members were a special case. Apparently the Party Control Commission (KPK) considered cases of party members' marital misconduct as serious moral lapses and expelled them.[89] D. A. Kirpichev left his legal wife and children during the war, claiming that he had been mobilized. In fact, he began working as the head librarian in a military school. Without getting a divorce, he "married" another woman. M. A. Pankov, a railway worker, married a woman during a business trip, without divorcing his wife. For several years his wife and daughter searched for him in order to demand material help. N. I. Smirnov also "married" a woman in 1945 without divorcing his prewar wife. After a while, he abandoned the new wife and their ten-month-old baby. He found yet another woman and started the cycle again. K. P. Berdennikov, secretary of Dzhambulskii gorkom in Kazakhstan, left with a coworker in 1946, abandoning his wife and two children.[90]

The party sought to punish such men on moral grounds for "inappropriate behavior in everyday life." In many other cases, especially when the man was not a party member, there was no systematic way to control such behavior nor any legal penalty to prevent it. Clearly, women, with few legal protections, bore the brunt of these serial liaisons. If a woman gave birth to a child in a non-registered marriage, she would officially become a single mother, but as long as she lived with the male partner she would not be eligible for state aid for single mothers. If her partner left, she would have no right to demand property or child support. She would instead become eligible for state aid, but many chose not to apply for aid to avoid humiliation and surveillance.

The 1944 law was designed to boost the number of single mothers and out-of-wedlock children, and this process of making and un-making marriage-like ties definitely accomplished this aim. But the process undermined other primary goals of the same law: increasing long-term population growth and stabilizing the Soviet family. The growing number of fatherless children meant at least a temporary increase in population, but A. Abramova, a party activist would soon point out that these children had special problems, both physical and psychological. The stability of the family could not be achieved in the way Soviet leaders had planned because instead of staying in legal marriage and taking responsibility for raising children, husbands in extramarital relationships simply walked out on their legal families. Moreover, some men avoided marriage altogether, so that they were never legally responsible for any family, even if they had fathered children. Their only responsibility under Khrushchev's reproductive system was to pay the bachelor tax.

From the viewpoint of the Soviet state, postwar family policy, having created millions of fatherless children, could be considered a success. However, this state "accomplishment" aroused great discontent, especially among women.[91] Considerations about children powered a moving communication from Sinel'nikova of Moscow in 1944, a 31-year-old widow without children. Her letter criticizing the 1944 Family Law articulated the illegitimacy of a law that crushed women "morally," leaving children "fatherless," although neither mothers nor children were responsible for the fact that there were no men to marry.[92]

One cautionary letter, concerned with the potential for incest, came from Kuzovkina of Komsomol'sk-na-Amure. She argued that if the law does not allow the child to carry the biological father's family name, in eighteen to twenty years, there would be marriages between brothers and sisters who did not know that they were related. Even worse, she argued, there might be marriages between fathers and daughters. "Therefore, children need to know their fathers and must carry their family name and patronymic, even if they do not receive support from fathers. . . . After all, children are innocent."[93]

One man, Sharikov (Engels, Saratov oblast), writing for his wife, posed this situation. The man and woman had lived together for ten years and had six children. They were expecting a seventh child. The wife asks, if she leaves her husband without registering the marriage and her husband takes the seventh child, why should the child have her family name?[94]

Party members who were responsible for women's issues heard about difficulties that the 1944 law had caused for women. In 1948, A. Abramova, a party activist, studied the condition of single mothers and their children using materials collected by the Ministry of Health (MZ), the Ministry of Internal Affairs (MVD), and the party.[95] She also interviewed single mothers. Based on this study, Abramova wrote a report addressed to Stalin, which described the "extremely grave" conditions that single mothers and their children were facing and proposed "immediate intervention."[96]

Abramova's report showed the rapidly increasing numbers of out-of-wedlock children. Her numbers were taken from ZAGS statistics, which, as she pointed out, were incomplete and probably underreported. In 1945, about half a million children, or 18.3 percent of all births in the Soviet Union, were out of wedlock. In 1946 and 1947 the absolute number of out-of-wedlock births was 50 percent higher than in 1945. Abramova predicted that the number would continue to grow as general living conditions among the population improved. The percentages were shockingly high in large cities. In Leningrad in 1945, 43.8 percent of all births were out of wedlock. In 1946, Moscow (29 percent), Kiev (28 percent), and Minsk (23 percent) all posted very high rates. Since such a large number of births were out of wedlock, Abramova thought it necessary for the state and party to consider the conditions of single motherhood an important factor in population recovery.[97]

The report showed that single mothers were psychologically and materially battered, and their children's health suffered as a consequence. Abramova discussed how single mothers were the victims of wartime demographic changes and of the men who betrayed them.

> During the Great Patriotic War, many women lost husbands. These wives, like most young women, sincerely wish to found a family, to have a husband and father for their children. However, they cannot realize their wishes because of the significant numerical superiority of the female population and unwillingness of some men to take on the burden of having a genuine family. . . . Among [single mothers,] of course, there are many women who became mothers due to the false promises made by men about a future life together.

Abramova's interviews with female factory workers provided numerous examples of those who became single mothers as a result of men's betrayal. To highlight her point that single mothers were not frivolous, Abramova mentioned that most of them had had a relationship with their partners for two to three years. But interviewees explained that male partners left the women as soon as they found out about the pregnancy and began going out with other women. The single mothers told Abramova that these "male butterflies" promised a wonderful life, using beautiful words, but all of this turned out to be "the conscious trickery of the immoral."[98]

Many women reported that once abandoned by their partners, they attempted abortion. Indeed, Abramova argued that this was reflected in the large number of abortions in Moscow; approximately 80,000 illegal abortions reportedly occurred between 1945 and 1948, but this figure was likely underreported. Abramova further argued that abortion both diminished the birth rate and harmed women's capacity to work. Every woman who had an abortion lost hours at work; plus, if the abortion led to physical damage or death, the total workforce was reduced. Abramova did not directly criticize current abortion policy, but the logical implications of her comments are that the only way to effect a significant reduction in underground abortion was to increase material support, including better housing conditions and a broader network of childcare facilities for pregnant women and mothers.[99]

Abramova's appeal for increased attention to the well-being of single mothers included a powerful discussion of the appalling health condition of out-of-wedlock children. The 1944 law stipulated that single mothers had the right to leave their children in orphanages and apparently many single mothers took advantage of this. In 1946, 20,007 children and in 1947, 35,790 children under one-year-old were sent to orphanages in the Soviet Union, many of whom contracted serious illnesses soon after being institutionalized. In 1946, 33 percent and in 1947, 44 percent of children placed in orphanages died. Probably based on this report, the MZ was required to study the health conditions of children in orphanages every month starting in 1948.[100]

Abramova suggested that the cause of this high incidence of disease and death was not a lack of material support for orphanages since the government provided sufficient funds. Rather, she argued, an orphanage child is "deprived of the most indispensable— maternal milk."[101] She also pointed out that children in orphanages, for whom the state was spending a per capita average of 7,435 rubles, were less healthy than fatherless children raised in single-mother families on whom the state spent 600 rubles.[102] Abramova proposed that orphanages refuse to accept children under one year of age, except when the mother had died or was ill.[103] Implicitly, she was also suggesting that the state provide more aid to single mothers to encourage them to raise their children at home, which would ultimately improve the health of fatherless children.

In addition to the physical health of mothers and children, Abramova argued that their psychological health was in danger. She was referring to the impacts of the new birth registration system in which fathers of out-of-wedlock children were not recorded anywhere in official documents; on birth certificates, the line for father would be simply crossed out. She argued that this registration system caused psychological damage to single mothers and possibly to out-of-wedlock children in the future.

> Sooner or later, either in school or at home, a child will face the question: who is your father? Therefore, we must change this condition and indicate on the birth certificate in the space labeled "father," his first name and family name, as reported by the mother. Such a record would relieve the single mother of the unnecessary and agonizing task of explaining to

her child. It will also protect the child from possible moral trauma, when the child for the first time sees the birth record without the first and family name of the father.[104]

Abramova also lamented the poor material conditions for single mothers, as the state aid to support them was, she implied, woefully insufficient and poorly administered. In order to qualify for state aid, a single mother had to obtain a certificate from the militia which indicated her age and the number of children living with her. The militia issued such a certificate, monthly, after visiting the family and conducting a personal investigation to ensure that she was not living with a male partner. Many single women considered this surveillance system humiliating because it resembled the police registration of "women of easy virtue" in Tsarist Russia.[105] Abramova pointed out that many single mothers consequently chose not to apply for aid despite their material difficulties; thus, the percentage of single mothers receiving aid remained low. In 1945, of 470,000 single mothers, 285,000 (60.6 percent) received aid. In 1947 out of 747,000, 482,000 (64.5 percent) single mothers received aid.[106]

Single mothers were also impoverished because they were not exempted from the taxes for citizens with few children. Abramova considered this practice wrong "from the viewpoints of both morality and material conditions." To improve living conditions for single-mother families, Abramova thought it important to stop militia surveillance of mothers, transferring this responsibility to house-management offices; and eliminate the taxes on single mothers for having few children, if they did not receive state aid or pension.[107]

Abramova emphasized the urgency of improving the physical, psychological, and material conditions of single mothers and their children, but in order to fundamentally resolve the problems with single motherhood, men's attitudes toward family had to change. To this end, the report proposed heavy taxes on single men, up to 45 percent of their wages. This she considered "just" since "many men using various excuses refuse to register their common-law marriages and completely abandon their children to the protection of their mothers and the state, avoiding all material and moral responsibility." The number "45," significantly higher than the 6 percent tax on salary paid by both male and female childless citizens, was rationalized as the average percent of wages paid by women to support their children, "not counting [the value] of personal labor, sleepless nights and all the stressful experiences" connected with the raising of children." [108] Whether as punishment or positive motivation, Abramova probably thought that increasing the financial burden might convince men to form a legal family and stop changing partners, the common practice of overlapping serial marriages, referred to in plaintive letters as "polygamy."[109]

Abramova's report recommended the formation of a special commission to discuss how to improve conditions of mothers and children. In response, the party formed the Commission under the Secretary of the Central Committee on the Question of Women's Labor and Improvement of the Protection of Motherhood and Childhood on December 10, 1948. Members included M. D. Kovrigina and Abramova.

This committee would become instrumental in generating reform ideas regarding the 1944 Family Law. Based on committee discussions and the Abramova report, members were asked to make recommendations for improvements in the working and living conditions of women. As issues such as the welfare of pregnant women and nursing mothers, abortion, and out-of-wedlock children's health fell to the Ministry of Health, M. D. Kovrigina, Deputy Minister of health, played a key role in this commission. Kovrigina, together with N. I. Smirnov, Minister of Health, represented the MZ on the commission and prepared an MZ recommendation on "improving the working and living conditions of women" some time in early 1949. Half of the measures concerned single mothers and half addressed the problems of pregnant and nursing mothers.[110] Regarding single mothers, the recommendations were extensive, including differentiated government aid to single mothers depending on the average income, extending government aid to single mothers until the child turned sixteen, and releasing single mothers from the responsibility of paying the small-family taxes.[111] One proposed new measure was to begin government aid for single mothers from the moment of confirmation of pregnancy. One can imagine that the authors were aiming for a preventive measure against abortion and an incentive for single mothers to carry pregnancies to term.[112]

Abramova's radical suggestion to levy high taxes on single men did not appear among the MZ recommendations. However, the document did echo Abramova by including an amendment to the 1944 Family Law to make "fathers become real fathers," if only in name. It said that if the father of the child wished, he could be recorded in the birth registration as the father either at the time of registration or at a later time, but without any ongoing financial responsibility for the out-of-wedlock child, even if the child used his patronymic. Such changes to birth registration were deemed important, because it "saves millions of children born of single mothers from moral trauma, when they first lay eyes on their birth registration lacking the first, middle and last names of a father."[113] Thus, health officials clearly understood the direct link between the 1944 Family Law and the unsecured welfare of mothers and children.

It is not clear whether these MZ recommendations, prepared for the party commission for women, were presented to higher levels of the party. However, a heightened concern for the well-being of single mothers and fatherless children was clearly in the air. In 1948–1950, special governmental legal commissions were preparing an amendment to the 1944 Family Law. The question of registering out-of-wedlock children—that is, making "fathers real fathers"—was one of the most contested issues being reviewed for amendment.[114] But no legal reform on the issue of paternity materialized during Stalin's or Khrushchev's reign.

Too Many Ways to Become a Single Mother

Home Again, a short 1947 novel by Zh. Gausner, mocks how women thought about marriage in the postwar marriage market. In this story, two mothers, each with a daughter of marriageable age, are concerned about finding partners for their daughters from a limited pool. There is an assistant manager of a factory, who is a legless demobilized soldier. Another is a widower who is much older and according to the young daughters "ugly" but materially well-off. Tellingly, the last contender is the district party secretary, who is married and lives with his wife and children. The daughters' first choice is the single, crippled man, but the mothers evaluate the situation differently. One even suggests that her daughter ignore the party secretary's existing marriage and lure him into a common-law marriage so that she would become the "first lady of the district."[115]

For many postwar women, finding a marriage partner was a serious challenge. Irina, born in 1929, said in an interview that half of her classmates in middle school remained single all their lives.[116] Lena, born in 1925, talked about how many women of her generation never married. Many women married much older or much younger men. In fact, Liudmila, born in 1923, married her husband, twelve years her senior right after the war. Some women who did not find husbands decided to become mothers anyway, like a friend of Irina who decided to have a child at age 37 when she got pregnant during a business trip.[117] As in *Home Again*, in reality, because of the gendered decimation of war, healthy, single, young, and "attractive" men were scarce. In this environment, many women had to think about marriage differently from the way it appeared in the prewar period.

Wartime relationships, the politics of demography, and the 1944 law shaped people's decisions and desires about postwar marriage and family. Demobilized men who had prewar families but had formed new liaisons usually did not want to return to their old households. If the prewar marriage was common-law, they were free to remarry, although the financial responsibility for earlier children remained. On the other hand, if they had registered prewar relationships, then they were now subject to new, stricter divorce laws. Getting the court, tasked with reducing the number of divorces, to grant one was no mean feat. The law generally did not allow easy divorce, even for marriages that had practically ended before the war began. However, this did not stop men and women pursuing new de facto marriages, family life, and personal happiness. This resulted in postwar de facto marriages and divorces, which had no legal significance but became the subjective reality of life for many.

As millions of demobilized men abandoned their former families, they created de facto single-mother families. The surplus of postwar women made it easy for single men and even men with de facto divorced status to find new partners. In a world without contraceptives, this was a simple recipe for more "single mothers." Women who had served at the front and had grown too close to their comrades-at-arms also found, often enough, that the relationship had been only temporary. The production of "single mothers" and the reproduction of "fatherless" children were both growth industries in the postwar Soviet Union.

State aid to single mothers was supposed to replace prewar child support by biological fathers, but the amount was continually reduced and was not always paid regularly.[118] On November 25, 1947, aid to mothers was cut in half on the grounds that since "the country's economy is expanding, the ruble is getting stronger, and its buying power has significantly risen, it would be unjust to preserve the high level of aid set up during the war."[119] Moreover, many single mothers chose not to apply for state aid because the qualification process was humiliating, or they were living with a partner. De facto single mothers, who were left by husbands without an official divorce, were not qualified to receive state support for single mothers. The 1944 law required enterprises to accommodate the children of single working mothers, but most factories did not have adequate childcare facilities. Thus, single working mothers were often forced to leave their children alone without regular nourishment or adult supervision. Both gradual deterioration in health and dramatic, even life-threatening, accidents were the predictable result. The alternative was state orphanages, where the mortality rate was much higher than average.

These varied life-courses produced tens of millions of unmarried mothers and out-of-wedlock children in the decades following World War II. The TsSU data for 1945–1963 show 13.6 million out-of-wedlock children over eighteen years of age. Partial data suggest slightly lower rates in the late 1960s, when changes in registration practices made identification of out-of-wedlock births more difficult.[120] Therefore, 15 million "out-of-wedlock" children between 1945 and 1968 seems a conservative estimate of "new single mothers," as well. In addition, in postwar society there were single-parent families, readily recognizable in public parlance as "single mothers," which included millions of war widows. Women who failed to obtain divorces but were abandoned by their husbands would also be counted as de jure married, de facto single. In total, it seems likely that between 1944 and 1968, Khrushchev's Family Law caused over 30 million Soviet mothers and children to experience the typical privations of the one-parent family under difficult financial conditions, even poverty. To this would be added the child's various traumas of growing to adulthood without a father. The bitter moments of single mother-life were more common in the postwar USSR than in any other country in the world.[121]

The Soviet government degraded the status of postwar women by identifying women's reproduction as a tool for the reconstruction of the Soviet economy and society, manipulating marriage and divorce laws in order to make reproduction easy for men to consider, creating a stigmatized group of out-of-wedlock children and unmarried mothers, and not providing sufficient support for women who brought up children alone. These negative social phenomena did not go unnoticed, but the expert commissions and committees learned that the top party leadership would not approve their recommendations. Although the policymakers had allowed this to happen in the name of pronatalism, eventually and ironically this would negatively affect the birth rate. Instability in Soviet families, driven both by the war and the 1944 Family Law, a reaction to the war, caused women to avoid pregnancy. For those who nonetheless became pregnant without the proper household conditions, illegal abortion beckoned. Abortion statistics continued their upward trend.

4

Who Is Responsible for Abortions?

Demographic Politics and Postwar Studies of Abortion

The number born in January–August 1948 is 22% lower than in the corresponding period in 1947.... In line with this, it should be noted that in 1948 the number of abortions went up. The data, received by TsSU from MZ for the first half of 1948, shows that the number of abortions is increasing.

V. N. Starovskii, head, Central Statistical Administration (1948)

Why isn't the husband held responsible [for abortion]?

M. D. Kovrigina, RSFSR Minister of Health (1950)

The growth in births from 4.03 million in 1946 to 4.45 million in 1947, was characterized by V. N. Starovskii, head of the Central Statistical Administration (TsSU), as "the postwar baby boom."[1] However, in October 1948, Starovskii highlighted the "falling birth rate crisis" in a secret report to top Soviet leaders, placing blame on the rising number of abortions. A. Abramova's August 1948 report to Stalin directly linked "difficulties with housing, crèches, and material conditions" to the rising abortion rate.[2] But Starovskii's report to the country's leadership did not make explicit the connection between real-life conditions for women and falling birth rate.

Starovskii was a shrewd statistician who understood that in order to survive under Stalin, statistics should follow Stalin's politics. In the late 1930s, Stalin had prominent demographers shot who presented census statistics that contradicted his predictions.[3] After Starovskii replaced a series of purged directors, he showed his loyalty by twisting the all-Union 1939 census to match Stalin's inaccurate views.[4] After this Great Purge of the profession in 1937–1938, the upper echelons of the Soviet leadership deprived themselves of key

Replacing the Dead. Mie Nakachi, Oxford University Press (2021). © Oxford University Press.
DOI: 10.1093/oso/9780190635138.003.0005

indicators and analyses for running an industrialized society, leaving what the best historical account calls "bureaucratic anarchism."[5]

Starovskii continued to focus on political survival rather than scientific development. In early 1944, when an initiative from a much-respected professor and authority on census evaluation, A. I. Gozulov, called for the re-opening of an Academy of Sciences demographic institute, Starovskii summarily dismissed it.[6] Gozulov had already enlisted the support of several other prominent academicians,[7] but Starovskii wrote back politely, yet bluntly on February 16, 1944, and said that no scientific institution should engage in the study of the current demography of the Soviet Union.[8] Starovskii wished to monopolize statistics so as to leave no room for "misuse." By practicing self-imposed censorship during thirty-five years of statistical authoritarianism under three general secretaries, he successfully covered up many devastating consequences of government policies.

During the evolving Cold War rivalry, Stalin wanted to make the Soviet Union look more populous, and therefore stronger, than it actually was. He had announced during his *Pravda* interview on March 13, 1946, that Soviet deaths in the war numbered only 7 million, although Starovskii was sure that the population level in 1947 was far lower than the level Stalin's comment implied. Instead of correcting Stalin, Starovskii advised against census taking. On July 14, 1947, he wrote to N. A. Voznesenskii, head of Gosplan, saying that census taking in the near future was inappropriate and instead proposing a one-time counting of the population.[9] Unlike census data, one-time counting data did not need to be published. In this way, statistics did not have to contradict Stalin's statement.

Moreover, Stalin introduced a further measure to strictly control statistical information. On March 1, 1948, he classified all key demographic information "state secret," cutting off industrial planners from estimates of key demographic data.[10] One of the key reasons for this was probably the desire to hide the effects of the 1946–1947 famine. Stalin's decision was diametrically opposed to the emerging world population control movement, for which the United Nations was urging every country to conduct a census around the year 1950.[11] Eminent British biologist and the first director general of UNESCO Julian Huxley wrote to UN Secretary-General Trygve Lie in 1948 that the contemporary understanding among the Western nations was that the Russian birth rate was still the highest in Europe.[12] By not conducting a census and keeping statistics secret, Stalin could let this myth prevail. In this environment, how to explain shifts in the birth rate was politically sensitive.

Starovskii would highlight positive signs of population growth, obscure true causes of negative trends, and avoid detailed analysis. In doing so, he identified abortion as responsible for the falling birth rate and never mentioned famine.

Globally, promotors of both anti- and pro-natalist demographic policies have often blamed women for what they consider an undesirable state of demography. In wartime Japan the pronatalist government encouraged early marriage and five children per couple on average. However, the birth rate was clearly falling, particularly in urban areas. Pronatalists identified the cause as "low moral character as a wife" and "lack of resolution and sense of obligation as the nation's citizen" among young women.[13] In the 1960s United States, population controllers blamed African American women for being "irresponsible" for reproducing "unwanted children" and causing many social ills.[14] In both cases women became easy targets. By blaming women, promoters of demographic policy could avoid discussing fundamental issues such as poverty, lack of childcare, inadequate housing, and racism that shaped "undesirable" reproductive practice among women. In the same way, Starovskii avoided discussing the famine, difficult postwar living and working conditions, and the ills of pronatalist policy.

Soviet doctors and lawyers would challenge this view that women were the cause of the falling birth rate by arguing instead that women were victims and providing detailed studies of women's abortion practices. The Ministries of Health (MZ) and Justice (MIu) conducted a study of abortion in late 1949–1950, the first comprehensive, large-scale study of abortion practice, including illegal abortion, since its criminalization in 1936. MIu, in line with its mission, limited its research to criminal abortion cases, while MZ studied the legal abortion system and illegal abortion practice, about which little was known. As Mariia Kovrigina noted, the result of this study challenged the notion that women alone were responsible for the rising number of abortions, an important recognition for the advancement of abortion policy reform.

This chapter discusses the way in which demographers reported the crisis of falling birth rate as a result of rising abortion, which led Starovskii to emphasize abortion as the main cause of demographic shrinkage. It will also cover the interministerial survey of clinical and non-clinical abortions to summarize legal and medical views, with a focus on the analysis of non-clinical abortions and the attempt to depict "typical" circumstances of underground abortions.

The group of women whom the MZ and the MIu studied sometimes over-lapped, since those questioned and prosecuted were primarily the ones hospitalized after botched abortion. However, the data compiled and the type of analysis diverged because of the different professional concerns and perspectives of the Soviet medical and legal professions. Collected survey data were also open to different interpretations depending on how the data were organized. Kovrigina took a decisive interpretive position and achieved unity among doctors and lawyers. Her views would eventually open the road to legalization of abortion after her elevation to USSR Minister of Health in 1954.

Demographic Approaches: Ignore the Famine, Blame Women

In the pronatalist state, demographic analysis of population growth directly affected the regime's expectations from and evaluation of the work of Soviet obstetrics and gynecology. According to Starovskii's projection in 1944, the number of births should have improved steadily after the war. Regarding abortion, there was an understanding that abortion surveillance stopped functioning during the war and non-clinical abortion became prevalent, though no statistics existed to prove this. After the war, it was expected that abortion surveillance efforts would resume and reduce the number of illegal abortions.

According to a TsSU report to the Soviet leadership, the number of births after the war showed an upward trend in 1946 and 1947. In 1946, there were 4 million births in the USSR, which was a significant rise from 2.5 million in 1945. In 1947 this number modestly increased to 4.5 million.[15] The number of births was expected to increase in 1948 as well, since the sex ratio in the villages had improved significantly since the end of the war, as Starovskii documented in a March 20, 1948, report to Molotov. Among the adult rural population of productive ages, the ratio of male and female rose from 37 to 100 on January 1, 1945, to 67 to 100 on January 1, 1948. Even in devastated Smolensk oblast the sex ratio improved from 19 to 100 in 1944 to 53 to 100 in 1948. This report circulated among the top Soviet leaders.[16] The TsSU's quarterly summary of demographic trends to the top Soviet leaders did not always include information on abortion although TsSU was receiving such data from the MZ.[17] In 1947, the number of all abortions was reported to be 581,000, down from 661,000 in 1946.[18] Thus, the trends exhibited by the 1947 data could be interpreted to suggest that the year 1948 would deliver a higher birth rate and decreased abortions, a victory both for Khrushchev's law and Starovskii's statistics.

Contrary to statistical expectations, 1948 brought bad news to the Soviet leaders. On October 9, 1948, Starovskii reported to Molotov that a comparison of the first eight months of 1947 and 1948 showed a 22 percent drop in the number of births. The "postwar baby boom," which he had trumpeted in 1946 and 1947, had ended prematurely.[19] Since the number of deaths for the first eight months of 1948, was 31 percent less than for the same period in 1947, Starovskii implicitly, but unmistakably, attributed the reduction in natural population growth to rising abortion rates:

> The number born in January–August 1948 is 22% lower than in the corresponding period in 1947, which coincided with the period of the postwar birth rate increase. In line with this, it should be noted that in 1948 the number of abortions went up. The data, received by the TsSU from the MZ for the first half of 1948, shows that the number of abortions is increasing.[20]

Starovskii's argument made women (and MZ) responsible for falling population growth. This may have even sounded convincing since, according to his data, the 103,000 loss of population growth for the January 1947–August 1948 period roughly matched the increase in the registered number of abortions (both legal and illegal) for the same period (98,000). An increase in the number of abortions in 1948 would have negatively affected the number of births not only for 1948 but also for 1949. In fact, the 1948 annual total of 885,000 was a leap from 581,000 in 1947, dashing hopes for a long baby boom and a further decline in abortions.[21] The Starovskii report set off perceptions of a 1948 "birth rate crisis."

However, Starovskii's presentation completely ignored the significant effects of famine in the winter of 1946–1947 on the trends in the 1948 numbers. If famine is factored in, the analysis of the same data can be quite different, both for births and abortions. Although the 1947 number of births (4.45 million) was higher than the 1946 figure (4.03 million), Starovskii ignored decelerating growth to emphasize "the postwar baby boom."[22] The rate of conception between March 1946 and February 1947, which was reflected in the number of births for 1947, should have been much higher than the conception rate between March 1945 and February 1946, the key indicator for births in 1946, especially since until September 1945 the USSR was still at war. One of the key factors must have been the famine.[23]

Because the famine occurred in late 1946, the number of births that year was largely unaffected. Instead, the full impact would show in 1947 through mid-1948, with the rate depressed by various famine-related conditions: amenorrhea, malnutrition and diseases, restraint in the face of hard times, and the overall high rate of mortality.[24] According to Starovskii's month-by-month data for January–August 1947, the number of births declined steadily from 458,000 to 369,000, continuing downward in early 1948 from 333,000 (January) to 255,000 (April), incorporating both the residual effects of famine and seasonality.[25] In May 1948, the number of births began to show an upward trend, but only in August did the absolute number of births recover to 405,000, the 1947 level. Any linkage to famine went unmentioned.[26]

Once the post-famine trend was established, it would have been possible to expect an upward trend for the number of births later in 1948, making the "crisis" of falling birth rate seem a temporary phenomenon at worst. In fact, the number of births for the entire year of 1948 was not much worse than the previous year, 4.12 million compared to 4.45 in 1947. In 1949, the number shot up to 5 million, as women who deferred having a child during the famine got pregnant.[27]

Some of the reasons for the sharp increase in the number of abortions in 1948 in comparison with 1947 also have roots in the famine. In 1947, many women who might have chosen to abort must have died or become temporarily infertile, driving the number of abortions down. Due to deteriorated health conditions, the conception rate in 1947 would have been lower, which would also have suppressed the overall number of abortions, even offsetting some increase in miscarriages and abortions. As health conditions gradually improved toward the end of 1947 and into early 1948, the rate of conception and the number of pregnancies gradually picked up. If pregnancies were not wanted, this would lead to an increase in abortion. In any case, it is possible to argue that one of the reasons that the 1948 abortion figure seems much higher than in 1947 was that the 1946 famine lowered conception rates, in turn reducing abortions.[28]

Of course, the fact that Starovskii did not want to discuss famine in relation to the 1948 basic demographic indicators was a conscious political decision. This did not mean that Starovskii and others never reported the impact of the famine on the demographic situation of the USSR. Khrushchev and

Kruglov reported directly to Stalin on the appalling situation created by the famine and the necessity of helping the population in affected areas.[29] In late 1947, Starovskii reported to Molotov on the numbers of deaths, births, and the natural population growth for January–July 1947 in comparison with the comparable figures for 1940 and 1946.

Here he focused on the significantly increased number of deaths (1.387 million) in 1947 compared to 0.924 million in 1946. He cited two causes: increased infant mortality, (up 132 percent from 135,000 to 314,000) due to "an increased birthrate" in 1947, and "a significant rise in the number of deaths in several regions." The affected regions were Ukraine SSR, Moldova SSR, Voronezh oblast, Kursk oblast, and Krasnodar krai.[30]

Starovskii did not say why there was a sudden increase of deaths in those particular regions, but there is no doubt that Soviet leaders understood that it was the famine. It would have been obvious to a demographer that such a sudden and large growth in deaths in a large area of the country that included key agricultural regions would have a negative impact on births and deaths at least until the early months of 1948. Starovskii was probably not wrong in reporting that the number of abortions in general was rising in 1948, but he avoided making a causal connection between the famine and the birth rate crisis.

This politically induced move resulted in directing Soviet leaders' attention to women's reproductive behavior. Once the main cause of low population growth was identified as abortion, it was not Stalin or leaders of agricultural industries but women and Soviet specialists in women's medicine who were at fault for the low birth rate. The MIu and the state prosecutor would also be forced to reexamine their work regarding abortion surveillance. In a sense, the ministries and their experts were taking the blame for the famine, but it did offer them a chance to do something about the precipitous increase in abortion.

In 1948, Soviet leaders were made aware of the rising number of abortions from several sources. The TsSU report was one of the earlier ones, but Abramova had already sent Stalin a report on August 14, 1948, about the rising number of abortions in connection with unstable gender relations and difficult living/working conditions, especially for single mothers. If, as the Abramova report suggested, rising abortion had a direct connection with the 1944 Family Law, it would be urgent to consider this factor in the creation of the All-Union Family Code, for which the drafting process was scheduled to begin in 1948.

With this bad news coming from multiple sources, in mid-1949 the Council of Ministers (Sovmin) criticized Soviet obstetricians and gynecologists for their failure to report directly on abortion to the Sovmin and to ask for help from other government organs. The MIu and the prosecutor's office were included among those blamed because of their role in abortion surveillance. Spreading responsibility among several institutions pointed the way to an interministerial study as a first step toward rectifying the situation.

The Battle with Abortion: The Interministerial Study Brigade Gathers All-Union Data

Medical professionals were fully cognizant of the rising number of abortions and surveyed illegal abortion practices toward the end of 1948.[31] Underground abortion rates had increased dramatically from 23.8 per hundred births (1947) to 43.5 (1948), with the highest rates in Moscow (97.6) and Leningrad (73.3) in 1948.[32] By 1949, the rate of abortion had surpassed the prewar levels of 1940.[33] Responding to the Sovmin criticism, at the MZ Collegium meeting on September 2, 1949, MZ SSSR officially called for the preparation of a comprehensive report to the Sovmin SSSR about the dynamics of abortion in the country by the MZ, the MIu, the state prosecutor, and the All-Union Central Council of Trade Unions (VTsSPS). [34] A special interministerial commission, headed by Mariia D. Kovrigina, was founded to prepare a report and proposal for the Sovmin. Not only medical experts but also representatives of the USSR State Prosecutor, the MIu, and the VTsSPS were included as members. Such a report would include diverse information on both legal and illegal abortion and general conditions of pregnant women and nursing mothers at work and at home. Court cases with regard to questions of alimony for children and divorce would also be incorporated.[35] The MZ, together with the VTsSPS, organized five brigades to study five oblasts.[36] A revised version of the 1948 MZ questionnaire was distributed and the survey was conducted for the fourth quarter of 1949 and the first quarter of 1950.[37]

As the number of incomplete abortions increased, the number of women reported to the investigator by doctors and then brought to trial increased as well, suggesting doctors' compliance with political pressure. Between 1948 and 1949 the MIu reported a sharp increase in the number of criminal cases of abortion. The general number of convicted (abortionists, women, and those who forced women into abortions) increased by 39.4 percent. Most significantly, the number of women who had self-induced abortion and were convicted increased by 66.9 percent, suggesting almost a doubling in many republics. Among various Soviet republics Tadzhikistan had the highest increase in convictions, with 168.6 percent, followed by Kirgiziia, 114 percent, Lithuania, 97.4 percent, and Belorussia, 91.9 percent. The most populous republics, RSFSR and Ukraine, had 69.6 percent and 73.8 percent increases, respectively.[38] The rise in the number of prosecutions probably not only reflected the rising number of illegal abortions but also increased alarm following the 1948 statistics from MZ.

Higher conviction rates put the spotlight on criminal abortion, so in late 1949, the MIu also launched a study of selected criminal abortion cases in various cities, oblasts, and republics. As mandated by the September 2, 1949, MZ Collegium, a commission was formed to study the battle with abortion in conjunction with the more general task of overseeing the implementation of existing legislation on motherhood and infancy. This commission, in turn, put together brigades with representatives from the MZ, the MIu, and the VTsSPS to collect the basic data in several locations, including Moscow, Saratov, Ivanovo, Sverdlovsk, and Khar'kov.

They were tasked with studying the support system for childbearing and childrearing, including medical, legal, and financial aid, as well as the working environment for women and housing options made available to mothers.[39] They also examined legal and illegal abortion practice by collecting and analyzing data about clinical abortions. Regarding non-clinical abortions, the brigade organized surveys among women who were saved from failed abortions at hospitals. The brigade asked specific local medical institutions to have such patients anonymously fill out a questionnaire.[40] The brigade further evaluated the abortion prosecution practice by examining selected local abortion cases as the MIu did. The survey study of illegal abortion provided data never before collected.

As of 1948 nearly 90 percent of all recorded abortions were estimated to be non-clinical, with only 11.3 percent legal, so the development of effective measures to reduce illegal abortion was clearly the key to the overall reduction of abortions.[41] The brigade surveys of women who ended up in clinics after botched abortions provided key materials for identifying the reasons and circumstances of those who sought underground abortions.

Many aspects of the brigade study of illegal abortions at the local level are unclear from available sources. However, the brigade and overall MZ reports and a set of 1948 and 1949 local reports from Saratov underscore key aspects and problems of the survey. By identifying differences and similarities between Saratov reports for 1948 and 1949, it is possible to deduce the MZ's evolving approach to the issue.[42]

Reports written by Professor M. A. Daniakhii, director of the women's clinic of the Saratov Medical Institute, detailed the results of 100 questionnaires.[43] The most important items highlighted in the conclusions included age, marital status, income level, presence of infant, housing, the number of abortions and pregnancies, and reasons for abortion. Postwar women in Saratov who had unsuccessfully induced abortions were most commonly between 20 and 30 years of age, followed by those between 30 and 40. Over 60 percent had between one and three children. Nearly 40 percent were childless.[44] The majority (around 70 percent) were married, but a third were single or in common-law marriages.[45] The addition of the category of common-law marriage is significant since that legal category had disappeared since the 1944 Family Law.

Since most women were either de jure or de facto married and already had a child or children, in the 1948 and 1949 surveys only thirteen of the 100 cases of abortion involved first pregnancies.[46] The 1948 and 1949 surveys indicated that although the majority of women who sought abortion themselves were making less than the 500 ruble average for a full-time garment worker, as a family they were often making more than 1,000 rubles. Unlike in the pre-1936 surveys that revealed poor material conditions as a common reason for abortion, poverty no longer seemed to be the decisive factor for postwar non-clinical abortions in Saratov.[47]

In the presence of a child or children, nursing was sometimes a factor affecting decisions about abortion, according to the brigade report. In Saratov, the percentage of nursing mothers among those who chose illegal abortions varied from year to year. While there were only two women in 1948 who had a child younger than 1 year old, in 1949, twenty-six had a child under 1 year, suggesting that this was not a consistent factor for increasing abortion.[48]

A more consistent problem was childcare arrangements. The survey revealed that very few children were sent to crèches or kindergartens. In 1948, fifteen of eighty-seven (17 percent) of those surveyed sent their child to a crèche. Children were mostly taken care of by mothers and grandmothers. Moreover, a surprisingly large number were also left without any care; 22 percent of respondents said that the child or children were without any supervision.[49] Of the fifteen mothers who gave reasons, nine said that they could not pay the fee and six said that childcare institutions did not provide good care. The 1949 survey produced similar results with regard to the number of children being sent to childcare institutions and the reasons for not sending them.[50] Perhaps the idea of babies left without care was politically too unpalatable to be presented, although it was not an uncommon option for single mothers.[51]

Insufficient childcare can be illustrated both quantitatively and qualitatively from other sources. On August 3, 1950, in a letter from Shabanov to N. S. Khrushchev, secretary of the Central Committee VKP(b) and Moscow Committee VKP (b), the number of crèches was reported as down 65 percent from the 1940 level. As a result, 11,000 children, mostly those of single mothers and war invalids, were on a waiting list. Shabanov continued, "Many single mothers have to leave children in a locked apartment without supervision." Concrete cases were provided. B. M. Poiasniuk wrote to the MZ that "her nine-month-old is tied up in the crib so that he does not fall out while alone all day." Many single mothers stopped working, leading to reduced income, poor material conditions, and impoverished diet both for the child and mother. Many working nursing mothers were losing milk. The report further connected material conditions with child health. According to a Moscow investigation, "30 percent of children entering crèche are in weakened health." Inability to place children in crèches had serious effects on the "material and moral conditions" of single mothers. Shabanov's letter asked for universal crèche access for all working mothers.[52]

The fact that most children were taken care of by mothers or grandmothers implied that unmarried mothers without their mothers to help them would have trouble working and raising a child. In the postwar period, orphanages were increasingly considered a depository for out-of-wedlock children. The percentage of children under the age of 1 housed in orphanages rose between 1948 and 1950 from 41 percent to 56.1 percent. At the same time, the percentage of out-of-wedlock children among all young children who entered orphanages steadily rose from 37.5 percent in 1947 to 62.8 percent in 1950.[53]

Free childcare and immediate access to orphanages for single mothers were stipulated in the 1944 Family Law, but this was not guaranteed in reality. The brigade reported that single mothers were often waiting for a long time before their children could be received at orphanages,[54] although the 1944 Family Law stipulated that they had the right to leave their children at orphanages whenever they needed. In Sverdlovsk oblast, twenty-four single mothers were reportedly rejected by orphanages because they had not adequately registered evidence of their husbands' deaths in World War II. In Khar'kov, single mothers had to sometimes wait two to three months before having their children accepted in orphanages, but some were still rejected. The VTsSPS was accused of doing nothing to resolve this problem.[55]

Probably based on the alarm expressed in Abramova's letter to Stalin and the statistical data therein, the MZ had been required to study the health conditions of children in orphanages every month since 1948. The quality of healthcare seems to have improved from Abramova's 1947 baseline. On July 12, 1951, Shabanov reported to the Presidium the Sovmin SSSR that, while in 1947 20.4 percent of all children in orphanages died, in 1950 the number was 6.9 percent. Also, the percentage of children dying before their first birthday fell from 36.8 percent to 13.9 percent.[56]

Housing was believed to be one of the major reasons for limiting the number of children. The Saratov survey showed that housing did matter, but it suggested that the amount of space was less important than the type of living space. The 1948 and 1949 results showed that there was a variety of housing available, so it would be wrong to conclude that women who tried to get an abortion did so simply because of lack of space. It is not surprising that women sharing a room in a dorm or apartment or living in one room were among the majority. However, in 1949 it is also notable that those who had two rooms or a separate apartment were not so rare (29 percent).[57] Bad housing conditions were not among the top factors on the list of reasons for abortion in Saratov.

The most illuminating information presented in the report was the reason for abortion. Each woman provided multiple answers, so the total is not known, making computation of percentages impossible. The Saratov survey showed that material difficulty (50) and relationship problems (35) were highest on the list in 1948. The presence of other small children (23) and bad housing conditions (10) followed.[58] By 1949, relationship problems had taken the lead; bad material conditions (35) and relationship problems (38) were the highest, while the presence of a small child was not far behind (32). "Relationship problems" included husband living with another wife, expected divorce, abandonment by the husband, a husband in hiding, or no husband.[59]

Even for those who were in stable relationships, low expectations of paternal help discouraged women from considering another child. The 1949 report specifically pointed out the fact that only 5 percent of women had no desire to have a child and that 95 percent of women answered that they wanted to have one more child but didn't consider it possible.[60] The first reason was "lack of confidence in childcare being shared by the father even at a minimum level."[61] With this perspective in mind, the 1949 report highlighted relationship problems, such as divorce plans, the husband's second family, and lack of husbands, grouping them into a category newly considered as the most important cause of illegal abortion. The second was identified as material difficulties, although these were rapidly declining compared to 1948. The third reason was the presence of children younger than the age of 3. The 1949 report noted that housing conditions were often combined with these reasons, but that basically material difficulties were less important than in the previous year.[62]

Similar brigade surveys were conducted, and reports were produced in Moscow, Ivanovo, Sverdlovsk, and Khar'kov. Based on them, the final brigade report was produced on March 20, 1950. The overall results on major reasons for abortion were similar to those of Saratov, although there was greater emphasis on housing and work environment in the final report. The five major reasons were listed as bad housing conditions (28.9 percent); instability of the family in various ways (existence of a husband's second family; marriage not registered; bad relationship with the husband; single) (27.5 percent); instability of family relationship and lack of appropriate housing (18.2 percent); the law on the protection of women not observed at workplace (15.4 percent); and bad material conditions (6.8 percent). Thus, the brigade report made the point that a combination of family instability and housing conditions led to underground abortion for all the localities where the survey had been conducted.[63]

The MZ produced a general conclusion to the study of illegal abortion using the local reports and brigade report. Interestingly, it showed a slight, yet significant shift in emphasis. Instead of simply copying the result of the brigade report, the MZ report supplemented it with other kinds of data from other parts of the USSR.[64] It stated that a "significant group of abortions fell upon the flower of young womanhood, having only one or two children or also childless," up to 30 years old. The basic characteristics of women having none, or one or two children, coincided with the case of Saratov, although the percentage of childless women and women with one or two children is higher in these additional oblasts (93.1 percent) than in Saratov (65 percent). The report said that the percentage of single women among women who induced abortion by artificial means varied depending on the city: 10 percent in Rostov oblast, 22.4 percent in Krasnodarsk krai, 12 percent in urban

Moscow, and 42 percent in Sochi. The percentage for Saratov was reported at 26 percent.

Finally, the MZ established the primary four reasons for abortion in the USSR: unstable family (45.7 percent); bad housing conditions (28.8 percent); hard physical work at enterprises (15.4 percent); and difficult material conditions (6.7 percent).[65] Nearly half of women asked listed the top reason for abortion as unstable family, which included several versions: husband's second family, unregistered marriage, and a bad relationship with the husband/partner. This meant that not only unmarried women chose to have an abortion for fear of becoming de jure single mothers, but married women also chose to terminate pregnancies lest they become de facto single mothers. It is important to note that the category "unstable family" is most likely a combination of the first two reasons for abortion presented in the brigade report. While the brigade report separated abortion performed due to family relationship difficulties from those due to both relationship problems and housing conditions, the MZ report combined the two.

"Hard physical work at enterprises" suggested that lack of support at work for mothers posed a significant reason for abortion. Unlike in Saratov, the general report did not include material difficulty as a primary cause for abortion, and this was confirmed by the fact that more than half of women who induced abortion by illegal means received between 300 and 500 rubles income per family member.[66]

It was important that family problems were reported as the primary reason, because this is how the cause of abortion would be explained at the highest level of government. Although government support and economic reconstruction could eliminate material problems for some women, they would not help the majority of women with family problems. Nor could the doctors of the MZ convince women to give birth without economic guarantees or supportive family relations.

The MZ result could be compared with the mid-1930s survey of reasons for abortion, which was probably the last survey officially conducted of abortion practice. This study questioned women who applied for clinical abortion under the legalized abortion system. Among 5,365 women, the number one reason (31 percent) for abortion was economic conditions, second (29 percent) was already large families, and third (20 percent) was pregnancy resulting from casual sex. Various family problems comprised only 8 percent.[67]

If the primary cause of illegal abortion was economic, it would have been possible to argue that no new policy was necessary because, as the Soviet Union rebuilt its postwar economy, women's economic conditions would gradually improve, so fewer women would choose illegal abortion. In this case, the war could be blamed for women's abortion practice. However, among the relationship problems, both de jure and de facto single motherhood and child-support issues could not be expected to fade naturally over time, especially since the number of out-of-wedlock children and the number of divorces were still increasing. By highlighting relationships as the major cause for abortion, doctors could also voice their concerns about irresponsible fathers, even though this problem was beyond the realm of their professional expertise.

In writing this report, the Ministry of Health, in particular Deputy Minister Kovrigina, must have been aware that medical experts could do nothing to eliminate the primary cause of illegal abortion. If so, doctors should focus on supporting, rather than prosecuting, women by expanding opportunities for legal abortion, making preventive means available, that is, education and contraceptives, and providing legal and economic support through the social-legal consultation office within women's clinics. These measures were pursued immediately after the study.

The MIu Analysis of Criminal Abortion: Why Are Only Women Prosecuted?

The MIu SSSR collected detailed reports from various cities, oblasts, and republics, including Ivanovo, Sverdlovsk, Khar'kov, and Saratov oblasts, and several raions (districts) of Moscow oblast and Moscow city (similar to the MZ study). The MIu prosecuted three categories of abortion crimes according to corresponding articles in the various republican criminal codes: abortionists, those who forced women into abortion, and women who underwent abortion. In the RSFSR, Article 140, part 3, 140-a, and 140-b of the Criminal Code corresponded to these crimes, respectively. It appears that all prosecutions under 140-a involved men, except for a few female friends who were also caught. Naturally, all 140-b prosecutions were women. Cases were examined by the categories of the Criminal Code, and other information was provided, such as what kind of sentence was given; person's class, age, party membership, and profession; the location of crime (urban/

rural); the accused person's past criminal record; reasons for abortion, place, conditions, method of abortion, timing of abortion within the pregnancy; and length of investigation.

An examination of criminal cases is helpful for learning about concrete cases of relationship problems that resulted in illegal abortions and for understanding who was prosecuted for abortions as opposed to who was responsible for abortions. Regarding the basic characterization of women who underwent illegal abortion, the MIu and MZ materials matched. In Sverdlovsk, Ivanovo, and Saratov, aborting women were not teenagers.[68] In Sverdlovsk, most aborting women had a child or children, and many of them had between two and four children. Few were childless. Regarding marital status, the MIu showed a higher percentage of single women, but with huge regional variations. In Kazakhstan, among the 263 cases of self-abortion examined, 70 percent were by single women. The rest were married.[69] In contrast, Ivanovo oblast was almost the opposite, with 79.5 percent married.[70] In Saratov, of 150 cases examined for a study of marital status, 65.3 percent were married, and 34.6 percent were either single, widowed, or divorced. Overall, single mothers were significant, but still not the majority: 41.2 percent were single, 58.1 percent were married, and 0.7 percent were widows.

Since most mothers had at least one child, this was rarely a case of first pregnancy. However, this did not mean that this was the first abortion. Women rarely confessed about past abortions, since they could receive a stiffer sentence than public censure for being recidivists. In some cases women did confess to past abortions for which they had not been caught, and such information provides an insight into millions of "successful" illegal abortions like Lena's in the Introduction, that would otherwise have gone unreported. For example, when Dubrovina was accused of having an abortion in January 1949, she admitted to having abortions twice before in 1939 and 1946. When she was caught in October 1948, Panacheva admitted to having had two abortions in 1941. In May 1949, Drankova said that she had had four pregnancies, two of which ended in abortion, the other two births.[71] None of these three had previously been convicted for criminal abortion.[72] In terms of the number or frequency of abortion, they are not likely to have been uncommon cases. Naturally, medical experts were concerned about abortion-induced infertility.[73]

Overall, criminal abortion was an urban phenomenon, both because the recorded number of botched abortion cases was smaller in the villages than in cities and because there were not many rural medical establishments for women to go to after failed abortion cases. The case of A. N. Filippova, a 35-year-old woman working in a kolkhoz (collective farm), can serve as an example. A widow and mother of a 12-year-old son, she tried to avoid the birth of a fatherless child when she was four months pregnant. But her attempt failed, and she was hospitalized with hemorrhage and stomach pain. The pregnancy was saved, but one evening Dr. Muzalevskii at the hospital gave her an abortion, without an agreement with Filippova's attending doctor, allegedly, at the request of Filippova's brother and sister. Both Filippova and Muzalevskii would end up as urban crime statistics, easily prosecuted and convicted, but the underlying cause and crime was a product of rural conditions and took place in the village.[74]

Identifying the reasons for abortion in the case of Filippova would not have been simple, especially because it involved her siblings. But even in cases where third parties were not involved, underlying causes were not thoroughly investigated. The Sverdlovsk report criticizes the People's court for often simply accepting the reasons given by the offenders. Nevertheless, causative factors in 306 cases were examined and listed as material difficulties combined with other reasons (49.6 percent); pregnancy from casual sex (15.6 percent); and nursing (4.3 percent). Material reasons were combined with presence of children, divorced from husband/abandoned by husband, husband is ill or imprisoned, and so on. However, following the method used by the MZ brigade, it would have been possible to group at least six reasons on the list with a clear "partner-relations" component and consider unstable relationship with the husband or other partner as being a significant reason for abortion. This totals 34 percent, putting "relationship issues" far ahead of "casual sex" as an abortion factor, though still lagging behind "material conditions."[75]

In places where single women represented the majority of abortions, the convicted had a more specific reason to abort. In Kazakhstan, where 70 percent were single women, the most common explanation was avoidance of out-of-wedlock births. This reason can also be viewed as a partner problem. Even among married women, relationship issues were common. In Kazakhstan, they often cited material difficulties, whether caused by the husband's low salary, illness or invalid status, and divorce from the husband.[76] In local societies where men were the main breadwinners, economics and relationships merged. In Ivanovo oblast the two major reasons were identified as poor material conditions (38.3 percent) and no husband (34 percent).[77]

"No husband" could encompass single women, married women with husbands who had abandoned them, and pregnant widows.

In Saratov, the four most common reasons were listed as the presence of one or several children, and no wish to have more; single status, pregnancy as a result of casual sex or brief de facto marital relations; poverty; and family discord. However, it is also possible to group several categories under problems with "husband."[78] Thus, the initial MIu analysis did not emphasize the significance of relationship problems as a major cause of criminal abortions, but this would be corrected by female participants at a MIu Collegium meeting.

Criminal cases incidentally provide some of the clearest examples of the male partner's decisive influence on abortion. For instance, E. A. Kurganova from Saratov had been in a registered marriage since 1937 and had two children. Her husband treated her poorly and betrayed her. When she became pregnant by him, her husband said to her, "Why do I need the child? Abort it."[79]

The case of A. P. Fedorova of Saratov was labeled "economic," but it also shows the deleterious effect of an unregistered marriage. Fedorova was 25 years old when she became pregnant by Citizen Voevodinyi, her de facto husband. Voevodinyi was conscripted to the army, leaving Fedorova with a two-year-old child, disabled parents, and a sister in middle school, all as her dependents. When six months pregnant, she was fired without warning. After several attempts to find a job, she decided to abort due to "difficult material conditions." She used a syringe to inject liquid manganese into her uterus. After this attempt failed, she took two airplane flights, thinking that might induce miscarriage. The child was born prematurely and died after twenty-one hours.[80] In this narrative, the departure of the de facto husband sounds innocent, but if he wanted, he could have registered the marriage and/or supported Fedorova and her family materially, even while in the army. What she considered "marriage" was a temporary relationship for him. As a de jure single mother who avoided having an additional child, she was prosecuted.

A case from Sverdlovsk presents a particularly tragic example of how unstable relationships involving single women could lead to multiple abortions. Riabov, a single man, who was without a full-time job, had sex with Pecherskikh and got her pregnant in 1946. Afraid of permanent ties to Pecherskikh, Riabov beat her and organized a scandal, pressuring Pecherskikh to get an abortion. He gave her 200 rubles, and she aborted. In 1947 Pecherskikh got pregnant again with Riabov and again aborted at his urgent request. In 1948, Riabov impregnated Valiavinaia. He insisted that she get an abortion, telling her the method of abortion that Pecherskikh had used. He told her, if she aborted, he would marry her, but if she didn't, he would not marry her. As a result, Valiavinaia intervened in the eighth month. Despite multiple offenses of the same crime, Riabov was given only a two-year sentence for forcing women into abortion.[81]

The majority of abortions took place between the second and sixth month of pregnancy. But some late-term abortions also occurred, and they often had especially tragic consequences. Valiavinaia's eight-month pregnancy seems to have ended in stillbirth, but there could have been even graver results from a late-term abortion. For example, T. E. Mironenko, a 28-year-old milkmaid at "Karamyshskii" sovkhoz, was single and, during her last trimester, she asked the accountant of the sovkhoz (state-owned farm) to give her an abortion. As a result, the child was born alive prematurely. Mironenko strangled the infant and threw it down a well. The dead child was found on July 8, 1949, the fifth anniversary of the 1944 Family Law. [82]

Cases involving pregnancy in an advanced stage also posed legal issues on the separation of abortion from murder. N. Ia. Papkina asked an abortionist Antonova to terminate her pregnancy when she was seven months pregnant. The attempt ended with a premature birth, and the baby was drowned in a dirty bucket.[83] M. V. Potanova's six- to seven-month pregnancy also ended with premature birth during an abortion attempt. The newborn soon died, and the mother buried him.[84] Based on such cases of abortion where the fetus was already capable of extrauterine life, the report asked to change either article 136 (murder) or 140-b (self-abortion) of the Criminal Code so that punishment for abortions after the sixth month could be made more severe.[85]

Many women also died in failed abortions. Less detail is provided on such women, since investigation was usually brief and muted. In Saratov, of the fifty-two women in thirty-nine cases studied, there were five deaths: L. M. Kostiukhina, weaver, age 23, died on December 9, 1948; M. F. Fadeeva, a kolkhoz worker, age 28, six months pregnant, died on January 24, 1949; P. P. Petrova, a factory inspector, age 30, three months pregnant, died on February 6, 1949; Z. I. Fadeeva, a worker at a sovkhoz, age 28, five months pregnant, died on August 13, 1949; and A. F. Shkolina, worker, age 44 (month of pregnancy not indicated), died on September 15, 1949.[86]

Despite the fact that forcing a woman to have an abortion was a criminal offense in all Soviet republics, men were rarely held legally accountable for such deeds. In Khar'kov oblast, there were three cases filed for 143-1 of the Ukrainian Criminal Code (equivalent of 140-a in the RSFSR Criminal Code).[87] In Sverdlovsk oblast, five cases were filed for 140-a, as opposed to 565 women prosecuted under 140-b. In Saratov, there was no filing for 140-a, although clearly the case of Kurganova should have been examined under this article. As the Saratov report criticized, "However, the prosecutor not only did not call Kurganov to account for this crime under Article 140-a, but he was not even interrogated." The People's Court also took no initiative.[88] In Ivanovo oblast, there were three cases under Article 140-a, as opposed to 535 cases under 140-b. However, there was one more case filed under Article 140-a. E. V. Belgradskaia, who attempted self-induced abortion, had explained that she decided to commit the crime under threat by her husband, who said he would leave her otherwise. However, the People's Court took no initiative in prosecuting her husband.[89]

Because of the difficulty in establishing a crime for 140-a, the number of cases in this category was usually negligible, and not much analysis or discussion was forthcoming. This lack of attention to the role of men in abortion cases would be criticized primarily by female legal experts at central meetings, who complained that those who encouraged abortion never received the attention paid to abortionists. When abortion was finally legalized, the criminalization of those who encouraged women to undergo abortion was also abolished, but uncertified abortionists remained illegal.

The brigade's evaluation of abortion prosecution, from the March 1950 report, not surprisingly presented similar conclusions. Here the criticism was mostly of the inadequate prosecution of criminals other than the women themselves and indifference of legal and medical professionals toward illegal abortion. It also criticized the court for handing down light sentences to abortionists, in particular medical doctors, who received only one-year sentences. Medical personnel were also attacked for becoming indifferent, even reconciled, to illegal abortion. Not much was said about those who encouraged women to undergo abortion. The report complained that prosecutors often used incomprehensible terminology, suggesting an uncooperative relationship between prosecutors and the brigades. Only a short discussion was dedicated to women's motivation for illegal abortions: "The numbing of Soviet and civil consciousness among the population has a great influence on the growth of abortions, . . . as does the instability of family life in a certain percentage of the cases."[90]

The 1950 MIu report on criminal abortion cases pointed out that the circumstances under which women chose criminal abortion had not been investigated properly. Based on the materials from the Ivanovo, Sverdlovsk, Khar'kov, and Saratov oblasts, and several raions of Moscow oblast and Moscow city, the conclusion stated that 63.1 percent, the "majority of cases, took place in the cities and workers' settlements." The report found that most women already had a child/children and that 42.8 percent were single women. Above all, it criticized inadequate punishment of abortionists. However, nothing was mentioned about those who encouraged abortion and were therefore eligible for prosecution under 140-a. Criticism of the investigation of abortion circumstances may explain the absence of an overview of causes.[91] The fact that the primary reasons for abortion were not identified and the role of men was not discussed would soon resurface at the MIu Collegium meeting, when female legal experts took up the case against irresponsible fathers and the 1944 Family Law and found themselves in accord with MZ Deputy Minister Kovrigina.

On May 10, 1950 the Collegium of the MIu SSSR met in Moscow to discuss the results of the abortion study and produced a resolution in the name of the presiding Minister of Justice K. P. Gorshenin. Not only legal experts but also representatives of public health, forged a joint policy on abortion. But the road to consensus proved rocky as discussions became heated at times. Both professional and gender perspectives clashed. The meeting began with a presentation by Comrade Sokolova, a representative of civil court organs of the Ministry of Justice.[92]

Sokolova's report is not filed in the archive, because it was probably distributed in advance in written form, but its main points are clear from the questions and comments that were recorded by the stenographer. Apparently, Sokolova discussed why women were aborting and how to stop them. She also talked about the fact that single women were a significant presence among those aborting illegally and proposed to increase punitive measures toward them. This drew criticism from Comrade Pashutina who noted, "It often happens that especially with single mothers, a number of circumstances force her to this path." Pashutina considered it more important to punish those who force women into abortion, whatever their relationship to the woman. She also suggested that single mothers should be exempted from the "bachelors" tax paid by those with zero to two children, because "all difficulties of raising children are on her."

In relation to single mothers, Pashutina mentioned out-of-wedlock children without registered fathers. "While the child is small, this does not mean much. However, when the child reaches school age and enters school, he will already understand that he has no father. In order not to force the child into such a trauma, we proposed that the mother could register the child with some kind of father, so that the child knows that he has both father and mother." Regarding the idea of increased aid to single mothers, Pashutina agreed with Sokolova that this was not good, because there were many problems administering aid to single mothers. For example, many single mothers rejected aid because of the humiliating process of check-up by the militia or housing administration. She considered that there should be another "path of government aid for raising these [out-of-wedlock] children" rather than through government aid to mothers.[93] In this way, female participants pointed to the connection between the creation of fatherless children through the postwar family law and women's decisions not to have another child.

At this point, MZ Deputy Minister Kovrigina presented the results of the recent study of anonymous questionnaires. She identified the major reason for abortion as "relationships within the family," referring to the general conclusion derived from the MZ study. What she considered most terrifying was that many women became infertile after their first underground abortion. "We must not cripple women. We need healthy women. However, we deprive women of health by our approach to these abortions." In order to save women's health, she considered that the husband's role was central to saving women from abortion and subsequent infertility, because the primary reason for abortion proved to be a poor relationship with the partner.

Kovrigina criticized the existing abortion surveillance system that made only women responsible, given that causes were shared by men and women. "Why isn't the husband held responsible [for abortion]?" Kovrigina asked rhetorically. She proposed that local party organs make husbands criminally responsible for forcing wives into abortion by taking away their party cards.[94] "This way, there will be an effect," she added. On this point Comrade Kliachko, the head of the social-legal office of the Moscow city public health administration, agreed because "penal policy has a great educational meaning" to help husbands learn not to force their wives into abortion. [95]

Public health officials' insistence on viewing abortion as a relationship problem between men and women and to punish men as well as women for their role influenced the MIu resolution. Although the general conclusion of the MIu study did not touch on the 140-a category, the resolution included a statement that said, "Trials of abortion cases at court are often conducted superficially. They do not clarify the real circumstances in which the abortion was attempted or reveal the people who necessitate and instigate women to abort." An example from Moscow was given to illustrate this point. Seminikhina, who was tried under 140-b, declared that her husband forced her to have an abortion, but her husband was not prosecuted.[96] The resolution included an order to the organs of the MIu to pay more attention to the protection of women's personal and property rights, especially timely and appropriate decisions of cases on child support, with strict enforcement of the decisions.[97] The idea that women alone were not responsible for abortion would be reflected in the 1954 decision that ended the criminality of women's abortions. Nevertheless, legal recognition of fathers' responsibility never entered the criminal code.

Medical Reforms: From Prosecution to Prevention, 1950–1952

Subsequent MZ measures for fighting abortion explicitly emphasized prevention of both undesired pregnancies and illegal abortions rather than prosecution. Some measures had already been proposed prior to the brigade study, but several novelties appeared afterward. In June 1950, the Collegium of the MZ SSSR discussed the results of the brigade study at a meeting to which representatives of the VTsSPS, the state prosecutor, and the MIu were invited. New measures for preventing abortion were issued in the June 30, 1950 *prikaz* (governmental order) and the July 27, 1950 instructive-methodological letter on the topic "public health work to fight against abortion." They included public health education, contraception, and consultation. General efforts were to be made to diversify media and expand audience for public education, to develop and increase production of contraception, and to improve consultation.

The new emphasis on understanding individual women's family circumstances and needs through individual consultation and identifying at-risk pregnancies was a clear outcome of the joint study. This understanding was most vividly expressed in the introduction of individual discussion in public education, as opposed to mass education through lectures and pamphlets. This was detailed in the 1950 instructive-methodological letter, which echoed medical experts' earlier laments that women did not register pregnancy as long as they were not sure whether to keep the pregnancy, and when women actually came to clinics to confirm their pregnancy, they often brought a fake identification or went to a consultation far from their residence, thus making medical monitoring nearly impossible. The 1950 prikaz again called on doctors to identify those who might abort from among those who came to confirm their pregnancies.

The instructive-methodological letter clarified how this should be done "most effective[ly]"during the doctor's individual discussions with patients, based on the doctor's abilities and authority. The instruction argued that most women visiting women's consultation do not need any "agitation for preserving pregnancy." These are people who "conscientiously relate to the questions of marriage, family, and motherhood." For such people, educational work would primarily entail imparting information to protect the health of mothers and children. However, "among the many pregnant women who visit woman's consultation," there "may be those for whom pregnancy is not desirable." In such cases, the important task for doctors and midwives was to "discover the reason" pushing the woman to seek interruption of pregnancy. Such a task could involve interviewing neighbors, friends, and/or the husband.[98] Unlike before 1949, the purpose of the doctor's investigation would be prevention of abortion rather than prosecution.

Since everyone knew that women who came to confirm an undesired pregnancy would disappear after confirmation, the instruction told the doctors to conceal the test result about pregnancy. This way there would be time to identify such women accurately, ascertain their reasons, and convince them not to interrupt their pregnancies.

In some cases such women clearly expressed the undesirability of having a child. In other cases, women listened to the doctor's confirmation of pregnancy nervously, in a state of heightened excitement, putting doctors on their guard. In such cases, doctors sometimes did not announce the pregnancy right away. Instead, they would recommend that the woman have a second examination in a couple of days. This created time for an investigation of the woman's living and working conditions involving doctors, nurses, and social-legal office consultants in order to help organize measures to support her pregnancy.[99]

Doctors were instructed to isolate at-risk cases. At the top of the list were "pregnant single women (not legally married)." The second group was pregnant women with traces of previous underground abortion. These two categories were at greatest risk, but a third group of concern included women who insisted on referral to an abortion committee without having the conditions listed in the criteria for clinical abortion.

In light of the brigade study's finding, the instruction said that doctors sometimes need to talk with not only the women themselves but also family members. Therefore, they would need to study in advance "individual family situations, including the relationship among family members, their knowledge of the pregnancy, and their relationship to the question of preserving the pregnancy."[100] In this way, doctors developed new measures to mitigate relationship problems and material difficulties, the two major reasons for abortion as identified by the study.

The renewed focus on the family relationship was also evident in the new measures for the work of the social-legal consultation office. This office employed consultants to discuss problems with the patient, and then contact workplace, housing administration, and trade union representatives to try to improve women's living and working conditions so that pregnant women would not be rejected or fired, and to ensure observance of labor laws concerning women, so that mothers could continue to work. It appears that except in large cities, social-legal consultation offices existed only on paper.[101] Due to the awareness that individualized support for women was the key to convincing them to keep their pregnancies, Kovrigina discussed the need to train consultants. This new approach was codified in the June 30, 1950, prikaz.[102]

The "new" measure of individualized discussion between a doctor and woman echoes the early postwar discourse of individual consultation that was later condemned as "private practice." In 1945–1947, this would allow individual doctors to adapt prewar criteria for legal abortion to the new women's health realities. In the post-purge context of MIGO, a proposal to influence patients in individual discussion is striking, for "individual discussion" in practice would probably function in the same way as "individual treatment." The difference was that this intimate space between a doctor and patient would be used not for providing a woman with an exceptional (or extralegal) permission for legal abortion but for identifying who she was in order to prevent her from undertaking abortion. In any case, similarities between these two approaches demonstrate that postwar medical experts consistently acknowledged that their effective participation in women's reproductive decisions was possible only when women shared with the experts their special circumstances.

To what extent doctors followed the instruction is not clear, but given the spirit of the period when doctors were trying to expand opportunities for clinical abortion, it is unlikely that doctors widely engaged in investiga-tive work through individual discussions in order to limit women's access to legal abortion. More likely doctors either helped women find a way to get a clinical abortion or helped them with financial, legal, and family problems through the consultation office. Of course, some doctors probably continued to use individual discussions in order to find ways for safe abortion, either by writing false diagnoses, offering an operation, or referring patients to an abortionist.[103]

The October 19, 1951 ukase promised more and improved contraceptive devices. In theory, the need for contraception for women whose conditions automatically qualified them for legal abortion existed as early as the 1936 criminalization of abortion.[104] However, the development of contraception was suppressed, since it would be counterproductive to the pronatalist goals. The brigade report also pointed out the chronic shortage of contraceptives for women who had conditions approved for clinical abortions and needed to practice contraception. Even in Moscow, "only a limited assortment of contraceptive devices was available," and so doctors' prescriptions could not be filled. This made it impossible to lower the number of legal abortion cases.[105] Thus, the brigade report offered a new opportunity to promote con-traception and the October 19, 1951 ukase codified this reform.

The new measure very clearly showed doctors' renewed commitment to improving the quality of contraceptives, in particular the kinds to be used by women. Those products included female condoms, intrauterine rings, cervical caps, and pessaries. Doctors justified the development of contracep-tion by arguing that "this (i.e, contraception) does not decrease birth rate, but saves the health of many thousands of women."[106] Their call for increased production of reliable contraception usually went unfulfilled because of lack of resources and poor quality control.[107] Doctors understood that in the planned economy, the investment necessary to increase the production of contraception depended on a leadership decision.[108] As long as that was not forthcoming, they could only develop technology and await the day when mass production would become possible.

The basic spirit of this reform was expansion and simplification of oppor-tunities for legal abortion. Here the brigade analysis became the basis for reform ideas. Under the 1936 law, when a woman who wished to have a legal abortion did not have conditions listed in the criteria for legal abortion, or the pregnancy was past twelve weeks, the local abortion committee was not allowed to grant permission. In such a case, she would have to submit her application for an exceptional permission, together with the doctor's diagnosis, to one of the central abortion committees, located in larger oblast-level cities. However, for a woman to be able to apply, she had to be a resident of that oblast. This highly centralized and rigid system created various delays in providing legal abortions to high-risk pregnant women, forcing them first to travel to seek exceptional permission and again to receive the operation.[109]

Another issue the brigade reported was that local doctors felt strongly that clinical abortion as a medical necessity should be free. Surprisingly, even after the 1936 criminalization of abortion, the fee for a legal abortion was determined locally. In the brigade study, it was revealed that in all five oblasts researched, the fee for clinical abortion was 50 rubles. According to the November 1936 instructions on legal abortion, collected fees were supposed to be used for improving women's health and material conditions, but in fact they were paid directly to the abortion committees. In Moscow, the chairman of the abortion committee received 15 rubles per hour, other members 10 rubles, and the secretary 3 rubles. The reason was that there was no other budget for the commission.[110]

Among various reform measures, the main ones were that abortion became free, abortion committee decision making was streamlined, and doctors were instructed to always refer women to an abortion committee, regardless of their health condition, whenever they so wished. In order to process permits for more cases of legal abortion, the ukase also stated that the number of abortion committee positions at gynecology and obstetrics hospitals and clinics should increase. Maternity homes and hospitals with a large abortion workload should also add a nurse to the staff for this specific purpose.[111]

Most important, the new measure expanded the list of criteria for legal abortion, as most medical experts were in agreement that serious new medical conditions had become common in the postwar period. One key issue was whether to include nursing (breastfeeding), one of the most common reasons for which women had been given exceptional permissions in the late 1940s. Even more controversial was the question of whether to allow other non-medical reasons. In light of the study of illegal abortions, which revealed that relationship problems, together with material and living conditions, were the major reasons for abortion, should these be included? Doctors and lawyers were fully aware of these causative links, but no available document reveals discussion of these issues.

On the new list of forty-nine criteria, some new categories of conditions are particularly noteworthy. Those who had seen the face of battle might well deserve abortion for the "absence of an extremity or lack of [an extremity's] movement," "blindness in both eyes," or "complete loss of hearing." An expanded list of tubercular and syphilitic conditions reflected those epidemics and a wide range of genetic diseases, such as myopathy, ataxia, deaf-dumb syndrome, and hemophilia, were also included as sufficient proof for abortion permission, if documented on either the maternal or paternal side.

As the result of this expansion, the number of legal abortions almost doubled between 1951 (130,440) and 1952 (240,309). The number could have been lowered significantly by making contraception widely available, but additional production and distribution remained blocked. As a result, the growth rate of clinical abortion continued to accelerate after the 1951 expansion of criteria.[112]

Although the absolute number of registered non-clinical abortions continued to rise between 1948 and 1954, the growth rate slowed after 1952. The expanded list of medical criteria, in the absence of contraception, produced a negative short-term result by increasing both legal and illegal abortions in absolute terms, but it appears to have been effective in slowing the rate of non-clinical abortions. As a means to prevent abortion, the MZ's measures were clearly insufficient, but doctors were aware of this in advance. For them, a 100,000-operation increase in clinical abortion could only mean an army of pregnant women saved from illegal, unsanitary conditions of abortion, women whose health and fertility might be preserved for future pregnancies. For the moment, this was all that preventive measures, widened criteria, and streamlined abortion decision making could achieve.

Thus, doctors' long-term desire to expand criteria for legal abortion was finally realized. However, inclusion of socioeconomic conditions (including nursing) was rejected at this time.[113] One important reason is probably that the MZ was simultaneously preparing a report and reform proposal to the Sovmin, together with the MIu, the VTsSPS, and the state prosecutor, based on the result of their joint brigade study, which would primarily cover the issue of improving socioeconomic conditions for pregnant women and mothers. Regarding the legal issues that particularly affected single mothers, the MIu was drafting reforms of the existing family law. Although the MZ had been central in raising consciousness among a range of professionals about abortion causes, the MZ reform of criteria left the largest issues for later, joint action. Underlying this caution might be the knowledge that the

1951 population level was still far lower than the 1940 prewar level, so that no one believed top leaders would allow radical reform that might endanger natural population growth in the short term.

New Knowledge and Heightened Professional Consciousness: The First Step Toward Reform

Even before the major study of illegal abortion, doctors and party activists understood that many single women resorted to illegal abortion to escape single motherhood. However, the more alarming and unexpected result was that married women were behaving as if they were unmarried. The study showed that the majority of women who sought clinical abortions, were actually in registered marriages, had a child/children, and even desired to have one more child. In contrast to de jure single mothers who were expected by the policy planners to have one child, married women were supposedly in stable two-parent families that might raise three or more children but they lacked confidence in their husbands' commitment to marriage and child-rearing. Many wives knew that their husbands had a second family and/or feared that they were about to be abandoned. Their children would carry the name of the father, but women were afraid that they would grow up practically fatherless, without material support from either the state or the father. Even some women in stable marriages avoided additional children, for they could not expect even minimal help in childrearing. When these problems were combined with poor material and housing conditions, as well as demanding jobs, married women resorted to illegal abortion, despite the risk of crippling, infertility, prosecution, or death.

This persistent practice of millions of women thwarted the postwar pronatalist policy and, when they conveyed their beliefs to the medical establishment, it became a powerful force for reform. If the major reason for abortion was gender relations in conjunction with bad material conditions, why should only women be punished? In this way, women's criminality was officially questioned by both Soviet legal and medical establishments, marking an irreversible shift from punitive to preventive approaches to abortion.

Neither making men responsible fathers nor increasing material help for mothers was in the realm of medicine. Accepting its own limited sphere of action, the MZ pushed for the expansion of criteria for clinical abortion and the development of effective contraceptive devices, arguing that damage to the reproductive health of the country could be limited. The culmination was the October 19, 1951, instruction that made legal abortion free of charge, significantly decentralized the abortion committee system, and expanded the list of criteria. This was the first major amendment to the 1936 Anti-Abortion Law.[114] It was also the direct, if delayed, answer to the postwar crisis in women's health.

Abramova's *cri de coeur* in August 1948 led to the establishment of a commission whose focus on women and children was somewhat derailed when Starovskii pointed the demographic finger at abortion. But this was a medical procedure and that made the MZ the dominant voice in the interministerial study that followed. Although the Justice Ministry was at first inclined to blame material conditions, Kovrigina convincingly argued for family relationships as the main cause and for more legal abortion and contraceptive opportunities to prevent illegal practices.

The in-depth studies of abortion in 1949–1951 were crucial for establishing the understanding among legal and medical professionals that women alone were not responsible for unwanted pregnancies and that they should have wider access to abortion. After Stalin's death in 1953, Soviet professions that had experienced the full ill-effects of the pronatalist policy on women and children would move the reform agenda forward.

5

Women's Reproductive Right and the 1955 Re-legalization of Abortion

I often think about the question: Do we have the moral right to force motherhood on a woman, if she cannot have a child at a given moment? It is not that she "does not want" [a child], as any normal woman wants to become a mother. But when she cannot, do we have the moral right to force this on her? If we propose to a man or woman to have an operation [for sterilization], but he or she refuses, we wouldn't forcibly put him or her on the operating table. Why should we force a woman to become a mother, when she cannot become one?

Dr. A. I. Dmitrieva,
Chairwoman, Moscow Central Abortion Committee (1955)

Although bearing children is a woman's social function, nonetheless it is also her personal matter. A woman should not be turned into a being that just keeps giving birth, again and again. Here, some reasonable idea should be formulated, that perhaps lifts the ban against the individual, that degrades a woman, by controlling her intimate life.

M. D. Kovrigina, USSR Minister of Health (1955)

After the 1949/1950 studies of abortion clearly showed that women alone were not to be blamed for abortions, medical professionals pushed for reform of the legal abortion system from within the Ministry of Health (MZ). Mariia Kovrigina took the initiative and went beyond the narrow boundaries of medical specialization to develop reform ideas for an improvement in women's general socioeconomic conditions. Together with the All-Union Central Council of Trade Unions (VTsSPS), the Ministry of Justice

Replacing the Dead. Mie Nakachi, Oxford University Press (2021). © Oxford University Press.
DOI: 10.1093/oso/9780190635138.003.0006

(MIu), and the State Prosecutor, she prepared recommendations for the battle against abortion. Some of Kovrigina's earlier proposals to the Party Commission reappeared almost verbatim in new drafts.

Kovrigina survived another round of postwar purges of mostly Jewish doctors in the "Doctors' Plot," but no major reform of Stalin's policy could advance until after Stalin's death.[1] When Kovrigina became the USSR Minister of Health the following year, she was able to resume reexamination of the abortion surveillance system. However, perhaps to the surprise of the reformers, Stalin had not been the biggest obstacle to an amendment of the 1944 Family Law. So long as N. S. Khrushchev, the initiator of the family law and the next leader of the Soviet Union, and other policymakers believed in the efficacy of the pronatalist law in repopulating the country, no change would be made.

The strongest defense of the status quo came in a 1954 report signed by the long-reigning head of the Central Statistical Administration, V. N. Starovskii. His conclusion was clear and simple: the 1944 Family Law had strengthened families by reducing divorce. Starovskii did not delve into how much unhappiness was buried in those constrained marriages. The report also claimed gains in the "out-of-wedlock" children category as a victory for pronatalism, but there were no previous statistics for comparison with the new category. This positive evaluation of the 1944 law's first decade meant that its provisions would remain intact for another decade. Kovrigina and her supporters shifted subtly away from opposing the 1944 Family Law toward a revision of the 1936 ban on abortion, successfully pushing first for decriminalization and then for legalization.

The legalization of abortion reflects several key characteristics of the early post-Stalin reform process that is often described as the "Thaw,"[2] or "de-Stalinization."[3] Demonstrating the intelligentsia's strong hope and belief in reforming Stalinist injustice to women and children, journalist Elena Serebrovskaia began a reform campaign in 1954. The attacks on abortion surveillance among doctors showed signs of the newly emerging discourse of "rights" in this period, as doctors and medical administrators expressed the idea that women had the right to make decisions about childbirth.[4] Legalization was also clearly an undoing of the 1936 Criminalization of Abortion under Stalin. Kovrigina's effort to undo Stalin's draconian criminalization of abortion succeeded. However, no "de-Stalinization" could undo the 1944 Family Law, Khrushchev's brainchild, so long as Khrushchev remained in power.

This chapter discusses the steps that led to the 1955 legalization. It shows how the MZ in coordination with the MIu, the VTsSPS, and the State Prosecutor, tried to develop a proposal to improve working conditions among pregnant women and mothers. One of the key issues was an amendment to the 1944 Family Law that was identified as a core cause of worsening gender relations. The MZ became involved in the MIu's reform proposals in which Kovrigina's 1950 recommendation to the Party Commission on the protection of women and children was repeated. But in 1952, as the medical profession came under increasing surveillance for its part in the Doctors' Plot, all forms of activity froze and no legislation emerged from the interministerial effort.

After Stalin's death in 1953, a group of intellectuals initiated a public campaign for a reform of the family law, a "thaw" moment to make fathers more responsible for their children. Journalist Elena Serebrovskaia published a famous letter to *Literaturnaia gazeta*, the main organ of the Writers' Union, calling for an amendment of the 1944 Family Law to end the plight of out-of-wedlock children. Many readers, particularly single mothers, responded positively and plaintively to her call.

In short, the central pillars of the pronatalist regime were called into question during the brief post-Stalin interregnum. Although this discussion generally focused on "fatherless" children and single mothers, women and doctors connected this issue with abortion. The momentum for change seemed to be strong, but despite the high hopes of cultural and literary figures, legal and medical professionals, and women from all over the Soviet Union, demographic politics would again block family law reform. In the end, it was Kovrigina who broke the deadlock by drafting abortion legalization in language that gave women a reproductive right in the name of a more farsighted pronatalism.

Reformist Intentions in Ministerial Corridors and Cultural Centers

As the MZ advanced its medical reforms of the legal abortion system, it also made recommendations for improving women's socioeconomic conditions. On July 3, 1950, Acting Minister of Health A. N. Shabanov reported to G. M. Malenkov, Secretary of the Central Committee VKP(b), that the MZ Collegium was preparing a recommendation to present to the

Central Committee of the VKP(b) and the Sovmin SSR.[5] The MIu submitted recommendations, which were then sent to Kovrigina in October 1950. The five items were all concerned with expanding privileges for pregnant women, mothers with many children, and single mothers in order to improve their working and living conditions. These included helping mothers with many children to obtain more living space, giving more days off from work for mothers with children under eight, and granting paid leave to mothers caring for sick children. Amendments to the divorce and birth registration dimensions of the 1944 Family Law were not mentioned, probably because the MIu had already been preparing separate reform proposals on these matters.

Nevertheless, legal experts clearly recognized the link between abortion and the legal status of marriage and children. The final item on the list recommended that the 1944 Family Law provide a single mother with government aid "regardless of whether she was in registered marriage with a person who is not the father of the child at the time of conception or whether the court decision on her divorce was [already] in force."[6] This recommendation aimed to help de facto single women who could not be divorced from their husbands because of the law's strict, time-consuming, and costly procedures. Trapped in a marital status with absent husbands, they were ineligible for government aid to single mothers, despite abandonment by the father of the child. They often chose to abort or else became de facto single mothers.

The MZ's draft proposal to the Sovmin consisted of twenty-three recommendations, primarily focused on three issues: working and living conditions for the pregnant and nursing women, medical care, and prosecution, particularly of abortionists. It called for the six-hour workday for pregnant and nursing mothers with full-time salaries, with the difference covered by the social insurance fund. Maternity leave would be extended up to 112 days and would be further extended if multiple children were born or medical complications resulted. All industries were to assure improved living conditions for pregnant or single mothers, or mothers with many children, giving them priority for distribution of living space, organizing special dorms for single mothers, and improving communal dining. Trade unions were asked to enforce labor laws, particularly for the benefit of pregnant and nursing women, such as organizing educational opportunities for workers about the importance of strengthening family and fighting abortion and offering sanatorium stays to pregnant and nursing mothers, with priority allotted to mothers with many children and single mothers.[7]

By the end of 1951, the joint effort produced a final recommendation with the Ministry of Social Welfare as a new participant. On January 24, 1952, Shabanov wrote to the Sovmin SSSR that the MZ SSSR would present a project in February 1952 for reduction of illegal abortion.[8] But the discussion died behind the closed doors of party and ministerial committees and never passed through the Sovmin; 1952 was not a year for reforms.[9] The eruption of the Doctors' Plot paralyzed the Ministry of Health, while Kovrigina, the guiding force behind medical reform, took refuge in a "study leave."[10] Instead of reform came a renewed emphasis on enforcement and punishment.

In this tense anti-medical atmosphere, insufficient prosecution of doctors for their involvement in abortions was highlighted. For example, on July 23, 1952, D. V. Boldyrev reported to Minister of Justice K. P. Gorshenin on the prosecution of abortion cases. Prosecutors' indifference to investigating abortionists and judges' light sentences were bemoaned, particularly in cases where women were killed. Similar cases were reported from many republics, krais, and oblasts, suggesting a Union-wide failing.[11] The cases reported in detail were primarily concerned with abortionists. Among many cases cited, some of the most alarming involved doctors as abortionists—for example, the case of Dr. N. V. Turbin, chairman of the abortion committee in the city of Proskurov in Kamenets-Podol'skaia oblast. He single-handedly signed permits for legal abortion, ignoring the conditions listed in the criteria. Dr. Mel'nichuk performed the abortions on fourteen women. Turbin and Mel'nichuk were each imprisoned for eighteen months.[12]

Although Kovrigina may have convinced the lawyers that male partners should take some blame as accomplices, no one seems to have been ready to apply Criminal Code Article 140-a to them. This left only the abortionists of Criminal Code Article 140, part 3, at whose expense both the MIu and the MZ could show their vigilance in 1952. Kovrigina must have had mixed feelings since the 1951 directive made it clear that a widening definition of clinical abortion was appropriate. Doctors could well have taken an expanded list as the opportunity to enjoy professional discretion again. The cases raised in 1952 seem to include doctors among the chief culprits. With the firing of Kovrigina's boss, E. I. Smirnov, in December 1952, she risked demotion with any misstep or could be offered a promotion, if she played her cards correctly.[13]

In 1953, there were few developments in the reform of abortion policy or family policy. At the beginning of the year, Soviet medical professionals were under attack for the alleged Doctors' Plot, and then there was great uncertainty about political directions and leadership after Stalin's sudden death. But this political vacuum also presented an opportunity. Citizens, especially intelligentsia and legal experts, continued to address the social and moral problems created by the incontrovertible existence of millions of distressed single mothers and fatherless children. By then, the first generation of out-of-wedlock children were already of school age, and the focus shifted from their health, physical and financial, to moral and psychological issues. At a time when the MZ and the MIu were reporting on difficult material conditions among mothers with small children, single mothers' downplaying of the economic factor was probably strategic. If single mothers had shown more interest in financial support, lawmakers might have been distracted from the amendment that would allow out-of-wedlock births to be registered under the biological fathers' name. For single mothers, the need to end illegitimacy was more important than improving their material circumstances.

The first public discussion of the problem of single mothers and fatherless children was ignited by a famous article by journalist Elena Serebrovskaia entitled "Life Calls for an Amendment, " published in *Literaturnaia gazeta* on January 16, 1954.[14] Serebrovskaia sympathetically depicted the out-of-wedlock children created by a wide range of postwar marriage conditions and the 1944 Family Law, pointing out the gap between law and life. Many out-of-wedlock children were raised without fathers. But others actually lived with their biological fathers, though without the right to bear their names. Still others were financially and morally supported by biological fathers who lived elsewhere. The "legal fine points," insisted Serebrovskaia, were beyond "common sense." She concluded that all children, regardless of parental marital status, should be allowed to have their fathers' names, so that no one should ever feel the shame of saying: "I never had a father."[15]

On August 28, 1954, *Literaturnaia gazeta* reported on the many reader responses to Serebrovskaia's article. Unlike her article, which focused on legal formulations and birth certificates, many readers discussed irresponsible fathers. The unidentified author of the report pointed out that children should not suffer for parents', especially fathers', immoral behavior. Many letters condemned fathers of out-of-wedlock children and discussed the necessity of bringing fugitive fathers to justice. Some demanded punishment for these fathers with "unclean consciences." The 1944 law itself was called into question when cited as the excuse for acts of cruelty. One anonymous woman's letter was printed "almost in entirety," but the brutal letter within the letter was written by the husband fleeing his responsibilities, flagellating his helpless "wife" and child. The "father" wrote:

> Have you not heard of the Law of July 8, 1944? According to Article 29 of KZOBS, since the child was born in an unregistered marriage, I owe nothing to you or your child. Extricate yourself as you wish. You are now an adult. No one asked you to bear children. Our socialist fatherland will direct and raise the boy in the Communist spirit.[16]

Some letters argued that single mothers were also to blame for their frivolous sexual behavior, but the reporter concluded that regardless of whether the father or mother or both were at fault, children should not suffer for it. The information contained in birth certificates should be uniform to prevent the trauma caused by the revelation of fatherlessness.

The second point that the author made was that single mothers did not consider themselves lonely, since they received support from the state and community. However, they suffered from the moral burden of having to someday tell their children that they did not have fathers. Letters from single mothers commonly expressed appreciation for material support by the state and psychological support from their bosses, colleagues, and neighbors, stressing that they were not seeking material gain. Yet they feared the moment when the child would learn the full truth. The author of the report acknowledged that changing the birth registration system would not erase the trauma of paternal abandonment, but removing the blank under "father's name" on the birth certificate would prevent accidental discoveries before the mother was ready to reveal this.

The two *Literaturnaia gazeta* articles invited many, particularly single mothers, to express their opinions about the family law. A group of single mothers wrote to Khrushchev asking for a change in terminology from "single mother to "childrearing mother."[17] A single mother Galiuga sent a letter to K. E. Voroshilov on September 7, 1954, after reading these two articles. She said that she did not feel lonely but had been suffering morally for the last ten years. In her case, she had been in a prewar common-law marriage and had had a child in 1944. In the postwar period, her husband refused to register their marriage and married another woman. Her mother accidentally lied and told her grandson that the father had died in the war.

She groaned, "I cannot imagine the moment when my son finds out that his birth certificate has that ominous dash in the column where his father's name should be. I am in pain and horror, wondering whether I will be able to explain to him without hurting his deepest feelings."[18]

The first public reform movement clearly conveyed single mothers' need to prioritize the registration issue. Next in importance came the matter of making men responsible for the consequences of their sexual behaviors. Economic factors were presented as a non-issue, because the Soviet government was presumably already investing much in support of mothers. The first issue, how to minimize the taint of illegitimacy, would be debated for the next fourteen years. The economic disadvantages of single parenting would never be seriously considered, despite many women asking, "Why are men responsible for nothing?"

Starovskii Celebrates 1944 and Undermines Reform

The tenth anniversary of the passage of the Family Law was considered a good time to reevaluate its results. One was that the number of abortions continued its sharp upward trend, as natural births fell after 1952.[19] By the end of 1953, recorded abortions reached 1,404,626, with urban abortions exceeding 1,381,437, the 1935 record.[20] Since the success and failure of the 1936 abortion surveillance system had been measured against the 1935 level, this figure crossed a symbolic threshold calling into question the efficacy of the abortion ban. The year 1953 also saw the annual number of births drop by approximately 0.2 million, causing a decrease in natural population growth for the first time since 1947.[21] On the other hand, there were some positive statistical indicators. For the first time in the postwar period, the population topped the prewar 1940 level.

Given that the results and analyses of abortion presented by the MZ and the MIu strongly suggested the negative effects of postwar pronatalist policy on abortions, a serious evaluation of the 1944 Family Law should have included an examination of the link between the two. Although TsSU Director Starovskii had sounded the alarm against abortion in 1948, abortion would not figure in a celebratory study. The final report on May 19, 1954, to G. M. Malenkov, chairman of the Sovmin SSSR, stressed the overwhelming success of postwar pronatalism, completely ignoring the concerns that mothers as well as medical and legal experts expressed about the negative influence of the law on women's reproductive lives and out-of-wedlock children.

The title of Starovskii's 1954 report was "On the Increase of Registered Marriages, Decrease of Divorce, and Increase of Births among Fertile Mothers and Single Mothers in the USSR in the Postwar Period." In his introduction, Starovskii stated that the 1944 Family Law included "significant changes in laws regarding marriage, family and guardianship that strengthened the Soviet family." Not surprisingly, he had carefully tailored the report so that the main message was that the law had strengthened marriages, increased out-of-wedlock births, and encouraged women to have second and third children. However, inspecting the data carefully suggests different possible interpretations. For example, while the number of registered marriages had indeed increased between 1940 and 1952 or 1953, the postwar trend did not show a steady increase.[22] Rather, registered marriages fluctuated around 2 million.[23]

Starovskii's positive evaluation of divorce data could also be contested. The divorce numbers in 1952 (86,100) and the 1953 estimate (98,100) were less than half those of 1940 (205,000), but the overall postwar tendency is an unmistakably steady increase from 17,400 in 1946 to 98,100 in 1953. Starovskii recognized this but stressed that the postwar numbers were significantly lower than in 1940. Given this general tendency, the report's title misleads by only mentioning "decrease in divorce."[24] Starovskii completely ignored the widespread phenomenon of de facto divorce, marriages that had dissolved without being registered as divorces.

To make the point that the family had become stronger, Starovskii used statistics showing that the percentage of marriages that ended within four years had significantly decreased, an argument that "frivolous marriages," often associated with youth, were decreasing. To support this statement, he even added a sentence (without data) that the number of divorces among people up to age 25 had fallen. However, the reason that divorce among the young had fallen was the lack of young men to marry due to increased deaths during the war and postwar period. Additionally, women who were lucky enough to be married would not have wanted a divorce, and the new law would prevent that from happening quickly. In addition, while stressing the idea of stronger marriage ties, Starovskii did not mention the impressive statistics for divorce within five to nine years (32 percent) and ten to nineteen years (29 percent) of marriage, despite the strict divorce procedure. The large number of divorces within ten to nineteen years probably represents a similar percentage of prewar marriages finally coming to terms with wartime and postwar realities.

Since one of the primary goals of postwar pronatalism was to increase out-of-wedlock births, Starovskii posited that the number of out-of-wedlock births (849,000 in 1952) was significant, if declining from 985,000 in 1949. To prove the policy's effectiveness, he presented data on maternal occupations, showing that the percentage of single mothers employed by collective farms, enterprises, and government increased from 72 percent in 1948 to 79 percent in 1952. Non-working mothers declined from 20 percent in 1948 to 16 percent in 1952. Further data showed the generosity of government policy, since aid recipients had increased from 2.52 million in 1952 to 2.84 million in 1953. This suggested that despite hardships and insufficiencies, more and more women were becoming single mothers and receiving government aid. Starovskii neglected to explain why only 2.52 million single mothers were receiving the aid, if 4.4 million out-of-wedlock children had been born between 1948 and 1952. This would certainly have begged hard questions about aid implementation, the same ones raised by A. Abramova in 1948.[25]

The other key reproductive goal of postwar pronatalism was to encourage all citizens to have three children. For this reason, since 1944 new incentives had focused on mid-size families. Starovskii argued that this was successful by presenting data on the increasing number of children born as the third or more child as a percentage of all children born between 1948 and 1952. By the end of 1953, more than 3 million women with four and more children had received government aid, and 705,000 mothers had received one-time government aid for those with three children. These numbers are impressive, although the decline of mothers with five and more children might suggest the more pessimistic interpretation that overall family size was actually falling.

Another potentially negative trend Starovskii did not mention was that the absolute number of mothers giving birth for the first time showed a decline from 1.81 million in 1948 to 1.78 million in 1952. This could suggest that childless women preferred to remain childless, a direct contradiction of the government's pronatal goal. This could have been a factor in the rising percentage of the number of mothers with three or more children.

Starovskii's summary listed only conclusions that supported a positive evaluation of the 1944 law: the number of registered marriages in 1953 was 1.9 times that of 1940, and the number of divorces "fell to a little less than half"; the number of mothers giving birth to a third child or more increased by 28 percent between 1948 and 1952, and the number of mothers giving birth to the fourth child and more increased by 26 percent; the number of out-of-wedlock children had been increasing, and there were 4.4 million such births registered from 1948 to 1952, inclusive; and the number of single mothers receiving government aid increased by 13 percent between 1952 and 1953 to reach a total of 2.8 million.[26] In the 1954 assessment of the 1944 Family Law, Starovskii strategically chose the time span for comparison, so he could always reveal optimistic trends.

There was also an important demographic trend of the postwar period that this report completely overlooked. That was the issue of regional differences and ethnic trends in birth statistics, which became one of the biggest political and economic concerns of the Soviet Union in the 1970s and 1980s. In the prewar period, fertility among Russian village mothers was still high, but in the postwar period, the rural birth rate dropped dramatically with the lack of men in the villages and out-of-wedlock births soared. This phenomenon was more prominent in some places than others. For example, Central Asian republics suffered much less from an imbalanced sex ratio, and fertility remained high, with a large percentage of the Soviet Union's Mother Heroines with ten or more children residing there.[27] However, Starovskii ignored this issue altogether.

Such an assessment of the 1944 Family Law by the TsSU, which focused on certain politically favorable demographic indicators, would have strongly promoted the law's efficacy to Soviet leaders, without probing more questionable outcomes. As Khrushchev would say almost a decade later, "We don't have any other numbers. Comrade Starovskii is a very careful man. I get my numbers from him. I don't have my own numbers."[28] If pronatalist policies were still desirable, there was no logical need to amend the law. The 1954 USSR population for the first time after the war exceeded the 1940 level, and both the number of births and natural population growth increased.[29] This was all good news, but the level was still lower than the 193 million of August 1940, the last number made public in the Soviet press.[30] Therefore, it was still too early to conduct a postwar census or declare a demographic recovery.

There is clear evidence that Soviet leaders still wanted a larger population. For example, in January 1955 Khrushchev mentioned that the USSR's population was 200 million. In the same month, Starovskii recommended to the Sovmin to plan the next all-Union census "no earlier than in 3–4 years, when the population of the USSR will significantly exceed

200 million."[31] Such a statement strongly suggests that pronatalism was still state policy as of 1955.

Last Lap to Legalization, 1954–1955

If the 1944 Family Law could be considered a successful pronatalist measure, the clear implication was that it should be continued until its goal was fully achieved: the replacement of the World War II dead. On the other hand, abortion policy could be reformed, since it was a Stalinist policy dating to the 1930s, not a part of postwar family law. Besides, unlike marriage, divorce, and birth rate indicators, abortion statistics unmistakably demonstrated a worsening trend. Moreover, punitive abortion policy was considered Stalinist, a cruel and repressive leadership style that would soon be repudiated. Even Khrushchev, who had called for increased punishment for abortion in early 1944, must have recognized the failure of the draconian approach.

Already in April 1953, the MIu and the State Prosecutor, at a meeting to discuss post-Stalinist amnesties, had suggested decriminalization of women undergoing abortion.[32] On August 5, 1954, this measure was enacted, annulling Paragraph 4, Article I, of the 1936 law. This change was not publicized, possibly to prevent a sudden leap in the abortion rates. The direct cause was probably the general reversal of Stalinist codes, although freedom from prosecution or punishment also made it easier for women to seek medical aid after failed abortions, to admit their guilt, and to name the abortionist.[33]

Annulment of criminal responsibility ended the punitive abortion policy but left a serious question as to why women were still condemned to dangerous underground abortions. The MZ data for 1949–1954 was clear: every year, roughly 4,000 deaths from illegal abortion were registered.[34] Kovrigina herself demanded that "the health authorities themselves . . . stop women from crippling themselves by turning to semi-literate, immoral people [for illegal abortions.]" Not everyone supported legalization, but most favored further expansion of criteria for legal abortion and the inclusion of socioeconomic reasons in the list, because "we have still not created the necessary conditions for women as mothers to raise children."[35] Medical opinion was divided on the issue of how to include non-medical criteria but not on the recognition that inadequate welfare for women made fertility control necessary.

On October 30, 1954, probably due to the number of abortions exceeding the 1935 level, the Sovmin ordered an interministerial commission to review abortion policy again.[36] In January 1955, a new study of illegal abortion practice was conducted; 3,242 women were asked to fill out a questionnaire anonymously after recovering from illegal abortions. On June 6, 1955, the results of the study were reported to Kovrigina by L. Grechishnikova, the head of the MZ administration for clinical-prophylactic service for children and mothers. Unlike in 1949, this time results were presented for three categories of women: women in registered marriages, women in common-law marriages, and single mothers. The commission clearly came to recognize that not only legal but also self-defined relationship status was the decisive factor in women's reproductive decision making. Of the 3,242 respondents, 2,352 (72.5 percent) were in a registered marriage, 471 (14.5 percent) were in a non-registered marriage, and 419 (13 percent) were single mothers. The fact that twenty-three women in registered marriages named "no husband" as a reason for illegal abortion probably means that they were de facto single, but this situation shows a complexity that could not be fully accommodated with these categories.[37]

Overall, the main conclusion of this study was that the primary reasons for abortion were bad material and living conditions, bad relations with "husbands," and the presence of small children, in that order. A look at individual categories provides specific characteristics of women choosing to undergo illegal abortion, broken down by eight questions: age, occupation, the number of previous abortions, ages of children, family income, childcare arrangements, housing, and reasons for abortion.

In addition to this second joint study of abortion practice, the MZ prepared a report on the history of abortion policy in the USSR in a comparative, international context.[38] Who conducted the study is not clear, but it is most likely to have been assigned by Kovrigina. The report became an argument for further expansion of legal abortion, soon to be presented to the Sovmin. The report compiled complete statistics of the registered number of clinical and non-clinical abortions between 1935 and 1954. The most significant argument, drawn from foreign examples, was that criminalized abortion policy was counterproductive in reducing illegal abortion. Regarding the British, US, and French experiences with sanctions, the report concluded that "illegal abortions were conducted secretly in completely unsanitary conditions mostly by those who had no medical training. . . . [A]t the same time, the numbers of abortions in all these countries are exceptionally high and steadily increasing. . . . Banning of abortions did not bring a decrease in their number."

The USSR's history was also reevaluated. The 1920 legalization of abortion was praised for lowering "abortion-related disease and death." In contrast, the criminalization of abortion in 1936 was portrayed as the beginning of a steady increase in illegal abortions. The dips of 1937 and 1947 were revealed as anomalies (although the Great Terror and postwar famine could not yet be mentioned),[39] with the general trend being unrelentingly upward. While 90 percent of registered abortions were labeled "non-clinical," that too was merely an indicator of magnitude, as many more abortions were completed successfully and without the intervention of the medical system, an unrecorded social fact involving millions of Soviet women. Abortion had become endemic during the two decades it had been illegal.

Aside from the reality that repressive measures had not been able to prevent illegal abortions, the next most important point of the report was the harmful effects of abortions on female reproductive health. The report presented non-clinical abortions as a mortal risk, based on the statistics of the registered annual number of maternal deaths from clinical and non-clinical abortions between 1949 and 1954, ranging between 3,716 (in 1952) and 4,302 (in 1951).[40]

If the approximately 4,000 annual maternal deaths from illegal abortions were not striking enough for the USSR leadership to reconsider current abortion policy, the report provided additional frightening figures. One-third of women with gynecological diseases had a history of abortion. Women who had a history of abortion had a three times greater risk of complications during delivery than women who had never had an abortion. A 1948–1949 study at the Institute for Gynecology and Obstetrics concluded that of 3,121 women who suffered infertility, 1,752 (56 percent) had a history of abortion, and 1,199 of the 1,752 said that they had had complications during abortion. Finally, many experts argued that between 18.5 percent and 35 percent of women who underwent abortions became infertile.

Such figures clearly showed the extremely harmful effects of abortions, especially non-clinical abortions, on both public health and demographic potential. Clinical abortion was a much better option than non-clinical. But even with the 1951 expansion of the list of criteria, it was noted that "a series of serious illnesses had not been taken into account, where continuation of the pregnancy would threaten the health of the pregnant woman."

In conclusion, the report stated that what the MZ could do to reduce the number of illegal abortions was "extremely limited," given the breakdown of women's reasons for abortions. Bad living and material conditions, relationship problems, and the presence of small children or an already large number of children identified abortion as a "social problem" to be dealt with only "by broad governmental measures" such as the construction of childcare institutions, increased living space, improved material conditions among women, and "permitting health services to carry out abortions from now on regardless of medical criteria." Thus, inclusion of non-medical reasons for legal abortion was presented as a temporary solution for countering social problems causing abortions. This blanket expansion of legal abortion criteria was the only way that medical experts could make an improvement, as long as improved welfare for women was not forthcoming.

The implications of such an expansion were enormous, requiring substantial increases in the number of beds and assigned staff in gynecological departments, as well as more staff in abortion committees. To cover some of these expenses, the report proposed charging fees for legal abortions when reasons were not medical. In order to evaluate social and material conditions of women, the involvement of representatives from local soviet and voluntary organizations would be necessary.[41]

On February 17, 1955, a commission consisting of Kovrigina, K. P. Gorshenin, the Minister of Justice, R. A. Rudenko, the State Prosecutor, N. V. Popova, the head of the VTsSPS, and N. A. Murav'eva, the Social Welfare Minister, wrote a report on the situation with illegal abortion and attached a draft law for further expansion of the list of criteria for legal abortion. This time, socioeconomic reasons were included. Timing, content, and language suggest that this document was probably drafted by Kovrigina based on the historical overview and then simply accepted by the other members.

Abortion continued to increase, the report began. The non-clinical operations, the overwhelming majority, resulted in cripples, infertility, deaths, and orphans. Analysis of causation followed the earlier document closely, with the percentages for material difficulties, relationship problems and young child matching exactly (60.5 percent, 30 percent, and 6 percent, respectively). The need to expand the criteria for abortion, to include socioeconomic reasons, personal medical conditions, and the medical conditions of family members, was the requested solution.[42]

Nineteen new items were proposed as additions to the forty-nine already on the list. Many of the new medical conditions were focused on the viability of the infant, whether for congenital reasons or due to the mother's question-able health. The upbringing of other children received attention for the first time. This could be a psychological effect, since the presence of a "disturbed" sibling could "have negative effects on the upbringing of other normal chil-dren." Physiological reasons were also adduced, as a child under 1 year of age might suffer a loss of mother's milk and associated "immunity" after the nursing mother became pregnant again. Stomach problems might also occur, especially in the summer, from drinking other kinds of milk. The mes-sage was that those already out of the womb should not be sacrificed to those within. It was a direct answer to the 6 percent who aborted due to having young children in the household. The most novel item, however, concerned housing conditions, specifying dormitories and lack of living space as abor-tion criteria, but only after a "special investigation." There was still no plan to offer women with relationship issues a legal abortion.[43]

The "joint" committee's proposal reflected the MZ's document directly, with no evidence of other government agencies' input. The MIu had made earlier proposals in 1951–1952 and was undertaking reform of the family law, but this was done separately. Lack of items that involved trade unions suggests their unwillingness to be involved with abortion issues. In fact, med-ical professionals complained that the VTsSPS, which should have been most concerned about protecting women workers, had no interest in improving mothers' lives. In the words of Professor V. I. Konstantinov, Deputy Director of the Khar'kov Institute for the Protection of Motherhood and Infancy:

> The practice has been established that we, doctors, are the only ones fighting for motherhood. Other departments have no idea about the tasks that they face. . . . We sent our observations to the central trade union. Our legal advisor made several legislative proposals. In his opinion, the present laws on the protection of maternity needed correction. Amazingly, the cen-tral trade union answered us that they did not consider it appropriate at the moment to make any legislative changes. And why? Because there were no economic reasons!![44]

That other government offices were not interested in the issue of improving mothers' well-being made doctors feel that it was their mission to provide legal abortion for those with socioeconomic problems.

But the path of expanding criteria remained blocked. Although the new list was sent to the Sovmin, it was not issued to replace the 1951 criteria. In the absence of archival materials, we can only speculate about the reasons. There may have been a disagreement in social principle at the highest level or over the details. As the report to Kovrigina argued, this policy would work only with a significant expansion of gynecological service and abortion committee work. Maybe the Sovmin was not ready to fund this. And the inclusion of socioeconomic factors would immediately require a range of evaluations that were not of a medical nature. What bureaucracy would undertake them?

Although the expansion of allowable abortion criteria might be seen more as a medical initiative, the MIu was actively undertaking reform along other lines as well. The time for reform seemed more favorable, following Stalin's death and the overwhelmingly positive response to the Serebrovskaia article. This prompted legal experts to resume preparations for amending the 1944 Family Law. In the context of abortion, medical experts primarily discussed the birth registration system and divorce law. For medical professionals, they were equally bad, causing instability to gender relations leading to abortions. For legal experts these were also the two key issues on the reform agenda. However, they had more difficulty forming a consensus on the birth registration system among themselves, due to issues of inheritance and child support, whereas they could reach an agreement about making divorce easier.

On June 8, 1955, Gorshenin sent a proposal for amending divorce procedure in the 1944 Family Law to the Central Committee. This proposal was made due to a number of citizens who complained to the MIu and other ministries about "the impossibility of ending a marriage, even if the family had fallen apart long ago. Both husband and wife already have new de facto families but cannot register their marriages, which is especially hard on children born juridically without fathers." The proposed measures included making it possible to divorce without the presence of one of the partners; allowing divorce through ZAGS without publishing an announcement in the newspaper when there was evidence that one partner was missing; obtaining divorce even if one of the partners did not show up for a hearing; and processing paperwork at the local court of either partner depending on the situation.[45]

This proposal to simplify divorce was not approved by the Sovmin.[46] Thus, by mid-1955 it was clear to medical experts that no other experts would or could develop measures for improving either material and living conditions or relationship problems for mothers. With expansion of criteria ruled out and divorce reforms also in limbo, medical experts, Health Minister Mariia Kovrigina in particular, realized that legalizing abortion was the last best chance to save abortion victims in the name of pronatalism.

The Right to Decide: Women's Voices

On January 7, 1955, Khrushchev made a speech to the Komsomol ranks of Moscow youth. Although the main topic was the Virgin Lands, other virgins were also targeted.[47] Khrushchev revealed that he was the one who proposed to Stalin the 1941 tax on single citizens, explaining that such a tax system was a necessary form of intergenerational financial justice.

> We have people who neither marry, nor have children after marriage. For the moment, we will not discuss why they don't. In any case, such people exist in our society, and they are taking advantage of all of our public weal. They will get old. We might ask, "who will take care of them when they can no longer work?" Of course, the answer is, those very young people who are being raised by our marvelous mothers with many children. That is why Comrade Stalin proposed to provide support for large families. At whose expense? At the expense of those who live without thinking about tomorrow.[48]

Khrushchev then went on to insist on three children per family, matching the language of the law he had authored.[49] Families with fewer children were considered worse than social parasites, even class enemies (bourgeois), undermining socialist society. Khrushchev's dream of a more populous country revealed his rampant pronatalism.

> The more people we have, the stronger our country will be. Bourgeois ideology has invented many cannibalistic theories such as the theory of overpopulation. They think about how to reduce birth rate and decrease population growth. Comrades, we are different. If we added another 100 million to 200 million, it would still be too little! . . . If every family has one or two children, the population of the country will not grow, it will decline. We must think about the development of society. That is why we must have at least three children in a family and raise them well![50]

Many women responded that their lack of children was not a sign of irresponsibility but because the war deprived them of future husbands. A group of single mothers wrote to Khrushchev, "After the war according to the statistics, there are more women than men. This means that not everyone can find a partner."[51] A childless woman wrote to Khrushchev directly criticizing the logic of his policy. She would have liked to become a mother, but because her partner already had a legal wife, she could not. She is currently paying the small family tax. If she becomes a mother, she would pay less tax and receive some state aid as a single mother, but she does not want to receive such aid paid by another childless woman who is in the same situation as herself.[52]

Understanding the pronatalist logic of Khrushchev's argument, some women demanded a "deal" where Khrushchev amended the 1944 Family Law, and in exchange, women would give birth to more children. A single mother wrote:

In my letter, not I alone, but those like me as well appeal to you with the request to make amendment to the 1945 Law concerning the payment of child support by the biological fathers of our children, who are considered illegitimate. We, healthy women, of course, will contribute to our Motherland and give birth to sons and daughters for our wonderful country. . . . You emphasized that we have to acquire family and have two-three children and that those who do not or do not wish to have children have no place in our society. As you know, it turns out that during the years of war our young people were a little spoilt, and they need to be tightened up. This regards men, who have no sympathy for women who give birth to children. A man lives with a woman, let's say, three to four years. For personal reasons he does not or is not able to marry legally and cheats on her. Then after some time, without feeling responsibility for what he has done, he looks for another woman, who has not given birth to his children and lives contentedly. He says that the government will help, because the son or daughter is not his, does not carry his family name, and is illegitimate. What a pity to hear those words when men become impudent and don't want to recognize illegitimate children, taking shelter in the 1945 Law. . . . We women of course, ask you, Comrade Khrushchev, to help us with amending the law. . . . If you comply with our request, which women await and watch closely, it will also be beneficial for the fertility of our generation.[53]

Criticisms of the 1944 Family Law aroused by Serebrovskaia's article and the abolition of criminal responsibility of women undergoing abortion in

1954 encouraged women to demand further expansion of legal abortion. At the final stages of abortion policy reform, women's voices became a key force. Between 1954 and 1955, many letters concerning abortion, everyday life, and marriage relations were written to Soviet leaders, such as V. M. Molotov, G. M. Malenkov, and K. E. Voroshilov, the MIu or the MZ, and the ones that mentioned abortion were forwarded to Kovrigina, too.[54]

Although public discourse on the family law did not touch on abortion, women and doctors understood the clear connection between the two. Thus, women's letters regarding abortion could be easily framed in the context of problems with the 1944 Family Law.[55] For example, E. N. Petrova, a pediatrician in Sverdlovsk, wrote to Molotov how most fathers had no time to participate in childrearing because they preferred drinking in their spare time. Men were also indicted for abortion: "Beating, insult, and humiliation necessitate [women] going for abortion." While the only real freedom from such a situation would be divorce, under the 1944 Family Law it was difficult to obtain. Petrova focused on relationship issues, making memorable points: "Why do we not ask fathers to provide the family's moral strength?" and "For the father, it is easy to find a new wife, but it's impossible for children to find a [new] father."[56] The choice of Molotov might have been made because of his visibility in "The Mother's Notebook (Pamiatka Materi)," a handbook issued to all mothers. The cover of the book had a quote by Molotov, which read, "We want public health to make great strides to strengthen labor and give birth to more Soviet knights."[57]

Using the critical logic of public discourse on the family law that emphasized the welfare of children, the 1954 decriminalization of abortion encouraged women to request an automatic legal abortion in order to save their lives either for existing or future children. Some of the letters were written by women who were denied legal abortion, appealing that decision and asking for permission again. As N. Voinova from Saratov wrote to Kovrigina on February 13, 1955, she had four children and did not want to have the fifth. Her only option was to "abort herself." She understood that "abortion was harmful for her health, but births are not always useful." She wanted to have a legal abortion in order not to risk death, which would leave her four children without a mother. Kovrigina granted her request.[58]

Buga Iaroslave of Baku also wrote to the MZ SSSR asking for a clinical abortion. The reason was that she already had two children, and the second child was six months old. She implied that she would consider having the third, but this was not the right time, by saying "I am only 25. What is the rush?" She was clearly responding to Khrushchev's speech, in which he blamed those who did not reproduce children. She agreed with Comrade Khrushchev that "our government needs children, who are builders of communist society." However, she felt that such blame should be addressed to women who "do not want to give birth, or who limited themselves to only one child, knowing how difficult it is to give birth and raise a child." But Buga believed that nursing mothers should get abortions. She complained that the abortion committee would not provide permission, even though it knew that she would not give birth. In this way, the committee is "forcing me to abort [illegally]." Further, she emphasized that the reason that she was asking for medical abortion was "not because I don't want to give birth any more," but because she wants to leave "the possibility of giving more births later," and only clinical abortion would protect this possibility. Kovrigina underlined this last argument. Buga was also granted permission for a legal abortion.[59]

A similar argument was made by other mothers who already had children. A. P. Konusheva wrote to K. E. Voroshilov on March 7, 1955, asking for permission for a clinical abortion. She was 28 years old and a mother of four, the youngest one being 5 months old. She also expressed the intention to give birth later, but she needed "a little rest. Indeed, I am not a machine for putting out children twice a year." She could induce abortion herself, but did not want to risk her life, since death would leave her children orphans.[60]

Some letters addressed relationship problems directly, the burden of child-rearing, and the creation of unsupervised delinquents. Others asked directly for amendment of the 1944 Family Law. An anonymous letter addressed to the Minister of Health said, "The main reason for poor upbringing is unhealthy family life, the [bad] relations of the couple, [including] unbridled behavior, cheating, polygamy and from these, scandals and sickness of which the innocent witnesses are the children. I want to wish for a revision of the law on marriage, family and support."[61]

A wide range of letters argued that abortion should be allowed and be conducted at medical facilities in order to save women's lives. A letter written by Burtseva, probably a medical worker, self-described as "an average Soviet woman," to the Minister of Health described how women's clinics were filled with women who had damaged their health by undergoing illegal abortion. The reasons given were material difficulties, the presence of a large family, an unhappy marriage and abandonment leading to the fear of having a fatherless child. In Burtseva's mind, the connection between pronatal policy and unnecessary death was clear.

Are there people so naïve that they believe that banning abortion will raise the birth rate and prevent abortions? A woman aborts nonetheless, often losing her health forever. Ask any gynecologist and he will tell you that most women suffering from women's diseases got them from underground abortions.... We must permit abortion, for operations in hospitals will save the lives and health of many thousands. It is time to reexamine this issue, so important for women.... Many women have been abandoned by their husbands. They go to the underground abortionist, contract an infection and are dead in a few days. The life of a young woman would have been saved by an abortion in the hospital. There are all too many such cases.[62]

These letters present important themes. In general, women were depicted as not wanting to remain childless. No one argued that women had the right to choose whether to become a mother. Many were already mothers of multiple children or were planning to have another child. They asked for the right to choose when to give birth. Determined to abort even if legal abortion would not be granted, they preferred not to risk their lives and health, because they were already mothers. Moreover, they suggested that legal abortion should be granted so that they would be able to become mothers in the future. Medical experts who supported legalization of abortion would use these themes to construct a language of women's reproductive right.

Legalization versus Further Expansion of Criteria for Legal Abortion

On August 23, 1955, an important meeting was held in the MZ SSSR where Soviet specialists of women's medicine discussed the MZ's new proposal for abortion policy to the Sovmin. Medical professionals frankly expressed their views, which influenced Kovrigina, who chaired the meeting. Soon afterward, she would propose legalization of abortion to the Sovmin. Significantly, at her opening speech she stated, "Unfortunately, we have dealt with [abortion] badly," with the number of non-clinical abortions continuing to increase. Punitive measures and educational efforts had failed. Now a drastic reform was deemed necessary, since the 1955 joint study of illegal abortion, showed "about the same results as in 1949."[63]

Kovrigina said that the proposal to the party and government would be "in general an expanded [list of] medical criteria," including socioeconomic reasons, but the discussion took a more fundamental turn to weigh whether to legalize abortion or simply expand criteria again. Of the nineteen participants who spoke up at this meeting and clearly expressed their position, ten were for legalization and nine for expansion. One person did not make a clear statement, though it seemed he preferred expansion.[64] With opinions evenly divided, no decision was made. Nonetheless, these discussions are important in understanding why Kovrigina proposed legalization in the fall of 1955.

Strikingly, both sides agreed on a range of positions that might be called the "medical consensus": the necessity of contraception, abortion's harm to women's reproductive health, orphans as the result of maternal death, women's double burden, the need for family law amendments, and the overall exigency of population growth. Both sides also considered it necessary to set some limits on granting legal abortion.

The subtle, but most important, disagreement was the principled position of whether to prioritize recognition of a woman's right to determine when to become a mother or the state's right to discourage abortion. In the language of Soviet doctors the concept of "women's rights" was phrased variously as "a woman should be given the right to decide herself," "giving women the chance to become mothers when they want," "women should decide when they want to become mothers," and "women's rights to abortion." Those who supported expanding criteria generally recognized that the existing list should be expanded to include socioeconomic reasons so that legal abortion would become available to a much wider group of women.[65] Some of them even specifically supported a woman's right to become a mother when she wanted and argued that contraception, but not legal abortion, should make this possible. Dr. A. I. Logutiaeva, head obstetrician and chairman of the Kalinin oblast abortion committee, who supported expansion of criteria, lamented the state of contraception as "worse than ever" and called for "women to be in control in this matter."[66] L. G. Stepanov, Director of the MZ SSSR Institute for Obstetrics and Gynecology, also argued for effective contraceptives to allow women to control the timing of pregnancies.[67] However, both believed that abortion should be illegal. Professor I. B. Levit, the head obstetrician in Ivanovo oblast, expressed the concern that the 1954 release of women from criminal responsibility for abortion gave women the wrong message that the government now allowed abortion. He and others who supported expansion were afraid that legalization would reconfirm this understanding, encouraging women to abort and working against the country's pronatalist policy.[68]

In contrast, those who supported legalization emphasized the principled position of giving women the right to legal abortion, although most of them also considered it necessary to set limits as well. Professor V. I. Konstantinov from Khar'kov contended that abortion was related to the fundamental fact that Soviet woman were unwilling to "blindly follow their natural maternal purpose," instead wanting to enjoy the opportunities of social and political life that flowed from the Bolshevik Revolution's promise of a better life for all workers. He supported legalization but with measures to prevent an irresponsible attitude toward motherhood.[69] A. I. Dmitrieva, the head doctor of Maternity Hospital no. 16 and chairman of the Moscow Central Abortion Committee, stated that doctors did not have the moral right to force women to become mothers when they were unwilling. Consequently, "it is necessary to legalize abortion." Yet she also considered it "necessary to have limits."[70] Restrictions were to be applied to high-risk cases such as late-term pregnancy and to first-time pregnant women to encourage births and to contain health damage.

Thus, both sides wanted much wider availability of legal abortion while still setting limits, but the dividing line was recognition of women's right to decide the timing of motherhood versus an anti-abortion position emphasizing state and professional control. The existence of the former position is significant, especially given the history of Soviet abortion. The 1920 legalization was realized not in support of women's reproductive rights but because of their difficult economic and cultural conditions, the legacy of pre-revolutionary Russia. It was also a way to "save" women from *babki* by employing modern medical science.[71] In 1936, the option of legal abortion was taken away from women due to the state pronatalist agenda. The 1955 medical discourse unmistakably addressed women's right to decide when to become mothers and questioned the government's right to impose motherhood on women. However, this was not a full recognition of reproductive rights of women. It assumed maternal desire, so it did not address women's right to decide whether or not to become mothers. Women's first silent, and then vocal, demands for sufficient medical support so that they could be healthy enough to give births to multiple children produced the language of rights.

Those who supported expansion stressed the logic of the state and the power of medical knowledge. They argued that state pronatalism and doctors were in basic agreement, since medical science concurred that abortions were harmful and that women should follow expert medical advice. In their view, women were passive actors, accepting the doctors' opinion. Professor V. P. Mikhailov said that 8 to 10 percent of women who were denied legal abortions later thanked the abortion committee for not having given them permission. Professor Kvater argued that "one should not legalize abortion. Many women can be convinced to reconsider and become mothers."[72]

In contrast, those who supported legalization often emphasized women's scornful words: "You, Soviet doctors, . . . should help us, but instead push us into underground abortions." Such doctors were labeled "bureaucrats," by women rejected for legal abortion.[73] In this narrative, women appeared to be determined individuals prepared to take the risk of illegal abortion to avoid unwanted children. Professor Konstantinov stated, "Women are fully aware of abortion's harm, but despite this, they do it, because often it is necessary." Dmitrieva echoed this sentiment: "I completely agree with those comrades who say that if a woman does not want the pregnancy, no prohibition or persuasion can help. She will not keep it and somehow she will get an abortion."[74] Just like the letters sent to the government leaders, female patients criticized doctors for not helping them, in the full knowledge that they would opt for an illegal abortion. No longer were Soviet women perceived as pitiful subjects who needed state protection, but as fully informed citizens who could make decisions for themselves. In this way, women convinced doctors that they were not "baby-making machines" and doctors should help women preserve their health until they chose the right time to have children.[75]

Kovrigina was also moved by women's voices as well as their widespread resistance demonstrated in statistics. She granted the requests of some who asked for legal abortion, even though they were denied by local abortion committees. Although Kovrigina did not take sides at the beginning of the meeting, as the discussion progressed, she sometimes made remarks such as "a woman should be given the right to decide herself."[76] When re-reading the stenogram, she marked "Important" next to Solnechnogorsk maternity hospital doctor G. A. Desiatov's comment describing a broad range of acceptable abortions: a Bashkir girl who became pregnant with a Bashkir partner who then married another woman; a 15-year-old girl who got pregnant either by rape or sexual dissoluteness; and a mother heroine who got pregnant with her twelfth child through casual sex. "I consider," said Desiatov, "that all these women are right to ask us for an abortion. And generally speaking, is this not some kind of violence against the individuals, if we tell them they must give birth? A woman says: I will not give birth, I cannot, and we say, no, give birth. From this point of view, this is unjust."[77]

The issue of contraception was raised frequently at the meeting. Many considered it much better that women use contraception rather than get pregnant and have an abortion. No one opposed the development of better products, increased production, and wider distribution of contraceptives as a way to limit demand for abortion. Comrade Karmanova of the Institute of Public Health Education even suggested that the USSR should learn from foreign countries in this area.[78] In general, doctors had blamed themselves for not developing effective contraception, but the comment that "we have not quite legalized contraception" pointed to political factors as well.[79] In her concluding remarks, Kovrigina encouraged the development of contraception as "a problem purely medical, and we must solve this problem. . . . If abortion is really as harmful as the obstetricians say, why do we not give women the means to prevent it? It seems to me that this was a big mistake of ours that we should overcome as quickly as possible."[80] In any case, the doctors were aware that their present decision should not count on the future availability of contraceptives, still a distant prospect.

From her comment it appears that Kovrigina was hopeful that if effective contraception could be developed, it would make a big difference in reproductive practice. It is hard to imagine that Kovrigina did not understand that contraception had been considered an almost illegal subject up to then. If so, she might have sensed at this time that the new Soviet leaders might react to the question of contraception, as well as abortion, differently than in Stalin's time. Her optimism emerged from the de-Stalinization environment, when the amnesty of Stalinist "criminals" and the abolition of some Stalinist criminal codes was taking place.

Toward the end of the August 23 meeting Kovrigina revealed her support for the legalization option, arguing that "although giving birth is a woman's social function, it is nonetheless her personal affair as well. We should not transform women into a being that only gives birth." However, the Minister was also of the opinion that some kind of limit was necessary, since abortion could be harmful to women's health. She considered that there should be a way to reconcile those positions. As the bureaucrat responsible for convincing Soviet leaders to legalize, she most likely thought that clear guidelines and limitations might help top decision makers agree to place abortion exclusively in the medical purview. She was also aware that public endorsement of women's rights risked encouraging abortion and was likely to meet strong opposition from Soviet leadership. In order to overcome these obstacles, she resorted to paternalistic language following historical examples.

Kovrigina's public language followed the developmental logic of previous abortion policies. In 1920, abortion, an evil practice of the past, was legalized reluctantly, due to the "fact" that abortion was "a moral legacy of the past" among working women who had lived under an oppressive state until 1917 and appropriate to "the difficult economic conditions of the present" in 1920.[81] The 1936 criminalization argued that "the destruction of capitalist exploitation in the USSR, better material conditions and gigantic improvement in the laborers' political and cultural level" had made abortion unnecessary.[82] Kovrigina took this rationale one step further to suggest that "cultural growth [and] a high level of consciousness among Soviet people had now made the ban on abortion unnecessary."[83] Although she avoided the language of women's right, her language clearly recognized women's ability to make good decisions for themselves. Once this framework was set, further content could reflect the true interests of the medical profession and their female patients. There were additional meetings to finalize their joint proposal to the Sovmin and the party, but Kovrigina's formulations and priorities remained intact throughout the process, except for the removal of all references to women's right.

By mid-October, Kovrigina's proposal to the Sovmin and the Central Committee of the Communist Party was circulated for discussion. Kovrigina included the following reasons for the necessity of abolishing criminalized abortion: statistics showed that criminalization was not effective in reducing abortion; most 1954 abortions were done in unsanitary conditions, whereas most of the 1935 abortions were clinical abortions; non-clinical abortions brought "irreparable" harm to women's health and often led to serious diseases and even death. Kovrigina also suggested improved material conditions for mothers as a way to raise the birth rate.[84]

No mention was made in any of the documents addressed to the Sovmin about problems with the 1944 Family Law, contraception, and women's right, the issues that were so important in the medical discussion and women's letters. Contraception was most likely omitted because it continued to be both controversial and unavailable. Kovrigina might have considered direct reference to rights not useful in securing approval from Soviet leaders, but the draft law clearly recognized that women should be able to decide the question of motherhood for themselves.

On October 28, 1955, the Presidium of the Central Committee examined Kovrigina's proposal to decriminalize abortion. It appears that most of the Soviet leadership accepted it, probably convinced by the statistical evidence that repressive measures had not worked and by the medical profession's concern that criminalization was crippling women and the future fertility of the population. Kovrigina was able to present abolition as a pronatalist measure to improve women's health. Also, the leadership was generally supportive of the abolition of Stalinist excesses in criminalization and coercion.

N. V. Popova, Secretary of the Central Trade Union and chairwoman of the Committee for Soviet Women in the Party, spoke about this Presidium meeting at the June 1957 Plenum.[85] Popova, together with Kovrigina, had submitted the proposal to the Central Committee of the Communist Party. She discussed how L. M. Kaganovich insulted her and Kovrigina and how A. I. Mikoian, who supported their initiative, warned Kaganovich that "this was exactly the way to discourage people from bringing [new] proposals." After reworking the proposal and making additions based on the criticisms of the Presidium, on November 16, 1955, the Presidium confirmed the abolition of criminalized abortion.

On November 23, 1955, abortion became legal. The law's preamble fully reflected Kovrigina's suggestions and language:

> The measures to encourage motherhood and protect childhood carried out by the Soviet state together with the steady rise in consciousness and cultural level among women actively participating in all sectors of the economy now make it possible to eliminate the legislative ban on abortions.
>
> From now on, lowering the number of abortions can be achieved by broadening state measures to encourage motherhood and of an educational and explanatory character.
>
> Removing the ban on abortions will also create the possibility of eliminating the great harm to female health caused by abortions outside hospitals, often by untrained individuals.
>
> With the aim of providing the possibility for women to decide themselves about motherhood[86] . . .

In addition to annulling the 1936 ban on abortion, two additional points were affirmed by the Presidium. First, all abortions must take place in medical facilities according to MZ instructions. Second, in cases of illegal abortions, those who carried them out, both medically trained doctors and non-trained ones, would be prosecuted. The criminality of those who encouraged women to have abortions was eliminated. Kovrigina and the medical establishment had long fought for their vision of abortion, even as it evolved. From now on, the MZ's views would become the new orthodoxy as abortion became one of the most practiced operations in the USSR. The number of clinical abortions continued to rise until 1965.

Remaining Issues

In a country where the paternalistic state considered itself the most important supporter of women's well-being, both the recognition of women's reproductive right—even if it was limited to the decision of when to reproduce—and Kovrigina's understanding of criminalization of abortion as "a prohibition on the individual that humiliates women, controlling the intimate side of their existence" were significant. The 1955 re-legalization of abortion also saved the lives of many Soviet women, both literally and figuratively. Legalization did not mean an easy, automatic clinical abortion on demand, as consultation with doctors and waiting in line became obstacles. Even so, for many women it became easier to obtain permission for clinical abortions for non-medical reasons, which was much less stressful and cheaper than having to arrange an underground abortion or trying to apply for a special permission, with the possibility of being denied and then having to go underground. Moreover, the rate of out-of-wedlock births went down after 1955. Most likely, one of the reasons for this was that women gained easier access to safe abortion.[87] In this way, re-legalized abortion improved women's ability to manage their own welfare in the face of unpredictable and often unstable family life in the environment where state support was insufficient. Since most women seeking abortion were already mothers, this decision also protected their first child(ren).

However, some issues and problems remained. As significant as the discourse of women's right was, this right was limited to choosing the timing of motherhood, but it did not extend to the decision to become or not to become mothers. The idea that women should have multiple births was never challenged. Moreover, the idea of women's rights or right was never widely accepted beyond the medical profession. In her presentation to the Central Committee, Kovrigina did not use the language of women's rights but stressed social reasons, in particular, the creation of thousands of orphans after fatally unsuccessful abortions. In the actual law legalizing abortion on November 23, 1955, it was not a woman's "right" that was provided but the state allowing the "possibility" of deciding the question of motherhood by herself. Thus, paternalistic language replaced the ideas of right and justice. The idea that criminalization had been an attack on women's private lives was also absent in the law. The language of women's reproductive rights would never appear in public under socialism.

Not surprisingly, medical professionals gained much from re-legalization. Because non-clinical abortions were replaced by clinical abortions, secondary damage to women's health was greatly reduced. As doctors predicted, legalization of abortion resulted in reversing the ratio between clinical abortions and non-clinical abortions, without affecting the birth rate. In addition, doctors no longer needed to play the role of investigators and could focus on their patient relationships. Without the fear of medical intervention to prevent abortion, women's participation in medical services would grow, enabling better medical research and public health.

Nonetheless, stronger medical control over women's reproductive health would only be possible when contraceptive devices became available. Preventing unwanted conceptions was far more desirable than performing clinical abortions. If doctors had no way of assisting women's control over the timing of conceptions, women would continue to get pregnant in undesirable conditions and subsequently get abortions. If this cycle was not broken, all medical efforts to maintain reproductive health would be in vain. In this way, the question of contraception became important both for women and doctors.[88]

The Development of Abortion Culture and Socialist Reproductive Practice

The Soviet Union's re-legalization of abortion became an important step toward the development of socialist reproductive practice beyond religious and national borders. Within the Soviet Union, women not only in predominantly Slavic-populated areas but also in republics where a significant percentage of the population was Muslim, would have expanded access to abortion. Compared with Slavic women, Muslim women generally had much lower rates of abortion and a higher birth rate, making many of them Mother Heroines. Nevertheless, use of abortion as a method of fertility control slowly expanded also among the titular nationalities in Central Asia, as an increasing number of local women received higher education. In Uzbekistan, for example, between 1956 and 1973 the number of abortions more than doubled.[89] Some scholars also suggest that ethnic and religious practice did not always define reproductive practice. For example, Kazakhstan, with a significant percentage of Russians living alongside the majority Kazakhs, set the stage for some local ethnic women to adopt the reproductive practices common among Russian women.[90] The United Nations 2007 abortion rate data continued to show the Soviet legacy, as the successor states to the former Soviet republics of Central Asia demonstrated some of the least restrictive abortion policies in the world and much higher rates of abortion compared to women from the very few other Muslim countries that provide abortion statistics.[91]

The effects of legalization went well beyond Soviet women, particularly in new postwar socialist nations in East and Central Europe. Following the Soviet lead, clinical abortion had become widely available in most communist countries earlier than in the capitalist "West."[92] After the February 1956 Soviet 20th Party Congress, which signaled both a definitive departure from Stalin's repressive approach to social issues and the removal of leaders in Eastern Europe who had followed Stalin's example in so many areas, most East and Central European countries legalized abortion. Bulgaria and Poland came first in April 1956, followed in quick succession by Hungary, Romania, and Czechoslovakia.[93] Interestingly, in Poland, wider access to abortion was partially justified by the claim that the Catholic Church, an institution antithetical to communist Poland, had supported criminalization.[94] But generally speaking, the reason for the change followed the Soviet official logic emphasizing the harm of underground abortion to women's reproductive health.

A few of these countries later restricted legal abortion when their governments recognized low birth rate as a problem, and notably, Romania criminalized abortion in 1966. But these reversals could not completely stop women from terminating unwanted pregnancies illegally.[95] Aside from legalization, women's participation in the economy and limited practical support for working mothers, combined with the general lack of safe, reliable, easy-to-use modern contraceptives made abortion the primary fertility control and the typical socialist reproductive practice.[96]

After the 1949 Revolution, Communist China initially adopted a pronatalist family policy and celebrated mothers with many children. But in the mid-1950s the Chinese government also increasingly expanded women's access to abortion and promoted contraception and sterilization through workplaces, although not so actively at this stage. Mao also spoke favorably about birth control.[97] Other Chinese Communist Party leaders also advocated abortion so that women could play their rightful role in revolutionary liberation. These included Deng Yingchao (the wife of Zhou Enlai), Deng Xiaoping, and Liu Shaoqi. But just as in the Soviet Union, in Mao's mind, abortion liberalization was not necessarily anti-natalist. In announcing the Great Leap Forward in 1958, Chairman Mao announced that a population of a billion would not be "cause for alarm."[98]

Two decades later China pursued a different socialist path and adopted an anti-natalist one-child policy, but abortion remained a common practice in a different context. Using a citation from Engels that left it to the communists of the future to decide demographic policy, China made reproduction conform to socialist production planning, including enforcement of delayed marriage ages, contraception, and abortion.[99] Chinese reproductive policies and practice diverged from Soviet ones in the late 1970s as China pioneered the road to "socialism with Chinese characteristics," including anti-natalist policies. But abortion culture remained as a punitive state practice in a new role.

East German abortion policy did not follow that of the USSR right away due to its central concern for repairing wartime demographic devastation. Nonetheless, a discussion of widening the criteria for legal abortion in 1961 led to an expansion of criteria in 1965. East Germany legalized abortion in 1972, when Walter Ulbricht was replaced by Erich Honecker, but around 100,000 East German women had illegal abortions every year before legalization. Beyond that number, there was also a significant group who made use of easy proximity to neighboring East European countries, such as Poland, where foreign women could also terminate unwanted pregnancies legally.[100]

Unlike most other socialist countries, East Germany introduced the pill in 1965, well before the legalization of abortion in 1972. Acceptance of the pill was slow initially, but then accelerated until it became the "default contraceptive choice" by the end of the 1970s. Not surprisingly, compared to the Soviet Union, where the number of abortions was consistently double the number of live births in the 1970s and 1980s, East Germany had lower ratios.[101] But access to contraception did not alter any of the other socialist reproductive traits. In the 1980s East Germany had approximately three times as many abortions as West Germany. East German women on average married at the age of 22, and their first child followed soon thereafter. In contrast, West Germans married six years later, on average, with more delayed first births. While childlessness among East German women was around 10 percent in the 1980s, 25 to 30 percent of all West German women were childless, and the number went up to 40 percent among the highly educated.[102]

This gap in norms of reproductive practice, in particular, the level of access to abortion, became an obstacle to reunification, as East German women insisted on their access to legal abortion, while West Germany allowed abortions only for limited circumstances and specific indications. Drafters of the Unification Treaty of 1990 generally had to adopt West German laws in case of conflict, but fearing that this issue might derail the unification process, they avoided making the decision then, entrusting the task to the wisdom of future policymakers in an already unified Germany.[103] Thus, the abortion rate in East Germany always remained much higher than in West Germany. Abortion culture, made in the USSR, became an enduring characteristic of socialist and post-socialist reproduction.

6

Beyond Replacing the Dead

Women's Welfare and
the End of the Soviet Union

The 1955 legalization of abortion was a significant achievement for Soviet women and medical professionals of women's medicine. Women's demands, the commitment among experts of women's medicine to improving women's reproductive health, and the personal interest of Health Minister Mariia D. Kovrigina made the legalization possible during the brief political interregnum between Stalin and Khrushchev. However, only after encountering inexplicable delays to family law reform, and the planned lack of modern contraception in a socialist economy run from above, did the medical and legal professions feel compelled to manage abortion in order to tame its worst ills.

In fact, doctors wanted to ensure that women did not misinterpret legalization as an encouragement or acceptance of abortion. A descriptive account of the abortion experience confirms that legal abortion for the millions was a painful and impersonal experience. The operation was performed by very experienced medical personnel and was completed within fifteen minutes, but anesthesia was rare and sanitary conditions were often wanting. In addition, medical personnel in abortion clinics were notoriously rude and unsympathetic to women, both unmarried and married. A woman wishing to have a clinical abortion would first obtain a note from a doctor, which entitled her to take three days off from work. She then completed paperwork and waited her turn. Abortion became a "conveyor-belt" operation in abortion clinics around the country. A large-scale abortion clinic operated on 200–300 women daily. Husbands and boyfriends were mostly indifferent about how many times their female partners were having abortions, and considered abortion women's business.[1]

Legalization triggered widespread anti-abortion propaganda campaigns, once doctors could better identify at-risk pregnant women.[2] Nonetheless, as had been expected, legalization resulted in a sharp rise in the total number

Replacing the Dead. Mie Nakachi, Oxford University Press (2021). © Oxford University Press.
DOI: 10.1093/oso/9780190635138.003.0007

of clinical abortions and a drop in the number of non-clinical abortions. Between 1955 and 1965, the total registered number of abortions more than tripled, from 2.6 million to 8.6 million per year. The figure peaked in 1965, declined until 1969, and stabilized at around 7.5 million until 1985.[3] Throughout the 1970s, Soviet doctors regularly performed 20,000 abortions a day. The Soviet Union had become a stable legal abortion regime.

The ratio between clinical and non-clinical abortions quickly flipped as well. In 1955, the ratio of clinical to non-clinical abortions was 23 to 77. Already by the following year, the same ratio was reversed to 70 to 30. From then on, clinical abortion as a percentage of all abortions gradually rose to 90 percent in 1989, reducing the percentage of non-clinical abortions to only 10 percent.[4] The 1955 legalization successfully achieved its goal of saving the thousands of lives previously lost to failed illegal abortions every year.[5] But the rise in the number of abortions from 1955 to 1965 had little influence on overall fertility in the Soviet Union because most abortions previously performed underground had become clinical abortions.[6]

During this decade, abortion became an almost universal female experience. Both legal and medical professionals continued feeling optimistic about the prospects of reforms in the context of "de-Stalinization." Some changes occurred, and medical professionals even launched a campaign for responsible fatherhood as a part of the anti-abortion campaign.[7] But the principle of one-parent pronatalism remained the same, and the contraceptive revolution was blocked. Part of the reason was that the creator of the 1944 Family Law, Nikita S. Khrushchev, took over leadership of the Soviet Union in 1957. Khrushchev did not allow major shifts in the existing policies toward population and reproduction. In the meantime, doctors of women's medicine focused on developing modern contraception, but this proved to be a dead end for both medical and ideological reasons.

This chapter first narrates the lack of family law reform in the Khrushchev era, followed by the promulgation of the 1968 Family Law. However, the new legislation still maintained the distinction between children born in wedlock and out-of-wedlock. Continuing coverage of the medical profession makes it clear that with abortion now legal and on the rise, doctors' efforts shifted to the development of modern contraception in order to reduce the number of abortions between the late 1950s and early 1970s. Like their foreign colleagues, Soviet physicians succeeded in creating effective pills and intrauterine devices, but the new pronatalism of the 1970s Soviet leadership blocked mass production and distribution of contraceptives. Common features of Soviet women's reproductive practice and the new population policies in the 1970s and 1980s increasingly encouraged women to take longer maternity and childcare leaves at home. This period saw the definitive formation of the distinctly socialist reproductive practice—young marriage and first births, high reliance on abortion for fertility control, and a very low rate of childlessness—diverging from the contrasting trends developing in the capitalist West.

Meanwhile, after several decades in disgrace, both demography and sociology had been resurrected starting from the late 1950s. As the Soviet population approached the prewar level, TsSU Director V. N. Starovskii informed Khrushchev that a new census could be conducted. In the run-up to this event, demographers gathered their forces. Their first big task after the 1959 census was to analyze the assembled data, but results remained inconclusive for lack of a reliable postwar reference point from which to extrapolate trends. In preparation for the next postwar census scheduled for 1970, an official party-government decree of 1967 called for the development of the social sciences, guaranteeing financial support for research on population at universities, in the Academy of Sciences and under various governmental organizations.[8] Especially after the results of the 1970 census became available, studies of family dynamics, sexual behaviors, and demographic trends revealed a dramatic decline in fertility, especially among Slavic women.

Having just recently proclaimed "developed socialism" in the Soviet Union and Eastern Europe, the Soviet leadership was troubled by the fall in fertility, since socialism was supposed to deliver demographic growth. They were now ready to listen to the policy-relevant advice of the new generation of Soviet social scientists, since the future growth of the planned economy depended on the future size of the labor force. Among the wide range of expert suggestions on offer, the Soviet government in the 1970s and 1980s would pursue its perennial goal of pronatalism by redefining women's role in socialism.

By this time all the advanced capitalist countries were also facing the same quandary as the Soviets—falling birth rate and rising divorce rate as women entered the workforce in ever greater numbers. Already in the 1960s, the women's rights movement inspired educational and career advancement. Accordingly, female participation in the workforce rose sharply first in the United States, Canada, Australia, Sweden, and Great Britain. France and Italy followed in the early 1970s with Japan and Germany marking significant increases from the late 1970s.[9] These society-shaking changes had important implications for family, labor force and social security. As social scientists analyzed these new issues and new data, policymakers everywhere had to re-think the new role of women in the family and society.

Missed Opportunities and Failed Legal Reforms in the 1950s–1960s

Even before Stalin's death in 1953, legal and medical professionals called for family law reform, but actual changes to the law had been blocked. The failure of the first public campaign for change proved that Stalin was not the only obstacle to reform. However, with the re-legalization of abortion and the gradual recovery from postwar demography, a new era of gradual, piece-meal reform began in the late 1950s and 1960s.

The first reform efforts focused on realizing welfare measures that the Health Ministry had already developed in the late Stalinist period to improve living and working conditions for all mothers. In 1956 the Ministry of Health issued two laws for improving the living and working conditions of working mothers. On March 26, a ukase was issued to set longer maternity leave for women.[10] On October 13, an additional directive was issued to help working women balance work and childrearing responsibilities, including improving after-school facilities for the children of working mothers.[11]

In the same year, tax reform reduced the financial burdens on mothers raising children. The family tax had been unpopular because it targeted all adults, married or unmarried, raising one or two children. Reform began in 1954 to exempt those whose salaries were small or who were widows of the Great Patriotic War.[12] It was broadened as part of Khrushchev's general effort to reduce the tax burden on low-income families and improve material conditions for workers, a goal set at the 20th Party Congress. The ukase of September 8, 1956, exempted all citizens whose salaries were below 370 rubles a month from both income tax and taxes on small families.[13]

Since the revenue from the small family tax funded postwar government aid to mothers, the change would affect them. In November 1957, a special commission proposed reducing small family taxes for adult citizens who had one child, as well as unmarried women and widows of the Great Patriotic War.[14] It also exempted single mothers. In this way, the primary payers of the infertility tax would become childless married men and women, and unmarried men.

The source of funding for government support for mothers was significantly cut as taxation became more progressive. However, the commission also wanted to increase government aid to mothers, especially to low-income urban mothers struggling to raise one or two children. The commission proposed disregarding marital status and creating new categories depending on income level, number of children, and their ages. Unmarried mothers who never applied for the special aid, married mothers whose husbands did not contribute to family income, and divorced women whose husbands refused to pay child support would have been the major beneficiaries of this new approach.

Another feature of this proposal was a new differentiation policy in state aid for mothers, because the new measure excluded mothers working on collective farms. Its significance lay in its contrast to the prewar pronatalist policy of celebrating large rural families and in reference to the growing fertility differentials among Soviet nationalities. Practically, the new scheme represented a shift away from encouraging mothers to have many children toward supporting all mothers, regardless of their marital status, to raise at least two children.[15] Thus, for the first time, support would be provided for the first or second child among low-income urban mothers, while ending support for affluent urban mothers, regardless of number of children.[16] This would also effectively increase support for more-urbanized Slavic women with relatively few children and reduce aid to less-urbanized Central Asian mothers with more children.

To make up the loss in small family tax revenue, estimated at 12.6 billion rubles, and to provide increased aid to mothers, the commission made this recommendation: "It will be appropriate to cover these expenses by adopting the proposal of the Finance Ministry to raise retail prices on vodka and hard liquor by an average of 20 percent in order to receive an additional 11.8 billion rubles annually for the budget." The rest of the deficit would be financed by improving the assortment of vodkas distributed to the public, which "should increase [sales] income by more than 800 million rubles."[17]

This could be understood simply as a fiscal technique, but it connected to Khrushchev's anti-alcohol campaign in the 1950s. The price increase was aimed at controlling alcohol consumption.[18] To further this goal, in December 1958 an additional decree was issued to prohibit the sale of vodka before 10:00 A.M., to limit the amount of vodka served at restaurants to 100 grams, and other measures.[19] In this way, alcohol, which was considered a major public health hazard, a source of family instability, and a cause of low productivity in the Soviet Union, particularly among the male population, would be used to fund government aid for mothers.[20]

The three proposed measures, however, were not all approved. While the tax cut and the price increase on alcohol were actually adopted, the differentiated restructuring of government aid to poor urban mothers, regardless of marital status, was not. Technically it was considered impracticable to introduce the new government support for lack of appropriate statistics to identify precisely who would be eligible for the aid.[21] Available archival records do not indicate other reasons, but there was resistance to changing support by differentiating between urban and rural mothers, while treating married and unmarried mothers equally.

Thus, differentiated aid policies for married and unmarried mothers continued under Khrushchev, as under Stalin. The needs of low-income urban women with one or two children, an important potential source of new births, were neglected, even as the urban population increased. In hindsight, this was a missed opportunity for demographic planning, since low fertility among urban Slavic working mothers became the biggest challenge to pronatalism in the late Soviet period. Only in 1974 would new aid to the children of low-income families be instituted, but again, without differentiating between the rural and urban poor.[22]

The reform of the small family tax in the late 1950s suggests Khrushchev's willingness and ability to revise the postwar population policy when he wished. However, his reluctance, if not resistance, is suggested by the non-revision of the most controversial legal measures regarding single mothers, out-of-wedlock children, and divorce procedures despite public campaigns initiated by the intelligentsia as well as many proposals submitted by legal commissions at this time.[23] Following the public efforts of journalist Elena Serebrovskaia, behind the scenes in the Ministry of Justice in late 1955 and early 1956 legal experts prepared drafts of a separate decree to improve the rights of out-of-wedlock children. All drafts stated that paternity could be registered for out-of-wedlock children when both parents agreed and that government aid for single mothers would be extended even after the child turned 12, suggesting that there was a consensus on this issue among legal experts. In 1956 and 1957, calls for change came from top officials at the Ministry of Education, the Ministry of Internal Affairs, the Latvian Sovmin, and the journal *Kommunist*, but nothing came of them.[24]

Public discussion reached its high point in the October 9, 1956 letter to the editor of *Literaturnaia gazeta*, initiated by the popular children's author and poet S. Ia. Marshak and signed by such luminaries as Ilia Erenburg, Dmitrii Shostakovich, and G. N. Speranskii.[25] As high-ranking men, they understood that "serious state considerations" might have lent the 1944 Family Law some validity in wartime conditions, but the title of the article stated that the law had now been "Repudiated by Life Itself." Any communiqué signed by these four men could be considered the voice of the intelligentsia. Possibly inspired by these ideas, legal experts again began to draft an All-Union family law. The Legal Commission under the Sovmin SSSR produced several drafts in the course of two years and submitted a final draft on October 6, 1959. However, for unknown reasons, it was not approved even in December 1961, two years after the submission.[26] It is not hard to imagine that Khrushchev, as the head of Sovmin from March 1958 to his ouster in 1964, had an influence on the fate of this proposal.[27]

Meanwhile, the intellectuals tried again. In 1961, Marshak mobilized young lawyer, Arkadii E. Vaksberg, as well as fellow children's poet Kornei Chukovskii and Veniamin Kaverin, an author who had spent the war as a frontline correspondent.[28] Vaksberg succeeded in getting Erenburg's signature, but the latter doubted that anything would come of it. Two years later, Vaksberg finally succeeded in publishing on this subject, but Erenburg again was pessimistic about legal change. Vaksberg's enthusiasm was met with a chilly proverb, "I'm not sure this matter will move, but 'water wears away stones.'"[29]

In the meantime, a joint legal commission under the Council of Unions and the Council of Nationalities of the Supreme Soviet prepared a draft all-union law, which was submitted to the Central Committee in July 1962 and prepared for publication in newspapers and magazines. However, publication never occurred due to lack of approval from the Central Committee. After that, several meetings took place to change the clause on out-of-wedlock children, suggesting that the Central Committee had expressed opposition on this issue. A further revised draft was sent to thirty-three universities, research centers, and institutes in January 1963, and members of the commission traveled to cities in Russia and other Soviet republics to introduce the draft and get feedback.[30]

In May 1963 the commission submitted a revised draft to the Central Committee, which asked the commission to revise again and resubmit. A new draft was submitted on June 19, but nothing happened. At the end of 1963, G. I. Vorobiev, chairman of the Commission of Legislative Preparation of the Council of Unions, announced the decision to publicize the draft all-union law. However, no draft was published in 1964.[31] Insiders predicted imminent promulgation, but in the end resistance at the highest political level blocked repeated initiatives.[32] Only after the fall of Khrushchev could the reform actually take place.

In light of the fact that the creation of fatherlessness in 1944 was a demographic measure, it is highly likely that Khrushchev's unwillingness to reverse the postwar policy was also based on the demographic situation at the time. In 1956 the population exceeded 200 million, the target level suggested by Starovskii as the moment to consider a first postwar census. However, Khrushchev was keen to see a further increase in the population as demonstrated in his 1955 speech. As the 1959 census had documented a serious reduction in fertility, especially among Slavic women, this would hardly have convinced Khrushchev to abandon the key component of his pronatalist policy.

Khrushchev aside, there must have still been strong opposition within the Sovmin and the Central Committee to the reform concerning out-of-wedlock children. After Khrushchev was ousted in 1964, the draft law publication did not take place in 1965, 1966, or 1967. Instead, there were piecemeal reforms in 1965 and 1967. On December 10, 1965, a ukase from the Presidium of the Supreme Soviet SSSR made divorce easier to obtain by ending the two-tier process and allowing the people's court to resolve all divorce cases. The proclamation also abolished the publication requirement. As a way to address the problem of divorced fathers failing to pay child support, on July 21, 1967, another ukase from the Presidium required those who failed to pay child support to receive a special stamp in their passports. Simplifying divorce procedure pushed open the floodgate for millions who lived de facto divorced lives. The divorce rate would soar from then on.

Finally *Izvestiia* and *Literaturnaia gazeta* published the draft USSR and Union Republic Basic Law of Marriage and Family (hereafter, the 1968 All-Union Family Law) in April 1968.[33] Public discussion of the draft would last until the end of June. *Literaturnaia gazeta* took special pride in having initiated the reform campaign in 1954. On April 10, 1968, the editorial board included a message on page 1, "the publication of the article in *Literaturnaia gazeta* by the Leningrad writer E. Serebrovskaia 'Life Calls for Amendment' began discussion of questions about the [1944] law on family and marriage. Writers, doctors, legal experts, teachers and many readers of the paper participated in this discussion. The conversation begun by us was continued in the pages of other publications."

Literaturnaia gazeta focused attention on the paternity issue and the treatment of out-of-wedlock children. In the proposed draft, paternity could be established either when the father wished to recognize it or through the court, when there was strong evidence of the parents living together and sharing a budget prior to the birth of the child, or joint childrearing after the birth. Fathers who wished to recognize paternity could do so for children born both before and after the promulgation of the proposed law. However, paternity suits could be brought to court only regarding children born after the law was introduced.[34]

The debate in the pages of *Literaturnaia gazeta* over this draft proposal approved of strengthening the rights of out-of-wedlock children but condemned unprincipled half-measures. A participant of the 1956 campaign, composer Dmitrii Shostakovich was basically content with the proposed measures. He characterized the 1944 Family Law as "contrary" to the "equal rights of women [with men], paternal responsibility for children, and the basic principles of raising a next generation." He was delighted that the new law would "finally resolve the problem of the dash in the birth record, set equal rights between wedlock and out-of-wedlock children, and reform the size and the procedure of child support." The point that he considered problematic was that the new law would not be applied retroactively for out-of-wedlock children. He rhetorically asked, "After all, why should they be responsible for the slowness of our lawmakers, who had worked on the new law for so long?"[35]

Another signatory of the 1956 petition, pediatrician, Academician, and Hero of Socialist Labor G. N. Speranskii, considered the new law a half-measure. Speranskii found it problematic that the draft law did not give full equal rights to out-of-wedlock children and wrote indignantly, "Why should a child's well-being be determined by the nature of the parents' relationship? I don't understand it."[36]

As Speranskii pointed out, this question of the rights of out-of-wedlock children was implicitly, but directly, related to the issue of how to understand the relationship of the parents to whom these children were born. In the postwar period, Abramova pointed out that out-of-wedlock births were often the result of women sincerely wishing to have a family and taking what was to become a temporary relationship very seriously as a "marriage." However, the later prevalent view was that they were born as the result of casual sex, chance acquaintance, or a frivolous relationship.[37]

Some legal specialists tried to refute this widespread assumption. V. Bil'shai asked, "With what logic can we evaluate a serious, but unsuccessful love, or even a casual relationship between a man and woman, which results in childbirth?"[38] Supreme Court RSFSR judge L. Anisimova also pointed out the law's inability to recognize and differentiate the complex and various relationships between the parents. She said that the proposed law intended to eliminate contradictions between law and life. For example, some couples might have had a long relationship without living together or sharing finances. Situations existed where a mother and her child live with a man who is not the father of the child. Therefore, she considered that the part of Article 16 that discussed the very limited conditions under which out-of-wedlock children could establish paternity through the court should be completely eliminated, so that judges could make conclusions based on law and evidence in each disputed case.

She was also opposed to Article 17, which said that where the father of an out-of-wedlock child does not agree to register his name for the child, the mother can use her family name and her choice of first name and patronymic to fill in the section on "father." She reasoned that both the child and people surrounding him or her would soon find out that the father's name was false, so this fiction was not much different from giving the child a dash on the birth registration.[39]

Some single mothers agreed with Anisimova's opinion. Single mother M. Volkova wrote, "If the blank in the birth record had provoked disgust in women, then not much better feelings will be produced by a fictitious record. This is also hypocrisy. My son will remain as hurt as before." M. Shternberg, a single mother, wrote: "The dash in [my son's] birth record kills me, literally kills me. The new law must give mothers the right to register the entire name of the real father [in a child's birth record]."[40]

Those who approved the limitation that the proposed law put on women bringing paternity cases basically made the argument that a single woman should be responsible for the consequences of having sex with a man who was not her legal husband. They also suggested that such a limitation, which kept the clear distinction between children born in wedlock and those born out-of-wedlock, was useful for encouraging young people to think seriously about having a family.[41]

Despite these timely critiques, the new family law ultimately maintained the proposed draft concerning out-of-wedlock births. In this way, the actual reform of the 1944 Family Law was kept to a minimum. There would no longer be blanks or dashes in birth certificates of out-of-wedlock children after the 1968 law, but, unless the father desired to recognize his paternity, the line for the "name of the father" could and often would be filled with a fictitious name. In this way, children's fates continued to be determined by the legality of their parents' marriage.

For adults, the results of 1968 were deeply gendered. Men retained the option of denying their out-of-wedlock children. Women, on the other hand, experienced change for the worse. The mid-1960s reforms condemned women's sex and reproduction outside marriage, which the 1944 Family Law had tried to promote in order to maximize the birth rate. The 1968 law required that one of three conditions be fulfilled to define a serious relationship: cohabitation while sharing all aspects of household management prior to the birth of the child, joint efforts at childrearing, or the father's clear recognition of paternity.[42]

Single motherhood would be officially associated with temporary, casual sex, leading to social shame and reduced opportunity for both unmarried mother and fatherless child. The agreement that out-of-wedlock children should not be blamed for the nature of their parents' relationship in turn meant that single motherhood was identified with the sin of the mother, as in most cases the father could not be identified and so would not be subject to social stigma. The 1968 law officially branded single mothers as morally questionable. If a man volunteered to recognize his paternity, he would become a responsible father. Only when the mother took the paternity case to the court against the will of the father would he be publicly identified as the father, but the 1968 law made sure that this was extremely difficult in practice. In this sense, the new law basically maintained the position of encouraging men to have non-conjugal sex without assuming any legal or economic responsibilities, as was intended in 1944. Again, this reform reinforced optional fatherhood.

The most significant change in the series of reforms following Khrushchev's ouster was the simplified divorce procedure of 1965, that drove the dramatic rise in divorce in the late 1960s. Unlike in the postwar period, the initiators of divorce were predominantly women, and the number one reason for divorce was infidelity, with alcoholism also ranking high.[43] As of the 1970s, the Soviet Union had the world's second highest divorce rate after the United States.[44] New marriage and sex patterns included younger marriage and younger first births, a trend beginning in the late 1960s. This new cohort, marrying young and divorcing quickly, had grown up in the postwar period, and many were from the 15 percent to 25 percent born out-of-wedlock, the first post-1944 "fatherless children."[45] Many others born in registered marriages on paper lived with de facto single mothers, such as war widows and women whose husbands left without official divorce, most often because husbands had formed a new "marriage" or family.

The direction of legal reforms regarding out-of-wedlock births and divorce in the 1960s was a welcome improvement for many, but it did not change the optional paternal responsibility for out-of-wedlock children. Unlike divorced men in the 1950s, divorced men in the 1960s often did not remarry and simply cohabitated with new partners, a practice that women preferred to call "common-law marriage," as "cohabitation" was considered a shameful practice.[46] Financially, single mothers, married or cohabitating women whose husbands or partners did not contribute to the family economy, and divorced women whose former husbands did not pay child support had to continue to make ends meet on their own. The fact that the government issued amendments in 1984 and 1986 regarding the failed child support payment system suggests that in times of high divorce rates, mothers were primarily responsible for childrearing.[47] In addition, unmarried mothers were at higher risk than before of being identified as morally corrupt, "loose women," if the biological fathers refused to recognize paternity.[48] If a woman made the decision to have an out-of-wedlock child, neighbors somehow found out, and the mother and the child faced discrimination.[49] The desire among women to give birth to a child in marriage or otherwise to abort would remain consistent as the postwar principle of one-parent pronatalism remained in effect.

Medicine's Dead End: Contraception by Abortion in the Late Soviet Era

With the 1955 legalization, the Soviet Union became one of the very few countries in the world to enact abortion on demand. However, it lagged behind in the development of effective modern contraceptives. An increasing number of Western women began to regulate fertility with oral contraceptives and IUDs, while pushing the government to regulate their safety and quality. Moreover, women's liberation movements succeeded in pushing forward women's demand to expand access to abortion in North America and Western Europe. In contrast, at the end of the 1970s, for Soviet women abortion still remained the only method of fertility control.

Although it had little impact on the birth rate, the successful implementation of the 1955 law led to a new reform consensus, one promoting contraception to make abortion less frequent and to improve the health of Soviet women. Under legalized abortion, each case of clinically performed abortion was recorded on the medical record, and large-scale studies documented statistical linkages between abortion and fertility.[50] As a result, doctors diagnosed various common short-term and long-term side effects of clinical abortion, such as perforation of the uterus, high fevers, and inflammation of the reproductive organs, reaching the conclusion that even clinical abortion carried health risks. In a local study conducted in Vitebsk, among 217 women who had had abortions over a five-year period, 12 percent suffered from irregular menstrual cycles, 11 percent from chronic inflammation of the reproductive organs, 9.9 percent from infertility, and 4.1 percent from reduced sexual sensitivity. Thus, more than a third of abortion patients developed symptoms associated with reproductive dysfunction. The most serious and long-term effects included miscarriages, premature births, and infertility. In another local study in Iaroslavl, doctors concluded that abortion was the number one reason for secondary infertility.[51] Clearly, according to these studies, alternatives were urgent for improving women's fertility.

Another large-scale study of abortion conducted in 1958–1959 also made it clear that contraception was necessary. In this survey, the Central Lenin Institute for Training Doctors distributed 50,000 questionnaires all over the RSFSR. Of these, approximately 20,000 were returned from urban areas and 6,000 from rural areas. The result showed important trends. Women who worked outside the home were two and a half times more likely to have an abortion compared to women who didn't work outside the home.[52] The most commonly expressed reasons for the decision to terminate were no childcare at home or no possibility of placing a child at a childcare institution, insufficient living space, material hardship, and absence of husband.[53] Relationship problems ranked lower than in the 1949 study. The average 1950s woman undergoing legal abortion revealed herself as employed, lacking childcare options, and with limited living space and income. The two most disturbing results of this study from the medical point of view were that 15 percent of urban women and 16 percent of rural women had more than one abortion in the same year, and 6.0 percent of urban women and 3.8 percent of rural women had terminated their first pregnancies.[54]

In addition, local surveys of those caught after undergoing a criminal abortion conducted in the 1970s revealed that unmarried young women constituted the largest group.[55] These abortions were generally the first pregnancy, which, Soviet doctors believed, often brought "irreversible harm" to reproductive health.[56] The rise in the number of young women terminating pregnancies called attention to the fact that women generally began such limited available contraceptive practices, as *coitus interruptus* and feminine douche, only after the first birth or abortion.[57] The logical conclusion was that in order to prevent abortions among young unmarried women, sex education in school to teach contraceptive methods should begin sooner, as sex lives were starting earlier.[58] According to one study, 66.7 percent of women experienced sex before marriage and 66.6 percent, before turning 20. Among working women, 15 percent had sex before turning 18. This caused a perceptible increase in the percentage of women who married young (before 20).[59] This tendency continued into the 1970s and was reflected in the younger ages of mothers at first birth, increasing numbers of teenage mothers, and more underground abortions.[60]

Thus, the scale of young women terminating their first pregnancy by underground abortion appears to have been higher than the reassuring official statistics suggested. One 1970s survey showed that the ratio of non-clinical to all abortions was 1 to 2.7, that is, around 30 percent illegal; and among criminal abortions, 70 percent in urban and 90 percent in rural areas terminated first pregnancies.[61] This practice alone was considered to be the primary cause of approximately 10 percent of infertile marriages and contributed to the high rate of premature births in the early 1980s.[62] Over the course of twenty years, medical researchers established that further improvements in women's health and fertility could only come with the introduction of mass contraception.

Toward this end, significant institutional developments for contraceptive research took place in the late 1950s and 1960s. Soon after the 1955 legalization of abortion an all-Union conference was organized at which Kovrigina emphasized the importance of teaching the population about the harm of abortion for women's health, of spreading knowledge about contraceptive methods and devices, and of training medical personnel regarding the reasons for abortions, including non-clinical abortion, even under a legalized abortion regime. A subsequent Academy of Medical Sciences (AMS) conference was held in April 1957.[63]

Multiple initiatives followed. In 1958, a new Scientific Research Institute for Physiology and Pathology of Women was founded in Tbilisi, Georgia, in order to study abortions and infertility. A special laboratory for research and approval of new contraceptive methods was created under AMS. In 1959, a "special expanded meeting" at the Institute for Obstetrics and Gynecology of

AMS was organized to discuss contraception and infertility. In 1960–1964 an experimental study on contraceptive devices was conducted in a Moscow woman's clinic by the Institute for Obstetrics and Gynecology. Media covered these issues as well. *Medical Worker* (*Meditsinskii rabotnik*), the main medical newspaper, and several medical journals published articles on contraception and abortion in the late 1950s and early 1960s.[64] The Soviet medical community was determined to develop contraception in order to decrease the rapidly rising incidence of abortions in the first decade after legalization.

Several contraceptive devices were available, with very limited distribution, in the Soviet Union in the late 1950s and 1960s. Condoms, cervical caps, and spermicide were all of poor quality and reliability. New products were under development. For example, the All-Union Scientific and Research Institute for Chemistry and Pharmacology introduced gramicidin, a contraceptive antibiotic.[65] Effectiveness was variously evaluated. For example, according to a study conducted by N. I. Sorokina, all of the methods listed above were considered equally effective.[66] But in general, barrier methods seemed more effective and reliable than chemical contraception.

In the 1960s, when oral contraception was becoming popular in the West, Soviet medical doctors eagerly followed the Western medical literature and conducted research on hormonal pills. East Germany had already begun production of hormonal pills and made them widely available in 1965, and the Soviet medical professionals would have had access to this information.[67] In the 1970s, at least one major symposium on hormonal contraception was conducted at the All-Union Scientific Research Institute for Obstetrics and Gynecology.[68] The enthusiasm of Soviet specialists of women's medicine for advancing reproductive medicine was reflected in the foundation in Moscow in 1972 of one of the four research centers for the Human Reproduction Project of the World Health Organization (WHO). In 1974, the WHO program in Moscow further expanded research on hormonal pills.[69]

The USSR's top doctors were well informed of the latest international developments in oral contraception, but generally Soviet doctors expressed concerns about safety. They had good reasons for this. After the hormonal pill was introduced in the United States as contraception in the early 1960s, it was believed to be safe, but later in the decade various side effects were revealed, leading 20 percent of women to stop using the pill. There was also strong criticism of the pill by some feminists in the late 1960s and 1970s. Nonetheless, the popularity of the pill remained very high among US and Western European women, because limiting the number of pregnancies was considered by many much more urgent than discomfort or a chance of later illnesses. As women complained about side effects, pharmaceutical companies also improved products and produced much safer low-hormonal dose pills.[70]

Thus it seems reasonable that Soviet doctors were cautious regarding mass application of the pill. But other aspects produced different developments in the West and the Soviet Union. In the West the contraceptive revolution began while abortion was still illegal. In addition, Western doctors and pharmaceutical industries were willing and able to respond to women's demands both to support women's well-being and to make profits. Also, in the West, large-scale trials were conducted on poor women at home or abroad to improve the quality and safety of the products.[71] In contrast, in the Soviet Union, where central planning determined production, there was no mechanism of responsive product-development based on consumer feedback and demand, since neither doctors nor women could decide investment and production priorities. Ultimately, in the Soviet system political choices overruled social needs, and renewed pronatalism was the most decisive factor in the fate of contraception.[72]

Postwar censuses in 1959 and 1970 continued to show declining fertility trends. For example, during the first postwar generation, the fertility level in RFSFR dropped to half of prewar levels.[73] Soviet demographers, whose field had only recently been rehabilitated, were forced to recognize declining fertility as an unmistakable trend.[74] Urbanization and the high rate of female employment contributed to the declining birth rate in the 1960s and 1970s. Urban population in the Soviet Union stood at 48 percent in the 1959 census, but grew to 56 percent by 1970.[75] The ratio of women among all workers of the Soviet Union, which shrank from an all-time high of 56 percent in 1945 to 46 percent in 1955, grew again to 51 percent by 1970.[76] This rise was due to the successful Soviet government campaign to mobilize housewives to join the labor force in the late 1950s and the 1960s, which achieved near universal employment of women by the end of the 1960s.[77] The difficulty inherent in the task was to encourage births without allowing women to leave their jobs, in order not to compromise the immediate need for their labor. In 1976, the 25th Party Congress for the first time called for effective demographic policy to aid further economic development in the Soviet Union by encouraging more births without losing women from the workforce.[78]

In this growing pronatalist atmosphere, some citizens suggested a new ban on abortions, but Soviet demographers openly opposed this, arguing that women would always find a way to terminate unwanted pregnancies illegally and that history had shown that a ban on abortion did not increase fertility in the long run.[79] Given their earlier views, doctors probably agreed with the demographers. Access to abortion was preserved, but contraceptive development stalled. In 1974, the Ministry of Health issued an instruction practically banning oral contraception by listing thirty contra-indications to its use. As a result, 80 to 90 percent of Soviet women became ineligible for the pill.[80] Officially, this decision was attributed to the questionable safety of the pill, particularly its long-term influence on the fetus. The Ministry of Health would continue to express caution toward the pill throughout the 1970s and the 1980s.[81] However, the fact that the government limited the production levels of contraception recognized as safe raises the question about the cause of the ban. Beyond the pill, all contraceptives were made deliberately scarce, as condoms and IUDs were produced at less than 40 percent of their officially estimated demand level in the 1970s and 1980s.[82] Only in the late 1980s and early 1990s did the possibility for mass introduction of oral contraception reappear in the Soviet Union.[83]

In the end, the Soviet government continued anti-abortion and pronatalist campaigns, while blocking the production and distribution of any kind of contraception. Women's limited control of their own fertility made no progress from 1955 on. Early 1980s studies showed that 70 percent of women in the RFSFR who came to a women's clinic had not been informed of contraceptive methods aside from the "rhythm method," *coitus interruptus*, and vaginal douches.[84] Twenty-five percent of women surveyed in Moscow preferred abortion and used no contraception.[85] Providing women with no effective means or knowledge to control their fertility other than physical intervention, contributed neither to raising the birth rate nor to lowering abortion, despite increased opportunities for open research and discussion. Contraception remained out of reach as the mass abortion regime put down institutional roots.

Denied condoms and the pill by pronatalist state imperatives, the medical profession had been forced to support the legalization of abortion. After 1955, it was logical that continuing limitations imposed on contraceptive devices would encourage doctors to widen easy access to abortion. This expansion reached its logical conclusion in 1987 with clinical abortion approved up to the twenty-eighth week of gestation.[86] An even more dramatic shift took place from the early 1980s, when vacuum aspirations, known as mini-abortions (*mini-abort*), became widespread in large cities as an out-patient procedure. Because this procedure was classified as "menstrual regulation" rather than abortion, the vast number of them performed until the twelfth week of pregnancy at non-state clinics were not even included in the abortion statistics.[87] In a classic irony typical of the Soviet regime, instead of providing alternatives to abortion, the doctors performed even more abortions while calling them something else. As easier and safer abortion became more widely available, fertility control became increasingly a woman's responsibility and obligation. The medical profession's emphasis on contraception as the future of reproductive practice had proved a dead end.

Social Science, Reproductive Practice, and Renewed Pronatalism after the 1960s

In the 1960s and the early 1970s, Soviet demographers had difficulty convincing policymakers that working women were having fewer children. This is because the original socialist vision of population growth posited that women under socialism would maintain high fertility because of the good working and living environment for women, state childcare support, and happy, equal relationships with husbands. As countries developed and reached communism, working women would desire many children. Therefore, no contraception or abortion would be necessary. This would assure a growing labor force, as well as the economic and military strength of the Soviet Union for years to come.

Of course, the Soviet government had had problems with low birth rates before. But when fertility declined in the early 1930s, the incomplete development of socialism was cited. In the postwar period, the war was blamed for the birth rate decline, but this argument was less and less tenable, once recovery was being trumpeted. Now that industrialization, urbanization, and the universal employment of women had been achieved, under the influence of Western demographic transition theory,[88] some demographers began to argue that all-round economic development and education of both sexes brought about cultural and social behavioral change, ultimately leading to lower fertility because women increasingly practiced fertility control.[89] In this vision, low birth rate was recognized as proof of Soviet modernization, and abortion was understood as a modern practice of fertility control. This interpretation also helped explain the fertility gap between Slavic women and women of other "less modern" Soviet nationalities, which became a growing concern for Soviet demography in the 1970s. If the maturing of socialism would not resolve the issue of fertility and labor, how could the Soviet government secure the future labor force?

Sociologists and demographers conducted many studies, identifying one of the reasons for limiting the number of children as women's difficulty balancing work outside the home, household tasks, and childrearing. Historically, the Soviet Union had pioneered the idea of ending women's double burden by socializing household work and childcare, but the original idea of developing a ubiquitous network of socialized canteens and laundromats did not develop beyond the revolutionary period. In the 1960s, a leading sociologist A. G. Kharchev wrote that dinners at home were essential for "domestic happiness."[90] The government did build thousands of childcare facilities, but never enough. As Khrushchev's famous 1959 "kitchen debate" with US vice president Richard Nixon showed, the Soviet position maintained the ideological orientation that the socialist system was superior to the capitalist system in supporting working women's double burden.[91]

However, most Soviet women did not feel that they received sufficient support. Despite all the pronatalist propaganda, expectant mothers, even legally married, were routinely treated without warmth or comfort by overworked doctors and nurses in maternity hospitals, unless they were able to make special arrangements *po blatu* (exchange of favors among a network of friends and family).[92] Despite the growing number of female workers, childcare facilities were not increasing apace. Soviet mothers were expected to return to work or school within two months after giving birth, but it was not always easy to find a vacancy in the nearest or most desired childcare facilities. Partial data for 1965 shows that 55 percent of urban children under 3 and more than 44 percent of those between 3 and 6 were waiting for vacancies in nurseries and kindergartens. Even after admission, mothers were not always satisfied with the quality of care.[93] Women generally preferred to stay home for the first years after giving birth to a child, even if that was detrimental to the family economy or the mother's career.[94] Tending to an infant while working was not easy in an economy of scarcity, as working women had to spend an enormous amount of time and effort searching for groceries, cleaning and cooking, without the benefit of electric appliances or semi-prepared meals.

Many cultural productions from the 1960s to the 1980s depict Soviet working mothers' mundane, yet frustrating, everyday life. The most famous one is the 1969 story "A Week Like Any Other Week" by Nataliia Baranskaia about Olga, a professional full-time worker. In the Soviet context, Olga has a good life—a job in her chosen field, a separate apartment, a loving husband, and two children, without any of the classic, statistically common problems, such as shared living space, an alcoholic husband, or lack of childcare. However, Olga suffers from the fact that all she can do is survive one day at a time, without any chance of accomplishing anything to her satisfaction, always falling a little further behind. She feels no control over her own life. Again and again, frustrations crop up. She misses work when a child gets sick; she has to get groceries in the middle of the workday and fails to complete professional tasks; and she comes home too late to prepare a meal before her children's bedtime. Olga's husband participates in dropping off and picking up children at nursery or kindergarten, but she cannot expect him to take over the cooking tasks when she works late.[95]

Similarly, Vera Golubeva's account of women's lives in Arkhangelsk suggests that real life in the heroic Far North was little different from Olga's daily treadmill in Moscow.

> Tired after their workday, they hurry [on the way] home to childcare centers. Bowed with the weight of grocery bags, they drag their children behind them. In a terrible crush of people, they wedge themselves into overcrowded public buses elbowing people aside and pushing their way through to an empty seat, if there is one. At last, they reach home. Here, new cares await them: Dinner must be prepared and the husband and children must be fed. The laundry and housecleaning still awaits because, for a working woman, there is no other time for these chores. She cannot depend on her husband for anything.[96]

In fiction and reality, working mothers rarely got any help from husbands with household work or childrearing. A study conducted in the late 1960s showed that only 7.7 percent of women said that their husbands helped them with household tasks, and 65 percent of women said that their husbands provided no help.[97] But women generally tolerated unhelpful husbands who at least contributed to the family budget, considering them much better than husbands who drank heavily and became violent. Many women endured even these all-too-common behaviors, while others left such husbands and became divorced single mothers.[98]

Grandmothers often provided essential help. In the 1930s, many young urban couples lived with a *babushka*, the archetypal grandmother, who helped with childcare and household work. In the postwar period extended households increased, due to the large number of widows who would cohabitate with their children's families. The formation of extended families was sustained throughout the 1980s, as high mortality among males produced new widows.[99] Demographer Boris Urlanis considered that babushkas could help raise Russia's birth rate by assisting young couples in raising multiple children.[100] But there were also changes to this practice of multi-generational female support. Demographers who studied family size in the Soviet Union wrote that the modern babushka is still working or, if retired, has her own pension, and thus is not always available or willing to be a helper of young families. A study in Leningrad showed that 87.9 percent of working women said that they alone did the household work, while 6.9 percent credited their own mothers, and 3.3 percent their mothers-in-law, as the main caretakers in the family. By the late 1960s, many babushkas did not want to participate in young couples' everyday household and childcare, unlike previous ones who often came from the village and were financially dependent on the young couple's income, while they helped the couple with household work and childcare. Even when babushkas wanted to help the young family, if they still worked and/or did not live nearby, they would not be able to provide daily help.

Women's full-time work and the shortage of help with childcare and household tasks at home continued to drive the birth rate down. It is no surprise that when Olga arrives at work on the Tuesday of her "Week Like Any Other," her female coworkers are arguing over Question Five on a questionnaire distributed by demographers: "If you have no children, then for what reason: medical reasons, living conditions, family situation, personal considerations, etc. (Underline your reason)."[101]

The Soviet Union was not alone facing the low birth rate problem in the 1970s. North America and Western Europe were seeing greater participation of women in the workforce. In addition to poor women who had always been in the workforce, inspired by women's rights movements, middle-class women en masse began to pursue higher education and their own careers outside the home. As women's participation in the workforce increased in the 1960s and 1970s, women were having fewer children.

In capitalist countries, a significant number of women remained childless by choice or delayed pregnancy until it was too late. Interestingly, Soviet women showed a different trend. Soviet demographers and sociologists studying family formation between the 1960s and 1980s found that Soviet women were marrying and having their first child at increasingly younger ages, by their mid-twenties. Except for the women whose reproductive years coincided with the wartime and postwar period, childless women were a very small percentage, possibly one of the lowest in the world. Even in Moscow, the late 1970s survey involving 2,000 women showed that everyone desired to have one child, regardless of their level of income, profession, age, educational levels, and living conditions, because all women considered that happiness as a parent could not be replaced by economic well-being.[102] Respondents also thought that women should have their first child by age 25. Indeed, the average marital age was 22–24 years old in the 1960s and 1970s, as women often felt pressure to marry by the time they turned 25.[103] Unlike in the immediate postwar period, childlessness was not a problem, but policymakers had to convince women to have second or additional children.

One sociological survey showed that a woman's desire for more than one child depended on the quality and amount of help she could count on. Women who could expect help from their own mothers were most likely to desire a second child. In the absence of reliable support, the demographers concluded that since women handle most childcare and household work, the more they enjoyed their professional work, the fewer children they desired.[104]

In a survey to investigate the reasons for regulating family size, the top answers included lack of childcare facilities and undesirable living conditions. However, demographers who analyzed the data argued that these should not be counted as serious factors, particularly the question of housing, because those respondents not planning to have the second child had better living conditions than those who were planning to have the second child.[105] Incidentally, this coincided with E. A. Sadvokasova's rationale not to consider living conditions or material difficulty as an objective reason for women to terminate pregnancy. Although surveys of women undertaking abortion highlighted such economic reasons, many poorer women, objectively measured, actually chose to give birth.

A different kind of survey revealed more objective reasons for limiting fertility. A late 1970s study of married women with two children living in Moscow showed that before the birth of the first child, almost all women desired to have two or three children. However, once the first child was born, many lost the desire to have more. They anticipated too much more housework, difficulties in coordinating work schedules, and lack of childcare. Nonetheless, they went on to have a second child because they desired a child of the opposite sex or wanted to have a surviving child in the unfortunate case of the first child's death.[106] Although a reduction in household work, a good childcare option, and a flexible work schedule were the measures Soviet working mothers considered necessary for having multiple children, the government pronatalist measures did not focus on women's needs.[107]

In the 1970s and 1980s Soviet policymakers regularly voiced their concern about women, children, and fertility. In 1971, the 24th Party Congress announced an increase in direct child support payments to families and a doubling of the number of eligible children. This initiative was treated coolly by leading demographers, who called it a step in the right direction that "ought to be followed by new decisions."[108] The 25th Party Congress in 1976 seemed to heed this advice by calling for demographic policy to support economic development.[109] In 1977, at the Trade Union Conference, the Soviet Communist Party's Secretary General Leonid Brezhnev went so far as to acknowledge that the "dual burden" had not yet received sufficient attention, blaming "us men."[110]

Top-level recognition of the problem led to an increase in socialized childcare, after-school activities, and holiday pioneer camps, but these measures failed to reduce women's domestic care work in the family, the heart of the "double burden." Instead, in 1981 the Soviet government proposed that women spend more time at home with children by introducing partially paid maternity leave for one year and offering the option of working fewer hours. The Soviet government also introduced more household appliances as well as semi-prepared and prepared meals as a way to reduce women's domestic labor. But the goods were not always available, and when obtainable, often of poor quality.[111]

Acknowledging the seriousness of the contradiction between production and reproduction also meant recognizing that targeted family support might be more effective, if inequitable. Geographically, the government now focused on industrial regions where fertility was low and predominantly Slavic. The traditional glorification of highly fertile mothers, predominantly rural or Central Asian, was significantly toned down. Instead, the new direction of pronatalism in the 1970s and early 1980s slowly focused on helping mothers of one or two children regardless of their marital status and on providing more aid to single mothers, a shift that had been suggested by the Mikoyan commission in the late 1950s but not adopted at that time. The honoring of mothers with many children became more perfunctory. A 1970 decree of the Sovmin SSSR instituted lump-sum payments for mothers on the birth of the first, second, and third child.[112] At the same time, government aid to single mothers was raised to 20 rubles per child per month rather than 5 rubles for the first child, 7.5 rubles for two children, and 10 rubles for three children, and the maximum period of aid was extended from age 12 to age 16.[113] A 1974 All-Union ukase provided low-income families with 12 rubles monthly support for each child up to age 8, more than the 10 rubles that a mother with the order of "Motherhood Glory" would receive monthly for her seventh or eighth child.[114] In 1980, the word "honorary" was omitted from the awards of Mother Heroine, Motherhood Glory, and Motherhood Medal.[115] The new tendency to shift the focus of support from large families to small families and to increase support for low-income working mothers and single mothers with only one or two children was very clear. Small families were finally the main beneficiaries.

The cultural representation of the Mother Heroine in the 1980s showed signs of her shifting position under the pronatalist policy. In the 1980 movie *Once, Twenty Years Later*, the main heroine Nadia (Slavic) is a Mother Heroine with ten children. One day Nadia and her high school classmates participate in a TV program where every participant individually answers such questions as "What did you accomplish in your life?" and "What else would you still want in your life?" Everyone talks about his or her professional life, but Nadia hesitates to answer. Eventually her husband shows up with ten children and everyone congratulates her on the great achievement. However, the film is not entirely celebratory of her life, as she is living for others most of the time and the family endured material difficulties particularly while the oldest children were still small. Nadia does not appear to be in control of what happens with her life, as she found herself pregnant again and again. At the end of the movie, she is pregnant yet again.[116] Nadia seems happy enough, but the film does not portray her fertile path as a model for every woman.

The shift from large to small families as the focus of pronatalist policy was also reflected in the development of regional demographic policy. In 1981, the adoption of a new pronatalist policy showed a clear intention to encourage births among working or student mothers in low fertility regions while delaying support for women in high fertility regions. "The measures for strengthening government support for families with children" of January 22, 1981, introduced preferential policies toward low-fertility regions. For example, it stated that working mothers or students who were on leave from production would receive partially paid maternity leave until the child became 1 year old, and the amount would be 50 rubles per month in the Far East, Siberia, and Northern regions, but only 35 rubles for the rest of the regions and republics. This support would begin with the Far East, Siberia, and

Northern regions and only later be applied to other areas[117] Since the indicated low–birth rate areas were largely Slavic, an unspoken prejudice against "southern" areas was implied. The geographic differentiation, rather than nationality based differentiation, was politically important. Even so, because such regional differentiations would have a differentiated impact on which nationalities' births would be supported, some considered it a direct violation of Soviet principles of equality among all nationalities.[118]

These measures aimed at gradual structural improvement in conditions that would take the sting out of the dual burden and thereby encourage additional births. But many pronatalist analysts did not think that these measures went far enough. They insisted on women's primary role as wives and mothers and identified the cause of low birth rate as the "blurring of sexual differences."[119] What this group stressed was the need for "normalizing" gender roles and reminding women of their biologically determined role in order to reverse their selfish "one-child family mentality."[120] In the late 1970s and 1980s a new educational campaign stressed the importance of traditional gender roles. Some teachers and sociologists argued that the reason the divorce rate was rising and birth rate declining was women's "loss of femininity" and a corresponding "loss of masculinity" among men. The cause for the loss of masculinity was identified as the demoralization of men, as their traditional role as family head was under attack by the state and women, who had cooperated in the multi-generational socialist promotion of women's status. According to this analysis, women's "problem" was their incorrect understanding of equality between the sexes, seeking public roles while abandoning their key role as the caretaker of the family and the household. Although Russian families were predominantly two-child families at that time, it was suggested that women with fewer than three children were not feminine. It was also considered wrong when women asked husbands to help with household work or childrearing, because men were supposed to lack the necessary skills, and if they developed them, they would become feminized.[121]

This discourse on femininity and masculinity apparently had an impact on policymakers and resulted in the adoption of sexual socialization education in 1984 in the European parts of the Soviet Union. Interestingly, Central Asia was excluded from this. The school course titled "Ethics and Psychology of Family Life" was offered for two hours per week for students in the ninth and tenth grades. Boys were taught to be honest, responsible, intelligent, brave, decisive, and noble, whereas girls were instructed to be kind, affable, tender, sincere, natural, trusting, and homemakers. Marriage and family were presented as the model for happiness, and motherhood and children were the most essential parts, not only because socialism brought ideal conditions for women, but also because of women's innate nature. It also taught children the harmfulness of one-child families, an expanding demographic phenomenon.[122]

Importantly, this education did not involve a discussion that women should stay at home. Since the war women had become too crucial a component of the Soviet labor market for politicians, economists, demographers, sociologists, educators, or anyone else to discourage women from working. Instead, social scientists and educational specialists argued for the legitimization of gender-specific roles for Soviet men and women, where women were expected to hold down full-time jobs, perform all the household chores, and take care of multiple children. Men should focus on their public work. Contemporary practice already closely followed this gender ideology.[123] What was new was the explicit message from the socialist government that the double or triple burden was "natural" to women, just when it was being called into question in the West. This tendency to reaffirm women's "natural" role as mother and wife was even endorsed by Mikhail Gorbachev, the last General Secretary of the Soviet Communist Party. In his 1987 book *Perestroika*, he argued,

> Over the years of our difficult and heroic history, we failed to pay attention to women's specific rights and needs arising from their role as mother and home-maker, and their indispensable educational function as regards children. . . . That is why we are now holding heated debates in the press, in public organizations, at work and at home, about the question of what we should do to make it possible for women to return to their purely womanly mission.[124]

The Soviet Union's reexamination of women's role in the family and society coincided with similar trends elsewhere. In the capitalist West, the postwar welfare state assumed the male-breadwinner model, where the stay-at-home wife took care of the household work, several children, the sick, and the elderly.[125] But starting in the 1960s, women, empowered by the women's liberation movement, began to pursue higher education, to work outside the home, and to contribute to the family income. As women delayed marriage and childbirth, or chose not to have children, fertility declined. These changes pushed many governments to reexamine the male breadwinner model and the existing welfare state structure, as a shrinking population impacted economic growth and the health of the social security system.[126]

Two types of welfare arrangements developed among capitalist countries. Countries such as Germany, Spain, and Italy (re-)designated women to be responsible for care work within the family, while making it easy for women to stay home and work only part-time. Longer maternity leaves and tax breaks led to women leaving jobs or switching to part-time employment, particularly after marrying or having a child in order to devote more time to care work at home. The government provided a limited number of public childcare facilities. In such a system, gender equality in the family is typically weak, and husbands' participation rate in the family care work is low.[127] Women's access to contraception and abortion in these countries remained restricted. This type of care arrangement was dubbed "familialism."[128]

The other group of countries, those that were "de-familializing," tried to move family care work, such as household work, childcare, and elder care, outside the family in order to realize women's fuller participation in the labor force.[129] Northern European countries and Anglo-Saxon countries belonged to this type, but in different ways. In the case of Scandinavian countries, to promote women's participation in the workforce, the governments socialized much of the care work and encouraged husbands' equal participation in household work and childcare at home. Anglo-Saxon countries did not socialize care work; instead, families purchased varying qualities and quantities of care work services from the open market according to their differing needs and economic abilities to replace care work traditionally performed by women at home.[130]

In both Scandinavian and Anglo-Saxon countries, the political empowerment of women influenced by feminist movements and women's increasing intellectual and economic power also helped promote women's working outside the home and having gender equality both outside and within the family, encouraging their husbands' participation in the household work and childrearing. Women in all these "de-familializing" countries typically had wide access to contraception and abortion and so were able to regulate fertility to suit their work and family lives. In the Anglo-Saxon variant, the quality of domestic care depended largely on income level.

In both familializing and de-familializing types, the capitalist market continued to provide families with improved time and energy-saving household appliances such as refrigerators, washing machines, and vacuum cleaners to ease the daily tasks of cooking and cleaning. In addition, unlike in socialist states, supermarkets provided one-stop shopping for frozen food as well as partially and fully prepared meals, to meet the demands of working parents,.

Importantly, among the capitalist countries where women's labor participation grew, those that chose "defamilialization" saw birth rates recover from decline, whereas familializing policies led to further declines in birth rate.[131] In fact, in Scandinavian countries where the female employment rate is high, birth rates were rising among the most educated couples in cases where the woman worked full time and made a significant contribution to the family income. In such cases, the husband's life course is most "feminized," and the gendered arrangement of domestic care work is typically most equitable.[132]

Following the classification outlined above, the Soviet Union might be classified as the "de-familializing" type in terms of the socialist government's encouragement of women's full-time work and commitment to providing public institutions for childcare.[133] But since the socialist government did not completely institutionalize care and did not have a capitalist market, care work not redistributed to public institutions could only remain in the family. If the government still wanted to support working women, household work had to be redistributed more equally among men and women, and the planned economy should have provided more adequately equipped housing, quality household appliances, and ready-made meals to help reduce the time spent on household chores and care work.

Some Soviet sociologists and demographers advocated more equitable sharing of family care work. Sociologist N. G. Iurkevich, for example, called for "men's return to the family" to the degree that women had taken up work outside the home.[134] Others called for more education and propaganda among young people to promote men's participation in household work, based on the finding that younger and more educated husbands tended to take up more household tasks than older and less educated ones.[135] Demographer K. K. Bazdyrov wrote that hypothetically the father could stay home with a baby as the "feeding father" while the mother fulfilled her social responsibilities, but Bazdyrov was uncertain about the practicability of such an arrangement, as he had never heard of such a case. Even the one who cares for a sick child at home was usually the mother, not the father.[136] But those who listened to women's voices knew that a fairer division of domestic care work was what the situation demanded. But their studies did not find favor among the policymakers.

Instead, the Soviet Union took a path toward more familialization, resisted "feminization" of men's role in the family, and betrayed the core socialist commitment to equality between the sexes. Further socialization of domestic care work, provision of housing, and production of consumer products would have required a substantial additional investment, but the 1970s oil bonanza was spent elsewhere. Not willing to commit resources to expand socialized welfare, policymakers allowed families to take care of their own needs in their own way, without insisting on strict adherence to the socialist ideology of women's liberation.[137] In the 1980s, the Soviet government showed commitment to familialism with a longer postpartum leave from work that encouraged women to stay home longer in order to take care of children and spend more time on household work, without providing full compensation for reduced salary. Moreover, gender education actively discouraged male participation in the household work; teachers told the boys not to share "feminine" duties and the girls not to let husbands help with "women's" work.

This is because policymakers and demographers considered that if women were given time off for a couple of years to take care of babies and received some cash, the birth rate would soon recover.[138] Indeed, in the short run the birth rate seems to have risen. But demographers argue that this did not mean that women decided to have more children. Rather, they achieved the number of children they were planning to have earlier than they had originally planned. In keeping with the explanation above, demographic data show the total fertility rate (TFR) for Russian women rising temporarily in the early 1980s, but declining steadily after 1987.[139]

The irony of Soviet reproductive politics was that although the socialist state was ideologically committed to becoming a country where workers could have as many children as they wanted by providing all the necessary conditions for it, in reality even after expansion of the welfare state in the 1950s, many Soviet women had fewer children than they had wished.[140] Late Soviet pronatalist policy failed to listen to women's voices and respond to one of the biggest factors for women to consider having more than one child: reliable and substantial help with domestic work and childcare at home. With fewer babushkas available to help young mothers and no capitalistic market to provide domestic services, encouraging husbands to become reliable partners in caretaking of the home and children could have been a cost-effective solution. Soviet women also did not have the modern conveniences of household appliances and prepared meals. Without these kinds of support, women had little incentive to consider additional births. Since there was no modern contraception, they continued to have multiple abortions to limit their family sizes. Familializing childcare and regendering domestic work moved away from socialist ideals of gender equality. Prioritized pronatalism also moved away from equality among different regions and nationalities. The 1944 Family Law had violated the socialist idea of equality among all children, and the 1968 Family Law did not reverse this situation. Having compromised its ideals of justice and equality, Soviet socialism itself would soon disappear.

Epilogue

Reviving Pronatalism in Post-Socialist Russia

> For Russia to be sovereign and strong, there must be more of us. . . .
> Our women themselves know when and what they need to do. . . .
> And despite the doubts of some experts—and I respect them—I am
> nonetheless convinced that a family with three children should be-
> come the norm in Russia.
>
> Vladimir V. Putin, President, Russia (2012)

Late Soviet pronatalism ended with the collapse of the Soviet Union in 1991. As Russia transitioned to a market economy, foreign contraceptive devices as well as high-quality household appliances became available to those who could afford them. Post-socialist women politicians attempted to re-form Russia's fertility control that relied on abortion by disseminating sex education and distributing modern contraception.[1] Under the presidency of Boris Yeltsin in the early 1990s, family planning programs were begun, as a part of a presidential program called "Russia's Children." Family planning centers were founded under the jurisdiction of the Health Ministry, and specialists designed sexual education programs for youths. Foreign and international organizations such as the US Agency for International Development (USAID) and the United Nations Population Fund, supplied medical institutions and obstetric clinics with state-of-the art medical equip-ment, contraceptives, and educational materials. About half of the family plan-ning budget for 1994–1995 was spent on the purchase of oral contraceptive pills, which were distributed gratis to young people.[2] The effects were clear. Although the government eased restrictions on abortion after the first twelve weeks in 1996,[3] the number of abortions and maternal deaths was quickly cut by almost a half in the 1990s and continues to decline.[4] Especially encour-aging, observes demographer Viktoriia Sakevich, are data for young women

Replacing the Dead. Mie Nakachi, Oxford University Press (2021). © Oxford University Press.
DOI: 10.1093/oso/9780190635138.003.0008

between 15 and 19, for whom "the Soviet 'abortion culture' is a bygone phenomenon".[5] But Russian women's dependency on abortion as a method of fertility control continues, especially among the older generations. Russia's abortion rate is still one of the highest in the world.[6]

Another area of reform was gender equality within the home. Liberal and feminist politicians actively participated in drafting the Family Law of 1995 and attempted to promote equality between mothers and fathers.[7] Minister of Social Protection Liudmila Bezlepkina, the Russian government's representative to the Fourth World Conference on Women held in 1995 in Beijing, made it clear that the family was a key arena in which Russia lacked full gender equality. Upon signing the Beijing Declaration, which committed Russia to promoting full equality between men and women in all fields and spheres of life, she stated, "Men in Russia are now ready to take on a significant portion of household work and childrearing."[8]

Such statements indicate the presence of new initiatives since 1991 to improve women's health and well-being, but the end of socialism also had profoundly distressing effects on the reproductive environment for post-socialist women. As the socialist state's commitment to providing childcare facilities and protecting women from discrimination at workplaces essentially ended, the quantity and quality of childcare institutions declined, women lost their jobs, and mothers with young children had a particularly hard time finding and keeping employment.[9] Private childcare services were still underdeveloped and too expensive for most people.[10] Still, the majority of post-socialist women simply wanted to work outside the home. One survey conducted in 1997 asked "Would you quit work if there is no financial necessity [to work]?" to which 54 percent of women responded that they would continue working, while only 24 percent responded they would quit.[11] Aside from having a genuine desire to work, the low level of childlessness and high probability of raising children alone made most Russian women consider an independent income crucial.[12]

With the economic situation looking unstable, the welfare system collapsing, and women having trouble getting paid, Russia's birth rate plummeted. The situation worsened further after the 1998 financial crisis. The number of children per woman in Russia declined from 1.892 in 1990 to 1.195 in 2000.[13] Among new births, the out-of-wedlock percentage rose quickly from 15 percent in 1990 to 30 percent in 2005.[14] With mortality among men also rising, reflecting the sharpest peacetime decline in male longevity ever recorded, Russia's depopulation began in 1992 and continued for twenty years.[15] The USSR's final census in 1989 tallied a population over 287 million, well ahead of the 247 million in the United States at that time.[16] A generation after Soviet implosion, the Russian Federation's 2020 population was 146.7 million, much closer to the population of Japan than the United States.[17]

Conservative and nationalist politicians recognized the shrinking population as a national crisis and considered economic reforms and foreign influences the likely main causes. They believed that if the economic situation improved, Russia's women would have more children. They also identified family planning as one of the causes of low birth rate and ended federal funding for family planning in 1998, thereby extinguishing many sexual education programs. To protect themselves from the growing attacks of conservative forces, public health educators who wanted to continue sex education among youth were forced to shift the focus of their work from enhancing young people' s ability to control fertility and protect their health with contraceptives to promoting anti-abortion and traditional family values.[18] The impressive post-Soviet revival of religious organizations, especially the Orthodox Church, led to a campaign against widespread abortion and promotion of families with many children as the truly traditional Russian and Orthodox family.[19]

In contrast, liberal Russian demographers argue that the primary cause of the low birth rate was a new phase in the "evolution of births" that began the mid-1990s; at that time the youngest reproductive cohort, born after 1970, started to delay marriage and first birth, and often formed families in cohabitation without official marriage. These demographers argue that this development was part of the second demographic transition in Russia, a process independent of the collapse of the Soviet Union.[20] This means that even if the economic situation improved, the general trend of low birth rate among Russian women would not dramatically change.

President Vladimir Putin, initially elected in 1999, works closely with the Orthodox Church and increasingly uses reproductive politics to demonstrate that his leadership can revive a strong Russia. He has regularly undertaken pronatalist measures. In the 2000s, a series of measures to restrict women's access to abortion were introduced: in 2003, the list of social criteria for permitting an abortion shrank to a third of its previous length; in 2007, an official order was issued requiring all women undergoing abortion be informed about possible complications and side effects of the operation; that year the list of medical criteria for abortion was reduced by two-thirds; and in 2009, a federal law limited advertisement of abortion services.[21] In July 2011, a federal law was issued to require that advertisements for abortion services use at least 10 percent of their space to describe dire consequences of abortion and never indicate that termination of pregnancies could be done safely. Also, a so-called "quiet week" was newly required before women could undergo the operation.[22] In 2013, the lower house of the Russian parliament discussed a bill on the exclusion of abortion from national medical insurance coverage.[23] In 2014, all advertisements for abortion services were banned.[24]

These successive restrictions on abortion go hand in hand with the government's official pronatalist measures to increase the birth rate in Russia. In 2006, Putin announced an initiative to improve Russia's demography and introduced a law on "motherhood (family) capital," which grants 250,000 rubles for a child born or adopted after January 1, 2007 as the second or subsequent child.[25] He tried to promote family values and celebrated 2007 as the Year of Children and 2008 as the Year of Family. Dmitrii Medvedev, who worked as the first vice premier under Putin on demographic policy, became the next president and continued the same line of policy together with Putin as prime minister. In 2008 Medvedev instituted the order "Parental Glory" to elevate family values, and he presented awards to eight families with four or more children at a January 2009 Kremlin ceremony.

The fact that motherhood capital has in parenthesis "family" and the medal is called "Parental" rather than "Mother," as in Soviet medals, suggests that post-socialist Russian government leaders are attempting to shift away from the mother-centric approach of the Soviet era to consciously promote fathers as the other responsible parent in childrearing. In fact, seeing the fathers on stage receiving the medal would have had a symbolic effect of marking a different approach from that of Soviet times. However, when the motherhood (family) capital is examined closely, fathers can receive the capital only in very exceptional situations, such as the death of the mother. Thus, it is essentially mother-centric.[26]

In the latter half of the 2000s, Russia's birth rate has risen, and the government widely advertises it as the success of pronatalist policy.[27] But demographers argue that, as in the 1980s, this rise occurred both because women had children earlier than they had originally planned and also because the birth rate was already predicted to rise because of the favorable postwar echo. Conversely, but also as predicted for the late 2010s, the generational echo of World War II losses is again driving the birth rate down starting in 2015.[28] The dead continue to depress fertility, even as the government strives to replace them.

Despite the Putin government's self-congratulations, many people criticize the inefficacy of the motherhood capital program for encouraging mothers to have one more unplanned child because the amount is inadequate; the way it can be used is too inflexible to help the mother raise children; and the paperwork for applying for the benefit is so complex that many mothers cannot complete it.[29] Some say that the budget for motherhood capital should be reallocated to building childcare facilities. Some positive effects exist, according to Tat'iana Maleva, director of the Institute for Social Analysis and Prognosis, who believes that motherhood capital changed the "social climate" by sending the signal that the government is serious about increasing the birth rate and encouraging some people who were considering a second child.[30]

During the decade after the introduction of the motherhood capital, the limits on the way the mother can use the capital have changed, and it is now possible to receive some of the capital in cash. But most parents who were not already planning to have an additional child do not seem to find the sum sufficient to change their minds. According to a survey conducted in 2011–2012, only 0.8 percent of those who became eligible for mother capital responded that they decided to give birth to an additional child because of the mother capital.[31] Also, although out-of-wedlock births are declining, a substantial percentage of children born annually are out of wedlock, in spite of the governmental policy promoting heterosexual two-parent families; this suggests questions about whether governmental policies are adequate in terms of target, content, and quantity for those who need the most support for childbearing and childrearing.[32] Not only among unmarried single mothers, the feeling of not being supported by partners who are the children's biological fathers is also common among the vast majority of women in post-socialist Russia. Since the post-socialist Russian government provides even less welfare support for women than the socialist government did, many women feel abandoned. Reliable support can come only from the babushka. However, just as in the late Soviet period, babushkas are not always available.[33]

In addition to official pronatalist policies, many half-official, nongovernmental organizations engage in activities to promote anti-abortion and family values. For example, since 2008, Svetlana Medvedeva, wife of the former president Dmitrii Medvedev, has headed a new initiative of the Socio-Cultural Fund celebrating July 8, the anniversary of Khrushchev's

1944 Family Law, as the "Day of Family, Love, and Faithfulness," which is followed by "Give Me a Life!" (anti-abortion week).[34] These actions are taken for "strengthening the family, and the preservation of family values and traditions." Since 2011, the organizing committee of The Day of Family began awarding the medal "For Love and Faithfulness" to couples married over twenty-five years, who are known as having had a loving and cooperative relationship and raised children who became good members of society. Clearly these organizations are working closely with the Orthodox Church. Importantly, the website for "Give Me a Life!" openly states, "What is important is not to criminalize abortions, but to make births desirable."[35] So far, Putin has stated that he would not criminalize abortion, as examples from other countries show that many women damage their health through illegal abortions while those with means go abroad to obtain legal operations.[36] But his pronatalist policy definitely combines mother-centric policies and restrictions on abortion.

Among former socialist states, low birth rate remains common.[37] While many have introduced pronatalist policies, some have gone further to scapegoat abortion. With the influence of the Catholic Church revived, Poland criminalized abortion in 1993, except for very limited cases such as when the pregnancy puts the mother's life at risk or the conception results from rape. Access to contraception has been restricted, and in 2017 the "morning-after pill" was made a prescription drug. This has caused a rise in illegal abortions as well as women traveling abroad for the operation. The goal of conservative politicians is to increase the number of women who will raise multiple children, while banning abortion completely, even in cases of rape and incest. In 2016 and 2018 such "Stop Abortion" bills were proposed, but mass protests and public demonstrations by women and men stopped the proposed legislation from going through.[38]

Post-socialist governments tend to attribute low birth rate to the socialist legacy of universal participation of women in the workforce, availability of abortion, and lack of religion. However, in Europe, the Nordic and other northern European countries have more women in the economy and politics than the rest of the world, and contraception and abortion are readily available there; these countries also have higher fertility rates than predominantly Catholic southern European countries, such as Spain, Portugal, and Italy, where the presence of women in public power is much weaker. This indicates that encouraging women to stay home, while restricting abortion and contraception, hardly guarantees a rise in fertility.

Within a country, most educated couples tend to achieve higher birth rates, while less educated couples tend to have lower birth rates. This is attributed to women's higher economic contribution to family income, which generally leads to greater participation of the husband in household and childcare work, as opposed to women with secondary education contributing less to family income, which leads to the husband's more limited participation in household and childcare work.[39] In Russia today women with higher education are demonstrating higher fertility than women with a lower level of education, which suggests that Russia follows this demographic pattern.[40]

On a number of occasions President Putin has appealed to Russian citizens and called for higher birth rates. In 2012 he announced that it should be the norm for Russian women to have three children, an echo of Khrushchev's attempts seventy years earlier to set new state aid for mothers who gave birth to a third child and glorify those with more, while maintaining criminalized abortion and restrictions on contraception.[41] Declining fertility since 2015 may alarm the pronatalist regime and trigger the urge to restrict further women's access to abortion and contraception. But history has shown that going back to such measures has little demographic effect in the long run because women make reproductive decisions not for the government, but for the well-being of themselves, their children, and their families.

Notes

Introduction

1. Lena is a pseudonym. In order to protect interviewees' privacy, throughout this book, I use common Russian first names that start with the same initial as the interviewee's own name.

2. From an interview with Lena (b. 1925) on November 27, 2002, in Moscow. The estimated average number of abortions for the late 1950s was based on the registered number of legal abortions after the 1955 re-legalization. A. G. Vishnevskii, ed., *Demograficheskaia modernizatsiia Rossii 1900–2000* (Moskva: Novoe Izdatel'stvo, 2006), 216.

3. The use of curettage under Soviet conditions of unsanitary environment and shortage of medicines, particularly antibiotics, made illegal and legal abortion more dangerous than necessary. Christopher Williams, "Abortion and Women's Health in Russia and the Soviet Successor States," in *Women in Russia and Ukraine*, ed. Rosalind Marsh (Cambridge: Cambridge University Press, 1996), 142.

4. Iu. A. Poliakov et al., *Naselenie Rossii v XX veke: Istoricheskie ocherki*, tom 2, *1940–1959* (Moskva: ROSSPEN, 2001), 25. The estimated number of women who served in the war ranges between 500,000 and 800,000. Mark Edele, *Soviet Veterans of the Second World War: A Popular Movement in an Authoritarian Society, 1941–1991* (Oxford: Oxford University Press, 2008), 143; Roger Reese, *Why Stalin's Soldiers Fought: The Red Army's Military Effectiveness in World War II* (Lawrence: University Press of Kansas, 2011), 257–258.

5. For this figure, see Rebecca Manley, *To the Tashkent Station: Evacuation and Survival in the Soviet Union at War* (Ithaca, NY: Cornell University Press, 2009), 1; From Moscow alone, by the end of November 1941, 2 million (44 percent of the prewar population) were evacuated. G. A. Kumanev, "Evakuatsiia naseleniia SSSR: dostignutye rezul'taty i poteri," in *Liudskie poteri SSSR v Velikoi otechestvennoi voine*, ed. R. B. Evdokimov (St. Petersburg: Russko-Baltiiskii informatsionnyi tsentr, 1995), 143. Mention should be made of the millions deported as "unreliable" ethnic minority groups in preparation for the war, but not included in the number of evacuees. For deportation, see Pavel Polian, *Against Their Will: The History and Geography of Forced Migrations in the USSR* (Budapest: Central European University Press, 2004).

6. On the tragically violent and complex history of the Soviet Western borderland during and after the war, see Alexander Statiev, *The Soviet Counterinsurgency in the Western Borderlands* (New York: Cambridge University Press, 2010); Timothy Snyder, *Bloodlands: Europe between Hitler and Stalin* (London: Vintage, 2011).

7. Mie Nakachi, "A Postwar Sexual Liberation? The Gendered Experience of the Soviet Union's Great Patriotic War," *Cahiers du monde russe* 52, no.2–3 (2011): 423–440.

8. Wendy Goldman and Donald Filtzer, eds., *Hunger and War: Food Provisioning in the Soviet Union During World War II* (Bloomington: Indiana University Press, 2015), 1; Edele, *Soviet Veterans*, 6. The historiography of wartime losses in World War II is almost as contentious as the discussion of "excess deaths" due to collectivization, famines, deportations, and purges, because together these issues provide the empirical basis for computing the demographic consequences of Stalinism. A full examination of this literature in English on World War II losses would include many articles by Barbara Anderson, Robert Conquest, Michael Ellman, Steven Rosefielde, Brian Silver, and Stephen Wheatcroft, all of them commenting, criticizing, and continuing the pioneering work of Frank Lorimer, *The Population of the Soviet Union: History and Prospects* (Geneva: League of Nations, 1946). A good introduction to the quantitative intricacies and political minefields is Michael Ellman and S. Maksudov, "Soviet Deaths in the Great Patriotic War: A Note," *Europe-Asia Studies* 46, no. 4 (1994): 671–680. For the estimate of 20 million, see Elena Zubkova, "Preodolenie voiny-preodolenie pobedy: Sovetskaia povsednevnost' i strategii vyzhivaniia (1945–1953)," *Pobediteli i pobezhdennye: Ot voiny k miru: SSSR, Frantsiia, Velikobritaniia, Germaniia, SShA (1941–1950)*, ed. B. Fizeler and N. Muan, (Moskva: ROSSPEN, 2010), 15.

9. The lowest 1944 rate (19 men per 100 women) was found in Smolensk oblast, and the highest rate (70 men per 100 women) was found in Tadzhikistan. RGASPI f. 82, op. 2, d. 538, ll. 40–43.

10. Stalin announced during his *Pravda* interview on March 13, 1946, that Soviet war deaths numbered 7 million. This was a correct estimation of military losses but did not include other categories of losses. G. F. Krivosheev, ed., *Grif sekretnosti sniat: Poteri Vooruzhennykh Sil SSSR v voinakh, boevykh deistviiakh i voennykh konfliktakh* (Moskva: Voenizdat, 1993), gives the total deaths for men in uniform at the front as 8.7 million (407). Ellman and Maksudov, "Soviet Deaths," 675, revises this down to 7.8 million, not far from Stalin's number.

11. "Ob uvelichenii gosudarstvennoi pomoshchi beremennym zhenshchinam, mnogodetnym i odinokim materiam, usilenii okhrany materinstva i detstva, ob ustanovlenii pochetnogo zvaniia 'Mat'-Geroinia' i uchrezhdenii ordena 'Materinskaia slava' i medali 'Medal' Materinstva,' Ukaz ot 8 iiulia 1944 g.," *Sbornik zakonov SSSR i ukazov prezidiuma verkhovnogo Soveta SSSR, 1938–1967*, tom 2 (Moskva: Izdatel'stvo Izvestiia Sovetov deputatov trudiashchikhsia SSSR, 1968), 409–417.

As others have argued, the Soviet attempt to control and manage the quality and quantity of the population should be understood in light of the broad development of modern governments' practice in and beyond Europe. In this development, individual reproductive and sexual practice became the object of government concern. On the analysis of Soviet reproductive policy in the interwar period, see David Hoffmann, "Mothers in the Motherland: Stalinist Pronatalism in Its Pan-European Context," *Journal of Social History* 34, no. 1 (Autumn 2000): 35–54. On the development of the modern state's attempt to control the population, see Marc Raeff, "The Well-Ordered Police State and the Development of Modernity in Seventeenth and Eighteenth-Century Europe: An Attempt at a Comparative Approach," *The American Historical Review* 80, no. 5 (Dec. 1975): 1221–1243; Michel Foucault, "Governmentality" in Graham Burchell, et al. ed., *The Foucault Effect: Studies in Governmentality with Two Lectures by and an Interview with Michel Foucault* (Chicago: University of Chicago Press, 1991). This essay was first published in 1978. See also Michel Foucault, "The Birth of Biopolitics," "The Birth of Social Medicine," and "The Politics of Health in the Eighteenth Century," in Paul Rabinow and Nikolas Rose, eds., *The Essential Foucault: Selections from Essential Works of Foucault, 1954-1984* (New York: New Press, 2003); James Scott, *Seeing Like a State: How Certain Schemes to Improve the Human Condition Have Failed* (New Haven: Yale University Press, 1999); Susan Gal and Gail Kligman, *The Politics of Gender after Socialism* (Princeton: Princeton University Press, 2000), 18–20.

12. Patronymics are very important in Russian, essential for adult conversations, so not at all like a middle name.

13. The 1950 official record counted approximately 4,000 women who died in non-clinical abortions in the Soviet Union. TsMAMLS f. 218, op.1, d.187, l.48.

14. In Imperial Russia, abortion was defined as murder in the Criminal Code of 1885. Wendy Goldman, *Women, the State and Revolution: Soviet Family Policy and Social Life, 1917-1936* (Cambridge: Cambridge University Press, 1993), 255. On prerevolutionary medical and legal debates about abortion, see Laura Engelstein, "Abortion and the Civic Order: The Legal and Medical Debates," in *Russia's Women: Accommodation, Resistance, Transformation*, ed. Barbara E. Clements, Barbara Alpern Engel, and Christine D. Worobec (Berkeley: University of California Press, 1991).

15. For discussion of abortion in the 1920s and 1930s, see Goldman, *Women, the State and Revolution*, 254–257; Elizabeth Wood, *The Baba and the Comrade: Gender and Politics in Revolutionary Russia* (Bloomington: Indiana University Press, 1997), 106–111; Alain Blum, *Rodit'sia, zhit' i umeret' v SSSR* (Moskva: Novoe izdatel'stvo, 2005), [a Russian translation of his *Naitre, vivre et mourir en URSS: 1917–1991* (Paris: Plon, 1994)]; Susan Solomon, "The Soviet Legalization of Abortion in German Medical Discourse: A Study of the Use of Selective Perceptions in Cross-Cultural Scientific Relations," *Social Studies of Science* 22, no. 3 (1992): 455–487; and Janet Hyer, "Managing the Female Organism: Doctors and the Medicalization of Women's Paid Work in Soviet Russia during the 1920s," in *Women in Russia and Ukraine*, ed. Rosalind Marsh (Cambridge: Cambridge University Press, 1996). On women's medicine in Central Asia, see Paula Michaels, *Curative Powers: Medicine and Empire in Stalin's Central Asia* (Pittsburgh: University of Pittsburgh Press, 2003).

16. Political interregnum refers to the period between Stalin's death in 1953 and Khrushchev's consolidation of power in 1957. *Molotov, Malenkov, Kaganovich, 1957: Stenogramma iiun'skogo plenuma TsK KPSS i drugie dokumenty*, ed. N. Kovaleva et al. (Moskva: Mezhdunarodnyi fond "Demokratiia," 1998). Although sometimes Khrushchev is given credit for the re-legalization, this book attempts to correct that misleading association. Rebecca Kay, "Images of an Ideal Woman: Perceptions of Russian Womanhood through the Media, Education and Women's Own

Eyes," in *Post-Soviet Women: from the Baltic to Central Asia*, ed. Mary Buckley (Cambridge: Cambridge University Press, 1997), 88.

17. M. D. Kovrigina, a trained pediatrician, was invited to Moscow from Cheliabinsk oblast in 1941 to become Deputy People's Commissar of Health SSSR. In 1954 she was appointed as the Minister of Health USSR and held the position until 1958. V. I. Ivkin, *Gosudarstvennaia vlast' SSSR: Vysshie organy vlasti i upravleniia i ikh rukovoditeli, 1923–1991 gg. Istoriko-biograficheskii spravochnik* (Moskva: ROSSPEN, 1999), 349–350.

18. Christopher Burton's pioneering study of the postwar abortion regime estimates 70–80 percent of doctors were women and links this fact with doctors' sympathies for women regarding abortion. "Minzdrav, Soviet Doctors, and the Policing of Reproduction in the Late Stalinist Years," *Russian History* 27, no. 2 (Summer 2000): 215. This corresponds well with the 74 percent female doctors mentioned as of December 1961 in *Zhenshchiny i deti v SSSR: Statisticheskii sbornik* (Moskva: Gosstatizdat, 1963), 118. Almost half of the participants of the 1955 medical committee meeting that decided in favor of legalization were women. TsMAMLS f. 218, op. 1, d. 188, l. 2.

19. Choi Chatterjee, *Celebrating Women: Gender, Festival Culture, and Bolshevik Ideology, 1910–1939* (Pittsburgh, PA: University of Pittsburgh Press, 2002), 149–152.

20. An excerpt from a statement by Dr. A. I. Dmitrieva. TsMAMLS f.218, op. 1, d. 188, l. 35. Other participants also shared the view that most women wanted to become mothers. TsMAMLS f.218, op. 1, d. 188, ll. 13, 24, 45.

21. In 1938, England allowed legal abortion for pregnancies as a result of rape. Judith Orr, *Abortion Wars: The Fight for Reproductive Rights* (Bristol: Policy Press, 2017), 23. In the same year, Sweden legalized abortion on medical, eugenic, and "humanitarian" (such as rape and incest) grounds. The Swedish Abortion Act of 1946 allowed socio-medical reasons. Lena Lennerhed, "Troubled Women: Abortion and Psychiatry in Sweden in the 1940s and 1950s," in *Transcending Borders: Abortion in the Past and Present*, ed. Shannon Stettner, Katrina Ackerman, Kristin Burnett, and Travis Hay (Cham, Switzerland: Palgrave Macmillan, 2017), 91. In Finland, in the midst of pronatalist policy, the 1950 Abortion Act made abortion legal for medical, ethical, or eugenic reasons. Miina Keski-Petäjä, "Abortion Wishes and Abortion Prevention: Women Seeking Legal Termination of Pregnancy during the 1950s and 1960s in Finland," *Finnish Yearbook of Population Research* (April 2012): 119. In Japan, the June 24, 1949, amendment to the 1948 Eugenic Protection Law made abortion available practically on demand, as it allowed economic reasons as the basis for legal access to abortion. http://www.shugiin.go.jp/internet/itdb_housei.nsf/html/houritsu/00519490624216.htm (last accessed September 1, 2020).

22. Great Britain (with the exception of Northern Ireland) practically legalized abortion in 1967, but abortion is still technically a criminal offense. Orr, *Abortion Wars*, 20, 67. Sweden introduced abortion on request in 1975. Lennerhed, "Troubled Women," 100. Finland legalized abortion on the basis of women's equality and self-determination in 1970. Keski-Petäjä, "Abortion Wishes," 132. In Japan, the women's rights movement defended abortion on economic grounds during abortion reform campaigns in the

1970s and 1980s. Miho Ogino, *Kazokukeikakueno michi: Kindainihonno seishokuo meguru seiji* (Tokyo: Iwanami shoten, 2008), 268–279. In the United States, the right to abortion was recognized as part of the right to privacy as the result of the 1973 Roe vs. Wade Supreme Court decision. See Linda Gordon, *The Moral Property of Women: A History of Birth Control Politics in America* (Urbana: University of Illinois Press, 2007), 301–302.

23. This study highlights the emerging concept of woman's right to abortion in the Soviet Union which led to legalizing abortion, the first country to do so. Throughout this book, I will refer to woman's "right" when I emphasize the limited nature of Soviet recognition of women's right to decide the timing of motherhood, but not the right to refuse motherhood outright. I will refer to "women's rights" in discussing women's rights more broadly. My focus on the issue of right/rights makes the 1955 repeal of the 1936 criminalization of abortion the high point of reproductive policy reform, a different type of legalization from the 1920 legalization, which was granted primarily from a medical point of view. It is true that the 1954 decriminalization freed women undergoing abortion from fear of arrest, but abortion, abortionists, and those who forced women into abortion were still illegal. Only the 1955 legislation was presented (behind the scenes) as a woman's right and only full re-legalization provided a stable legal basis on which to institutionalize the Soviet abortion empire that outlived the Soviet Union itself. "Ob otmene ugolovnoi otvetstvennosti beremennykh zhenshchin za proizvodstvo aborta," ukaz ot 5 avgusta 1954," and "Ob otmene zapreshcheniia abortov ukaz ot 23 noiabria 1955," in *Sbornik zakonov SSSR i ukazov prezidiuma verkhovnogo soveta SSSR, 1938-iiul' -1956gg* (Moskva: Gosudarstvennoe izdatel'stvo iuridicheskoi lieratury, 1956), 401-402. For more detail on the legalization and rhetoric of rights, see Chapter 5.

24. Historians have argued that women's rights were not part of the motivation for Soviet re-legalization. See, for example, Alena Heitlinger, *Women and State Socialism: Sex Inequality in the Soviet Union and Czechoslovakia* (London: Macmillan Press, 1979), 129. The notable exception is Deborah Field, who noted the re-legalization's invocation of motherhood as women's own decision, rather than their social obligation, as a "real innovation." Deborah Field, *Private Life and Communist Morality in Khrushchev's Russia* (New York: Peter Lang, 2007), 58.

25. "Ob otmene zapreshcheniia abortov, ukaz ot 23 noiabria 1955," *Sbornik zakonov SSSR i ukazov prezidiuma verkhovnogo soveta SSSR, 1938-1967 t. 2* (Moskva: Izdatel'stvo Izvestiia sovetov deputatov trudiashchikhsia SSSR, 1968), 423.

26. Amy Randall, "'Abortion Will Deprive You of Happiness!': Soviet Reproductive Politics in the Post-Stalin Era," *Journal of Women's History* 23, no. 3 (2011): 13–38.

27. Here I am building on the theory of the politics of reproduction and its application to both global processes and everyday life, as presented in the pioneering article by Faye Ginsburg and Rayna Rapp, "The Politics of Reproduction," *Annual Review of Anthropology* 20 (1990): 311–343.

28. In 1950, 47 percent of the workforce was female. Gail Lapidus, "The Female Industrial Labor Force: Reassessment and Options," in *Industrial Labor in the USSR*, ed. Arcadius Kahan and Blair Ruble (New York: Pergamon Press, 1979), 237.

29. Elaine Tyler May, *Homeward Bound: American Families in the Cold War Era* (New York: Basic Books, 1999); Susan Hartmann, *The Home Front and Beyond: American Women in the 1940s* (Boston: Twayne, 1982).

30. On postwar women's difficult everyday life, see Greta Bucher, *Women, the Bureaucracy and Daily Life in Postwar Moscow, 1945–1953* (Boulder, CO: East European Monographs, distributed by Columbia University Press, 2006); Gregory Smith, "The Impact of World War II on Women, Family Life, and Mores in Moscow, 1941–1945" (PhD dissertation, Stanford University, 1990). For a discussion of war invalids, see Beate Fieseler, "The Bitter Legacy of the 'Great Patriotic War': Red Army Disabled Soldiers under Late Stalinism," in *Late Stalinist Russia: Society between Reconstruction and Reinvention*, ed. Juliane Fürst (London: Routledge, 2006), 46–61; Edele, *Soviet Veterans*, 81–101. For a literary representation of women as healers, see Anna Krylova, "'Healers of Wounded Souls': The Crisis of Private Life in Soviet Literature," *Journal of Modern History* 73, no. 2 (June 2001).

31. Donald Filtzer, *Soviet Workers and Late Stalinism: Labor and the Restoration of the Stalinist System after World War II* (Cambridge: Cambridge University Press, 2002); Donald Filtzer, *The Hazards of Urban Life in Late Stalinist Russia: Health, Hygiene, and Living Standards, 1943–1953* (Cambridge: Cambridge University Press, 2010).

32. On wartime and postwar emergence of vegetable plots, see Charles Hachten, "Separate Yet Governed: The Representation of Soviet Property Relations in Civil Law and Public Discourses," in *Borders of Socialism: Private Spheres of Soviet Russia*, ed. Lewis Siegelbaum (New York: Palgrave Macmillan, 2006), 65–82; Stephen Lovell, *Summerfolk: A History of the Dacha, 1710–2000* (Ithaca, NY: Cornell University Press, 2003), 163–178; Goldman and Filtzer, *Hunger and War*, 18–20.

33. On self-censorship, see Alen Blium, *Rodit'sia, zhit' i umeret' v SSSR* (Moskva: Novoe izdatel'stvo, 2005), 40.

34. Mie Nakachi, "Population, Politics and Reproduction: Late Stalinism and Its Legacy," in *Late Stalinist Russia: Society between Reinvention and Reconstruction*, ed. Juliane Fürst (London: Routledge, 2006), 38–40.

35. Galmarini-Kabala's study focuses on the crucial role of Soviet professionals in mediating between social deviants and the state in the prewar and the postwar periods. Maria Cristina Galmarini-Kabala, *The Right to Be Helped: Deviance, Entitlement, and the Soviet Moral Order* (DeKalb: Northern Illinois University Press, 2016), chapter 6.

36. An earlier version of this analysis appeared in Mie Nakachi, "Liberation without Contraception? The Rise of the Abortion Empire and Pronatalism in Socialist and Postsocialist Russia," in *Reproductive States: Global Perspectives on the Invention and Implementation of Population Policy*, ed. Rickie Solinger and Mie Nakachi (New York: Oxford University Press, 2016), 293–299.

37. Kent Geiger, *The Family in Soviet Russia* (Cambridge, MA: Harvard University Press, 1968), 44–49. On the women's liberation movement and changing attitudes toward sex and gender in the late imperial and early Soviet period, see Richard Stites, *The Women's Liberation Movement in Russia: Feminism, Nihilism and Bolshevism, 1860–1930* (Princeton, NJ: Princeton University Press, 1978); Laura Engelstein,

The Keys to Happiness: Sex and the Search for Modernity in Fin-de-Siècle Russia, (Ithaca, NY: Cornell University Press, 1992).

38. Thomas Malthus, *An Essay on the Principle of Population; or A View of Its Past and Present Effects on Human Happiness: With an Inquiry into Our Prospects Respecting the Future Removal or Mitigation of the Evils which It Occasions*, Selected and Introduced by Donald Winch (Cambridge: Cambridge University Press, 1992 [1803]), 23–24, 368–369.

39. K. Marks i, F. Engel's, *Sochineniia*, vol. 20 (2nd ed.) (Moscow, 1961), 69; and Ronald Meek, ed., *Marx and Engels on Malthus* (London: Lawrence and Wishart, 1953), 59–62, 122–123.

40. "Population and Communism," in Engels's letter to Kautsky of February 1, 1881, in Meek, *Marx and Engels*, 108–109.

41. August Bebel, *Woman in the Past, Present, and Future*, translated from *Die Frau in der Vergangenheit, Gegenwart und Zukunft*, trans. H. B. Adams Walther (London: William Reeves, 1893), 255.

42. V. I. Lenin, *Polnoe sobranie sochinenii*, vol. 23 (Moskva: Gos. Izd-vo politicheskoi literatury, 1961), 255–257, 488, 530.

43. On changing and unchanging attitudes toward sex among young people in the early Soviet period, see Sheila Fitzpatrick, *The Cultural Front: Power and Culture in Revolutionary Russia* (Ithaca, NY: Cornell University Press, 1992), in particular chapter 4. Dan Healey's study of forensic medicine in the 1920s and 1930s shows that women workers and their family members asked forensic medicine experts to establish sexual innocence, demonstrating that women's sexual promiscuity played an important role in establishing female and family reputation. Dan Healey, *Bolshevik Sexual Forensics: Diagnosing Disorder in the Clinic and Courtroom, 1917-1939* (DeKalb: Northern Illinois University Press, 2009), 56-57.

44. Beatrice Farnsworth, *Aleksandra Kollontai: Socialism, Feminism, and the Bolshevik Revolution* (Stanford, CA: Stanford University, 1980), 399. On Kollontai's view of the family, marriage, love, and sex, see Barbara Clements, *Bolshevik Feminist: The Life of Aleksandra Kollontai* (Bloomington: Indiana University Press, 1979), 56–59; and Farnsworth, *Aleksandra Kollontai*, 164–168.

45. There were physicians who considered contraception even harmful, although they generally accepted that abortion was worse. Frances Bernstein, *The Dictatorship of Sex: Lifestyle Advice for the Soviet Masses* (DeKalb: Northern Illinois University Press, 2007), 167.

46. Sheila Fitzpatrick, *Everyday Stalinism: Ordinary Life in Extraordinary Times, Soviet Russia in the 1930s* (New York: Oxford University Press, 1999), 142–143.

47. Wendy Goldman, the top expert on this period, argues against this simplistic Stalinist logic, concluding that "legalized abortion was not the cause of this [demographic] fall—it was simply one of several methods women used to keep from bearing children." Goldman, *Women, the State and Revolution*, 291.

48. As historian David Hoffmann has argued, pronatalist policymaking was a global trend in Europe and Japan in the 1930s. Hoffmann, "Mothers in the Motherland."

49. "O zapreshchenii abortov, uvelichenii material'noi pomoshchi rozhenitsam, ustanovlenii gosudarstvennoi pomoshchi mnogosemeinym, rasshirenii seti rodil'nykh domov, detskikh iaslei i detskikh sadov, usilenii ugolovnogo nakazaniia za neplatezh alimentov i o nekotorykh izmeneniiakh o zakonodatel'stve o razvodakh" (Postanovlenie TsIK i SNK SSSR ot 27 iiunia, 1936), in *Postanovleniia KPSS i Sovetskogo pravitel'stva ob okhrane zdorov'ia naroda* (Moskva: MEDGIZ, 1958), 264–265.

50. Alan Ball, *And Now My Soul Is Hardened: Abandoned Children in Soviet Russia, 1918–1930* (Berkeley: University of California Press, 1994).

51. Many regarded the 1936 law as a retreat from or betrayal of the revolutionary vision of socialized childrearing. Nicholas Timasheff, *The Great Retreat: The Growth and Decline of Communism in Russia* (New York: E. P. Dutton, 1946); Leon Trotsky, *The Revolution Betrayed: What Is the Soviet Union and Where Is It Going?* (London: Faber and Faber, 1937).

52. The many millions of Stalin's victims by dekulakization, GULAG, deportations, and purges remind us that neither the preservation of human lives nor the enhancement of social welfare was the dictator's priority. Stalin, who believed in the socialist theory of population growth, adopted pronatalist measures to increase the number of births for the purpose of securing the workforce for the future economic growth and military strength of the Soviet Union. In line with this Stalinist thinking, this book defines "pronatalism" narrowly to refer to state efforts to increase the number of births. I thank Vladislav Zubok for pointing out the oxymoronic nature of the phrase "Stalinist pronatalism" during my presentation at the 2008 Conference on "Northeast Asia in the Cold War: New Evidence and Perspectives," at the Slavic Research Center, Sapporo, Japan.

53. Post-1944 one-parent pronatalism should not be confused with either the idea of state alliance with mothers or the state's "marginalization" of fathers, views that are more relevant for the 1920s and 1930s. Olga Issoupova, "From Duty to Pleasure? Motherhood in Soviet and Post-Soviet Russia," in *Gender, State and Society in Soviet and Post-Soviet Russia*, ed. Sarah Ashwin (London: Routledge, 2000), 38; Sergei Kukhterin, "Fathers and Patriarchs in Communist and Post-communist Russia," in *Gender, State and Society in Soviet and Post-Soviet Russia*, ed. Sarah Ashwin (London: Routledge, 2000), 78. My research shows that the Soviet state failed to replace fathers, while many fathers happily avoided paternal responsibilities. Only a generation later, in 1968, the state allowed fathers who so desired to take some paternal responsibility for their out-of-wedlock children.

54. Fitzpatrick, *Everyday Stalinism*, 143–147; Lauren Kaminsky, "Utopian Visions of Family Life in the Stalin-Era Soviet Union," *Central European History* 44 (2011): 63–91.

55. An earlier discussion of this theme appeared in Nakachi, "A Postwar Sexual Liberation?" 423–440.

56. A translation of "Zhdi menia" appears in Vera Dunham, *In Stalin's Time: Middleclass Values in Soviet Fiction* (Durham, NC: Duke University Press, 1990), 71.

57. "No. 67. Iz dnevnika moskovskogo vracha E. Sakharovoi," in *Moskva voennaia 1941/1945: Memuary i arkhivnye dokumenty* (Moskva: Izdatel'stvo ob'edineniia Mosgorarkhiv, 1995), 657–687.

58. Ilya Ehrenburg, *The War 1941–1945*, trans. Tatiana Shebunina (London: MacGibbon and Kee, 1964), 191. I use "Ehrenburg" only in reference to his publication in English, where he is spelled that way. Otherwise I use "Erenburg," the Library of Congress transliteration of his Russian name.

59. Ehrenburg, *The War*, 123.

60. These behaviors were recorded by venereologists who were concerned with the growing rate of venereal disease in the military and civilian populations, particularly after late 1943. GARF f. 8009, op. 1, d. 489, ll. 4-5.

61. RGASPI f. 17, op. 122, d. 72, ll. 39, 100.

62. On attempts to discipline cohabitation, see Roger Markwick and Euridice Cardona, *Soviet Women on the Frontline in the Second World War* (New York: Palgrave Macmillan, 2012), 199–200.

63. Svetlana A. Alexievich, *U voiny ne zhenskoe litso. Poslednie svideteli: povesti* (Moskva: Sovetskii pisatel', 1988), 169. Her work encompasses different genres of writing. Oleg Budnitskii analyzed wartime sexual relationships within the Red Army using diaries and memoir materials. Oleg Budnitskii, "Muzhchiny i zhenshchiny v Krasnoi armii (1941–1945)" *Cahiers du monde russe* 52, no. 2-3 (avril–septembre 2011): 405–422.

64. Before July 8, 1944, such a union, even without registration of marriage, would have carried legal meaning. In this sense, the use of the term "marriage" did reflect the legal reality. As we will see, despite the 1944 law's non-recognition of common-law marriages as legal, women especially continued to refer to such unions as "marriage."

65. Alexievich, *U voiny*, 170, 225.

66. Interestingly, Anna Krylova's study claims that Soviet women in combat, who comprised about a quarter of all women who served in the Red Army during World War II, constructed a puritanical narrative about themselves arguing that only non-combatant women engaged in military sex. Anna Krylova, *Soviet Women in Combat: A History of Violence on the Eastern Front* (Cambridge: Cambridge University Press, 2010), 282–283.

67. PPZh also stands for *pokhodno-polevaia zhena* (field campaign wife). In return for their service to male officers, PPZh were privileged in their living conditions, getting better access to supplies and transportation. Barbara Alpern Engel and Anastasia Posadskaya-Vanderbeck, eds., *A Revolution of Their Own: Voices of Women in Soviet History* (Boulder, CO: Westview Press, 1998), 197–198; Edele, *Soviet Veterans*, 73–74. Most commanders seemed to have taken a PPZh. Reese, *Why Stalin's Soldiers Fought*, 299.

68. Reese, *Why Stalin's Soldiers Fought*, 303; Mark Popovskii, *Tretii lishnii: On, ona i sovetskii rezhim* (London: Overseas Publications Interchange, 1985), 93–102. Popovskii, who served in the war as a medic, writes that he was asked to facilitate abortions by women or their sexual partners and that he also conducted a number

of medical examinations to establish pregnancy, then used to dismiss female soldiers from the army.

69. In September 1942, there was a series of decrees and orders regarding state aid for pregnant women who worked in the military both as civilians and service women. They were published in Iu. N. Ivanova, *Khrabreishie iz prekrasnykh: zhenshchiny Rossii v voinakh* (Moskva: ROSSPEN, 2002), 241–243. One of them—the September 1, 1942 decree on "the procedure of wartime payment of state aid for pregnancy and birth among the enlisted and junior officers who were discharged from the Red Army, Navy, and NKVD troops"— stipulated that discharged pregnant service women would receive state aid (*posobie*) for thirty-five days before birth and twenty-eight days afterward. In addition, at birth there would be an additional sum for the child. Ivanova evaluates these decrees and orders quite positively as "measures for the preservation of women's health and restoration of the country's population" (171) and never mentions that discharged pregnant service women were often stigmatized. However, many such women never even applied for such aid due to the stigma and the brief duration of benefits.

70. GARF f. 8009, op. 1, d. 489, l. 5.

71. Karel C. Berkhoff, *Harvest of Despair: Life and Death in Ukraine under Nazi Rule* (Cambridge: Belknap Press of Harvard University Press, 2004), 114–115.

72. Berkhoff tells how young Ukrainian girls often sought a German partner on the street in the hope of getting material help and protection. Berkhoff, *Harvest of Despair,* 182–183.

73. Ehrenburg, *The War*, 94.

74. Also discussed in Edele, *Soviet Veterans* 73–78.

75. Competition between capitalist and socialist regimes contributed to the expansion of welfare states under both systems. Herbert Obinger and Carina Schmitt, "Guns and Butter? Regime Competition and the Welfare State during the Cold War," *World Politics* 63, no. 2 (April 2011): 246–270.

76. Fitzpatrick, *Everyday Stalinism*, 142. Due to limited budgets for building facilities and providing resource for the protection of motherhood and infancy, propaganda functioned as a cheaper alternative in promoting better hygiene practices among nursing mothers. Tricia Starks, *The Body Soviet: Propaganda, Hygiene, and the Revolutionary State* (Madison: University of Wisconsin Press, 2008), 139-140.

77. *Byvshie, kulaki* and *lishentsy* were excluded categories involving millions of souls not protected by incipient Soviet welfare in this period. Golfo Alexopolous, *Stalin's Outcasts: Aliens, Citizens, and the Soviet State, 1926-1936* (Ithaca, NY: Cornell University Press, 2003).

78. For the first comprehensive study of Soviet social policies, see Bernice Madison, *Social Welfare in the Soviet Union* (Stanford, CA: Stanford University Press, 1968). Mark Edele, *The Soviet Union: A Short History* (Hoboken, NJ: Wiley Blackwell, 2019) provides an overview of Soviet welfare development. On the development of welfare policies in the 1920s and 1930s, see David L. Hoffmann, *Cultivating the Masses: Modern State Practices and Soviet Socialism, 1914-1939* (Ithaca, NY: Cornell University Press, 2011). On a discussion of housing as a welfare project, see Mark

B. Smith, *Property of Communists: The Urban Housing Program from Stalin to Khrushchev* (DeKalb: Northern Illinois University Press, 2010). On pension reforms, see Mark Smith, "The Withering Away of the Danger Society: The Pensions Reforms of 1956 and 1964 in the Soviet Union," *Social Science History* 39 (Spring 2015): 129–148. On the development of public health in the postwar period, see Christopher Burton, "Soviet Medical Attestation and the Problem of Professionalization under Late Stalinism, 1945–1953," *Europe-Asia Studies* 57, no. 8 (December 2005): 1211–1229. For a discussion of welfare policy development for the deaf, see Claire L. Shaw, *Deaf in the USSR: Marginality, Community, and Soviet Identity, 1917–1991* (Ithaca, NY: Cornell University Press, 2017).

79. Linda Cook, *Postcommunist Welfare States: Reform Politics in Russia and Eastern Europe* (Ithaca, NY: Cornell University Press, 2007), 31-37. Linda Cook, "Eastern Europe and Russia," in *The Oxford Handbook of the Welfare State*, ed. Francis Castles et al. (New York: Oxford University Press, 2010), 672–673; Smith, "The Withering Away of the Danger Society," 129–148; Susan Gal and Gail Kligman, *The Politics of Gender after Socialism* (Princeton, NJ: Princeton University Press, 2000), 63–64.

80. Hoffmann, *Cultivating the Masses*, 50.

81. Wood, *The Baba and the Comrade*; Wendy Goldman, "Industrial Politics, Peasant Rebellion and the Death of the Proletarian Women's Movement in the USSR," *Slavic Review* 55, no. 1 (Spring 1996): 52–54.

82. The official reason was that women no longer needed special assistance because they had become equal to men. On details of the conflicts between the women's department and the party leadership during the period of the New Economic Policy, see chapters 5, 6, and 7 of Wood, *The Baba and the Comrade*, and Goldman, "Industrial Politics," 72–77.

83. Hoffmann, *Cultivating the Masses*, 57–64; Edele, *The Soviet Union*, 112–114. Hoffman dates the beginning of the Soviet welfare state to the mid-1930s when the Constitution expressed the idea of universalized social welfare system, while Edele sees this development through "the prism of socialist realism" (Edele, *The Soviet Union*, 113). Both agree that actual delivery of benefits was inadequate, not universal, and not up to the level of the propagandistic discourse.

84. Fitzpatrick, *Everyday Stalinism*, 74–75.

85. Mark Edele, "Veterans and the Welfare State: World War II in the Soviet Context," *Comparativ: Zeitschrift fur Globalgeschichte und Vergleichende Gesellschaftsforschung* 20 (2010): 28–29. On the disenfranchised, see Alexopolous, *Stalin's Outcasts*.

86. "O naloge na kholostiakov, odinokikh i bezdetnykh grazhdan SSSR, ukaz ot 21 noiabria 1941," *Sbornik zakonov SSSR i ukazov prezidiuma verkhovnogo soveta SSSR, 1938-1967* t. 2 (Moskva: Izdatel'stvo sovetov deputatov trudiashchikhsia SSSR, 1968), 304-305.

87. I. Z. Vel'vovskii, working in Kharkov, Ukraine, developed psychoprophylaxis, a psychological method for painless labor shortly after World War II. Paula Michaels has written a fascinating history of the transformation of this new practice into the Lamaze method outside the Soviet Union. Paula Michaels, *Lamaze: An International History* (New York: Oxford University Press, 2014), chapter 2. In contrast to some other

innovative ideas developed in this period but rejected for implementation, the Soviet government officially adopted psychoprophylaxis for Union-wide practice in 1951 as the method met the needs of pronatalist policy and required little material commitment. Michaels, *Lamaze*, 42-43.

88. For similar development of reform ideas in the postwar Stalinist period and attendant disciplining, see A.V. Pyzhikov, "Sovetskoe poslevoennoe obshchestvo i predposylki khrushchevskikh reform," *Voprosy istorii*, 2 (2002): 33–43; Julie Hessler, "A Postwar Perestroika? Toward a History of Private Trade Enterprise in the USSR," *Slavic Review*, 57, no. 3 (1998): 516–542; Elena Zubkova, *Russia after the War: Hopes, Illusions, and Disappointments, 1945–1957*, trans. and ed. Hugh Ragsdale (Armonk, NY: M. E. Sharpe, 1998); Edele, *Soviet Veterans*.

89. Housing reform was an example of major post-Stalin reforms that took place based on the ideas developed in the postwar period. See Smith, *Property of Communists*; Stephen Harris, *Communism on Tomorrow Street: Mass Housing and Everyday Life after Stalin* (Baltimore: Woodrow Wilson Center Press and Johns Hopkins University Press, 2013); and Christine Varga-Harris, *Stories of House and Home: Soviet Apartment Life during the Khrushchev Years* (Ithaca, NY: University of Cornell Press, 2015).

90. See "Ob otmene ugolovnoi otvetstvennosti . . . " and "Ob otmene zapreshcheniia abortov . . ."

91. Elena Zdravomyslova, "Gendernoe grazhdanstvo i abortnaia kul'tura," in *Zdorov'e i doverie: Gendernyi podkhod k reproduktivnoi meditsine*, ed. Elena Zdravomyslova and Anna Temkina (St. Peterburg: Evropeiskii universitet v Sankt-Peterburge, 2009), 120.

92. Randall, "Abortion Will Deprive You"; Field, *Private Life*, 58.

93. Natasha Maltseva, "The Other Side of the Coin," in *Women and Russia: Feminist Writings from the Soviet Union*, ed. Tatyana Mamonova (Oxford: Blackwell, 1984), 114–116; Carola Hansson and Karin Liden, *Moscow Women: Thirteen Interviews*, trans. Gerry Bothmer, George Blecher, and Lone Blecher (New York: Pantheon House, 1983), 63–64.

94. Oleg Kharkhordin, *The Collective and the Individual in Russia: A Study of Practices* (Berkeley: University of California Press, 1999); Field, *Private Life*; Brian LaPierre, *Hooligans in Khrushchev's Russia: Defining, Policing, and Producing Deviance during the Thaw* (Madison: University of Wisconsin Press, 2012); Edward Cohn, *The High Title of a Communist: Postwar Party Discipline and the Values of the Soviet Regime* (DeKalb: Northern Illinois University Press, 2015).

95. The family law reform was blocked because Khrushchev was the creator of the law and continued to believe in the law's demographic efficacy. In other areas, Robert Hornsby's study argues that Khrushchev's regime was willing to improve material conditions to prevent discontent among workers, particularly after the Novocherkassk disorder in 1962. However, the regime often ignored or suppressed intellectual and political dissent, as neither of these was likely to be satisfied by material improvement. Robert Hornsby, *Protest, Reform and Repression in Khrushchev's Soviet Union* (Cambridge: Cambridge University Press, 2013), 4–5.

96. Gail Warshofsky Lapidus, *Women in Soviet Society: Equality, Development, and Social Change* (Berkeley: University of California Press, 1978), 290–292.

97. Lynne Attwood, *The New Soviet Man and Woman: Sex-Role Socialization in the USSR* (London: Macmillan, 1990), 184–191.

98. For his essentialized view of gender, see Mikhail Gorbachev, *Perestroika: New Thinking for Our Country and the World* (New York: Harper and Row, 1987), 116–118.

99. Michele Rivkin-Fish, "From 'Demographic Crisis' to 'Dying Nation': The Politics of Language and Reproduction in Russia," in *Gender and National Identity in Twentieth-Century Russian Culture*, ed. Helen Goscilo and Andrea Lanoux (DeKalb: Northern Illinois University Press, 2006); Michele Rivkin-Fish, "Pronatalism, Gender Politics, and the Renewal of Family Support in Russia: Toward a Feminist Anthropology of 'Maternity Capital,'" *Slavic Review* 69, no. 3 (Fall 2010): 701–724; Mie Nakachi, "Roshiano fukushito jenda," in *Shin sekaino shakaifukushi 5 Kyusoren too* ["Welfare and Gender in Russia" in *Global Social Welfare*, vol. 5, *Former Soviet Union and East-Central Europe*], ed. Manabu Sengoku (Tokyo: Junposha, 2019), 127–180.

100. Magali Barbieri, Alain Blum, Elena Dolkigh, and Amon Ergashev, "Nuptiality, Fertility, Use of Contraception, and Family Policies in Uzbekistan," *Population Studies* 50, no. 1 (March, 1996):69-88; Victor Agadjanian, "Is 'Abortion Culture' Fading in the Former Soviet Union? Views about Abortion and Contraception in Kazakhstan," *Studies in Family Planning* 33, no. 3 (September 2002): 237-248.

101. Tyrene White, *China's Longest Campaign: Birth Planning in the People's Republic, 1949-2005* (Ithaca, NY: Cornell University Press, 2006), 20.

102. A useful survey of Eastern European abortion policies can be found in Henry David, *Family Planning and Abortion in the Socialist Countries of Central and Eastern Europe: A Compendium of Observations and Readings* (New York: Population Council, 1970). In particular, see p. 64 on Bulgaria, pp. 81–82 on Poland, pp. 103–105 on Hungary, p. 128 on Romania, and p.162 on Czechoslovakia. In the mid-1950s, China also liberalized restrictions on abortion and contraception. Tyrene White, *China's Longest Campaign China's Longest Campaign*, 35; and Masako Kohama, "*Chugoku kingendaini okeru boshieiseiseisakuno kenkyu* [A Study of Public Health Policy toward Mothers and Children in Modern and Contemporary China], A Research Report," published as the result of a 2002~2005 project funded by the Japan Society for the Promotion of Science (March 2006), 12–15.

103. See Sergei Zakharov, "Russian Federation: From the First to Second Demographic Transition," *Demographic Research* 19, article 24 (2008): 916–918. Tomas Sobotka argues that convergence of reproductive behavior among East and Central European countries continued until 1970. Tomas Sobotka, "Fertility in Central and Eastern Europe after 1989: Collapse and Gradual Recovery," *Historical Social Research* 36, no. 2 (2011): 250–257.

104. Data come from different years depending on the country. http://data.un.org/Data. aspx?q=abortion&d=GenderStat&f=inID%3a12 (last accessed September 1, 2020).

105. Jay Winter and Michael Teitelbaum, *The Global Spread of Fertility Decline: Population, Fear, and Uncertainty* (New Haven, CT: Yale University Press, 2013); Ann Buchanan

and Anna Rotkirch, *Fertility Rates and Population Decline: No Time for Children?* (Houndmills, UK: Palgrave Macmillan, 2013).

106. Ann S. Orloff, "Gender and the Social Rights of Citizenship: The Comparative Analysis of Gender Relations and Welfare States," *American Sociological Review* 53 (June 1993): 303–328.

107. Gøsta Esping-Andersen, *The Incomplete Revolution: Adapting to Women's New Roles* (Cambridge: Polity Press, 2009), 79–83.

108. Ann S. Orloff suggests two basic approaches: one is the Nordic model of high subsidy, high quality, and high cost, and the other, the American model of stratified quality and quantity care. Ann S. Orloff "Gender," in *The Oxford Handbook of the Welfare State*, ed. Francis Castles et al. (New York: Oxford University Press, 2010), 261.

109. Stephen Kotkin, "Speaking Bolshevik," chapter 5 of *Magnetic Mountain: Stalinism as a Civilization* (Berkeley: University of California Press, 1995).

110. Nikolai Krementsov, *The Cure: A Story of Cancer and Politics from the Annals of the Cold War* (Chicago: University of Chicago Press, 2002).

111. As discussed above, prior to the 1944 law, it was common for men and women to identify any type of sexual relationship as a de facto marriage or common-law/civil (*grazhdanskaia*) marriage. Therefore, those who would be regarded as "unmarried mothers" after 1944 could previously have claimed to be married or divorced. This practice led to widespread de facto bigamy and polygamy. For a discussion of this in the prewar period, see Fitzpatrick, *Everyday Stalinism*, 145–146.

112. The ministries were called people's commissariats until 1946.

113. On May 23, 2003, I interviewed Dr. O. G. Frolova, head of the Department of Socio-Medical analysis at the Research Center for Obstetrics, Gynecology, and Perinatology in Moscow. She showed me her recent analysis for the Putin government, where she compared the postwar demographic problems, namely, low fertility and few healthy men, with the current (2003) crisis of low fertility and early mortality, especially among men. Frolova argued that the 1944 Family Law was a success and should become the model.

Chapter 1

1. Nobel Lecture by Svetlana Aleksievich, NobelPrize.org. Nobel Media AB 2018, Sunday December 23, 2018. https://www.nobelprize.org/prizes/literature/2015/alexievich/25414-nobel-lecture-by-svetlana-aleksievitch-in-russian/.

2. RGASPI f. 82, op. 2, d.538, ll. 40–43. Both the statistics and citation are from this file.

3. Political scientist Peter Juviler had revealed the fact that the 1944 Family Law was initiated by N. S. Khrushchev based on interviews with insiders in the Soviet Union, but he did not have any details or written evidence on how this came about. Nor could he cite his sources by name. This chapter provides exhaustive documentary corroboration of his fifty-year old claim. Peter Juviler, "Family Reforms on the Road to

Communism," in *Soviet Policy-Making: Studies of Communism in Transition*, ed. Peter Juviler and Henry Morton (London: Pall Mall Press, 1967), 31.

4. GARF f. 8009, op. 1, d. 497, l. 164.

5. The US baby boom period lasted from 1946 to 1964. Cheryl Russell, *The Baby Boom: Americans Born 1946 to 1964* (Amityville, NY: New Strategist Press, 2009). Fertility rose between 20 and 40 percent between the 1930s and 1950s, depending on exactly which indicators are used. Jeremy Greenwood, Ananth Seshadri, and Guillaume Vandenbrouske, "The Baby Boom and Baby Bust," *American Economic Review* 95 no. 1 (March 2005):183.

6. The term "baby boomlet" appeared in *Encyclopedia Britannica*'s "Population: The Industrialized Countries since 1950" to describe the much lower and shorter level of rise seen in most Western European countries, https://www.britannica.com/science/population-biology-and-anthropology/The-developing-countries-since-1950#ref366965. Japan's fertility rise in the late 1940s is similar. Naikakufu (Cabinet Office of the Japanese Government), "Shusshosuu・shusshoritsuno suii (Changes in the number of births and the birth rate)," https://www8.cao.go.jp/shoushi/shoushika/data/shusshou.html.

7. Miho Ogino, *Kazokukeikakueno michi: Kindai nihonno seishokuo meguru seiji* (Tokyo: Iwanami, 2008), 142.

8. Elena Zubkova, "Preodolenie voiny-preodolenie pobedy: Sovetskaia povsednevnost' i strategii vyzhivaniia (1945–1953)," in *Pobediteli i pobezhdennye: Ot voiny k miru: SSSR, Frantsiia, Velikobritaniia, Germaniia, SShA (1941–1950*, ed.B. Fizeler and N. Muan (Moskva: ROSSPEN, 2010), 15.

9. "Bebi-bum," in *Demograficheskaia entsiklopediia* (Moskva: Izd. Entsiklopeidiia, 2013), 46–47; and A. Vishnevskii, ed., *Demograficheskaia modernizatsiia Rossii 1900–2000* (Moskva: Novoe izdatel'stvo, 2006), 164.

10. The goal of the 1941 tax was mentioned in The State Archive of the Russian Federation (GARF) f. 8009, op. 1, d. 497, ll. 171–174.

11. Nicholas Timasheff, *The Great Retreat: The Growth and Decline of Communism in Russia* (New York: E. P. Dutton, 1946); Leon Trotsky, *The Revolution Betrayed: What Is the Soviet Union and Where Is It Going?* (London: Faber and Faber, 1937).

12. Some scholars use such terms as "marginalization" of fathers, stressing the sense that the government and mothers excluded fathers from a role in the family. For example, Olga Issoupova, "From Duty to Pleasure?: Motherhood in Soviet and Post-Soviet Russia," in *Gender, State and Society in Soviet and Post-Soviet Russia*, ed. Sarah Ashwin (New York: Routledge, 2000), 39. Instead, "optional fatherhood" emphasizes the point that fathers often chose to exclude themselves from their roles in the family.

13. Various scholars have suggested parallels between the Soviet/Russian family and African American families in the United States, where young mothers give birth to and raise children in the absence of fathers. For example, see Brienna Perelli-Harris and Theodore P. Gerber, "Non-marital Childbearing in Russia: Second Demographic Transition or Pattern of Disadvantage?" *Demography* 48 no. 1 (February 2011): 317–342.

14. An earlier version of this discussion appeared in Mie Nakachi, "N. S. Khrushchev and the 1944 Soviet Family Law: Politics, Reproduction, and Language," *East European Politics and Societies* 20, no. 1 (2006): 40–68. Copyright © 2006. DOI: [https://doi.org/10.1177/0888325405284313].

15. Ilya Ehrenburg, *The War 1941–1945*, trans. Tatiana Shebunina (London: MacGibbon and Kee, 1964), 109.

16. Ehrenburg, *The War 1941–1945*, 99.

17. A. L. Perkovskii and S. I. Pirozhkov, "Demografichni vtrati narodonaseleniia Ukrainskoi RSR u 40-kh gg," *Ukrains'kii istorichnii zhurnal* 2 (February 1990): 23. It should be remembered that the demographic woes of Ukraine, Holodomor (man-made famine), deportations and outright slaughter, were inflicted both by Germans and Russians.

18. Nikita S. Khrushchev grew up in Ukraine and began his political career in the Donbass. He climbed up the party structure in Donbass, and then Kiev. In 1928 he became the deputy chief of the department of organization at the Central Committee of the Communist Party of Ukraine. In 1929 he moved to Moscow to study at the Industrial Academy and took up various party positions there. After working in Moscow for several years, most memorably as the builder of the subway, he was sent back to Ukraine in 1938 as the first secretary. During the war and German occupation, he stayed in Ukraine as a member of the military council. After the war, he was chairman of the Council of People's Commissars of Ukraine between 1944 and 1949. He devoted himself to the postwar reconstruction of Ukraine until 1949, when Stalin suddenly recalled him to Moscow to head the Moscow party organization. V. I. Ivkin, *Gosudarstvennaia vlast' SSSR: vysshie organy vlasti i upravleniia i ikh rukovoditeli 1923–1991* (Moskva: ROSSPEN, 1999), 578; Nikita S. Khrushchev, *Khrushchev Remembers: The Last Testament* (Boston: Little Brown, 1974), 93–95.

19. United Nations Relief and Rehabilitation Administration (UNRRA) European Regional Office, "Operational Analysis Papers, No. 39: Economic Rehabilitation in the Ukraine" (April 1947), 3.

20. UNRRA, "Operational Analysis Papers, No. 39," 7–8. The director of UNRRA, Fiorello Laguardia informed Stalin of the situation during a meeting on August 29, 1946. RGASPI f. 558, op. 11, d. 374, ll. 138–142.

21. For example, see *Sovetskaia Ukraina v gody Velikoi Otechestvennoi Voiny, 1941–1945: Ukrainskaia SSR v period korennogo pereloma v khode Velikoi Otechestvennoi voiny* (Kiev: Naukova Dumka, 1985).

22. Perkovskii and Pirozhkov, "Demografichni vtrati," 16, Table 1. A large percentage of the 2 million driven to Germany as forced laborers would return or at least survive, but they are not registered yet in 1944.

23. See the proposal to accommodate 300 orphans from Ukraine in an orphanage in Omsk oblast in *Sovetskaia Ukraina*, 378–379.

24. *Sovetskaia Ukraina*, 15.

25. See Alexander Statiev, *The Soviet Counterinsurgency in the Western Borderlands* (Cambridge: Cambridge University Press, 2010).

26. Donald Filtzer, *Soviet Workers and Late Stalinism: Labour and the Restoration of the Stalinist System after World War II* (Cambridge: Cambridge University Press, 2002). Chapter 2 is particularly useful in understanding how the postwar Soviet government tried to solve the problem of labor shortage.

27. In May he reported to Stalin that a group of Ukrainian men who had just been mobilized into the Red Army, was being escorted by twenty Soviet troops, either military or NKVD, when they were suddenly attacked by more than 100 men, resulting in six deaths and two wounded among the escort. The mobilized men escaped. Nonetheless, Khrushchev wrote as if armed opposition was in decline, although in fact armed resistance would continue until the end of the decade. *N. S. Khrushchov i Ukraina* (Kiiv: Academy of Sciences Press, 1995), 163–164, 170.

28. Bohdan Krawchenko, "Soviet Ukraine under Nazi Occupation, 1941–44," in *Ukraine: The Challenges of World War II*, ed. Taras Hunczak and Dmytro Shtohryn (Lanham, MD: University Press of America, 2003), 49.

29. UNRRA, "Operational Analysis Papers, No. 39," 8–11.

30. "O naloge na kholostiakov, odinokikh i bezdetnykh grazhdan SSSR," ukaz ot 21 noiabria 1941, in *Vedomosti verkhovnogo soveta SSSR* 42 (December 1941): 3; Khrushchev later admitted that this had been his initiative. *Izvestiia*, January 8, 1955.

31. GARF f. 8009, op. 1, d. 497, l. 171.

32. On Ptukha, see T. V. Ryabushkin's obituary, "Mikhail Vassilievitch Ptukha, 1884–1961," *Revue de l'Institut International de Statistique / Review of the International Statistical Institute* 29, no. 3 (1961): 111–112; and the biography introducing his famous article, Mikhail Ptukha, "Naselenie Ukrainy do 1960," a paper published in 1930 (in French) and reprinted in T. V. Riabushkin et al., eds., *Sovetskaia demographiia za 70 let: iz istorii nauki* (Moskva: Nauka, 1987), 46.

33. GARF f. 8009, op. 22, d. 28, ll. 20–21.

34. RGASPI f. 82, op. 2, d. 538, ll. 41–42.

35. RGASPI f. 82, op. 2, d. 538, ll. 24–27.

36. RGASPI f. 82, op. 2, d. 387, ll. 35, 90.

37. Who initially proposed this ukase is not clear. Molotov's correspondence with A. Gorkin, secretary to the Presidium of the Supreme Soviet SSR, regarding various drafts of the ukase, does not include any discussion about how the ukase was conceived. RGASPI f. 82, op. 2, d. 387, ll. 18–34.

38. RGASPI f. 82, op. 2, d. 387, ll. 38–39. I will use the word ukase and law interchangeably.

39. RGASPI f. 82, op. 2, d. 387, l. 35.

40. TsMAMLS f. 218, op. 1, d. 45, ll. 1–3.

41. GARF f. 8009, op. 1, d. 497, l.184.

42. Two sets of these materials were found in two archives: one in GARF and the other in RGASPI. I am indebted to Charles Hachten who drew my attention to the RGASPI file.

43. In the Soviet context, the language of the caring state was a practice of "speaking Bolshevik." Chapter 5 "Speaking Bolshevik," of Stephen Kotkin, *Magnetic Mountain: Stalinism as a Civilization* (Berkeley: University of California Press, 1995),

198–237. Clearly, the Soviet leadership was aware of when and where it was appropriate to use it or not.

44. GARF f. 8009, op. 1, d.497, l. 185.

45. GARF f. 8009, op. 1, d. 497, l. 185, details 150 rubles per month for the first child, 225 rubles per month for the second child, and 300 rubles per month for each additional child.

46. GARF f. 8009, op. 1, d. 497, l. 187.

47. GARF f. 8009, op. 1, d. 497, l. 188.

48. GARF f. 8009, op. 1, d. 497, l. 188.

49. GARF f. 8009, op. 1, d. 497, ll. 185–186.

50. GARF f. 8009, op. 1, d. 497, l. 186. The literal translation of the Russian original "*s prisvoeniem emu otchestva po ukazaniiu materi*" would be "with conferring of the patronymic as instructed by the mother." This expression is slightly different from the one used in the *spravka*, "*s prisvoeniem otchestva po ee vyboru*," which matches the title of this chapter. GARF f. 8009, op. 1, d. 497, l. 167. In Russian conversation adults address each other using the first name and patronymic, e.g., Ivan Denisovich (Ivan, son of Denis). Therefore, patronymics are culturally very important, and not like middle names.

51. GARF f. 8009, op. 1, d. 497, ll. 193–195.

52. GARF f. 8009, op. 1, d. 497, l. 191.

53. GARF f. 8009, op. 1, d. 497, l. 190.

54. Both men and women and their spouses whose reproductive health conditions were diagnosed as preventing procreation (*protivopokazano detorozhdeniiu*) by the medical commission were exempted from the taxes in the 1941 law. See "O naloge kholostiakov, odinokikh i bezdetnykh grazhdan SSSR."

55. GARF f. 8009, op. 1, d. 497, l. 192.

56. Jeffrey Brooks, *Thank You, Comrade Stalin! Soviet Public Culture from Revolution to Cold War* (Princeton, NJ: Princeton University Press, 2000), especially, pages 89–93. In the case of the draft ukase, the new subsidies were also presented as gifts. The comparison between *spravka* and draft ukase demonstrates that this representation was chosen deliberately.

57. GARF f. 8009, op. 1, d. 497, l. 165.

58. GARF f. 8009, op. 1, d. 497, l. 165.

59. The suggested "birth bonus" for a third child was 500 rubles. For the fourth child and up it ranged between 1,500 and 5,000 rubles. GARF f. 8009, op. 1, d. 497, l. 165.

60. The average number of children per married peasant woman, including stillborns, in Russia between 1897 and 1917 was nine. Iu. A. Poliakov et al. ed., *Naselenie Rossii v XX veke: Istoricheskie ocherki, 1900–1939*, t.1 (Moscow: ROSSPEN, 2000), 60. R. I. Sifman's 1960 study of family size based on three generations of women shows that the average number of children that peasant women bore was shrinking steadily: born to peasant women between 1890 and 1894: 5.54 children; born between 1895 and 1899, 5.43 children; born between 1900 and 1904, 4.86. Poliakov, *Naselenie Rossii*, 205. According to oral interviews conducted in the 1990s, peasant women born before 1912 gave birth between six and twenty times and lost one-third of the babies.

David Ransel, *Village Mothers: Three Generations of Change in Russia and Tataria* (Bloomington: Indiana University Press, 2000), 103. In 1945, the average number of children per peasant family was 3.5. Iu. A. Poliakov et al., ed., *Naselenie Rossii v XX veke, Istoricheskie ocherki,1940–1959,* t. 2 (Moscow: ROSSPEN, 2001), 243.

61. Mark Edele, "Veterans and the Village: The Impact of Red Army Demobilization on Soviet Urbanization, 1945–1955," *Russian History* 36 (2009): 159–182.

62. GARF f. 8009, op. 1, d. 497, l. 164.

63. There is no discussion of the human rights of the fetus in any of the documents concerned with reproduction. Because all policymakers agreed that population increase was the key goal, prevention and termination of life at any reproductive stage was considered harmful.

64. GARF f. 8009, op. 1, d. 497, l. 177. Due to venereal disease prevention measures, some condoms were made available to soldiers; however, in general, citizens had very limited access to contraceptive devices. In 1936, a secret directive was issued by Minzdrav ordering contraceptive devices to be withdrawn from sale. Peter Solomon, *Soviet Criminal Justice under Stalin* (Cambridge: Cambridge University Press, 1996), 212. However, this was apparently not enforced, as there were advertisements for contraception in the late 1930s. On this, see Sheila Fitzpatrick, *Everyday Stalinism: Ordinary Life in Extraordinary Times, Soviet Russia in the 1930s* (Oxford: Oxford University Press, 1999), 244, n13. Khrushchev's proposal makes it clear that no official ban on the production, advertisement, or sale of contraception existed prior to 1944.

65. GARF f. 8009, op. 1, d. 497, ll. 175–178.

66. E. A. Sadvokasova, *Sotsial'no-gigienicheskie aspekty regulirovaniia razmerov sem'i* (Moskva: Meditsina, 1969), 116. Clearly many Ukrainian women also gave birth to mixed children. According to a German report, Germans fathered 10,000 children with local women in Ukraine. Karel C. Berkhoff, *Harvest of Despair: Life and Death in Ukraine under Nazi Rule* (Cambridge, MA: Belknap Press of Harvard University Press, 2007), 182.

67. Under the new proposal, doctors would be sentenced to prison confinement for three to five years. Abortionists without special medical training would receive a five- to ten-year prison sentence. GARF f. 8009, op. 1, d. 497, l. 177.

68. "O zapreshchenii abortov, uvelichenii material'noi pomoshchi rozhenitsam, ustanovlenii gosudarstvennoi pomoshchi mnogosemeinym, rasshirenii seti rodil'nykh domov, detskikh iaslei i detskikh sadov, usilenii ugolovnogo nakazaniia za neplatezh alimentov i o nekotorykh uzmeneniiakh o zakonodatel'stve o razvodakh" (Postanovlenie TsIK i SNK SSSR ot 27 iiunia, 1936) in *Postanovleniia KPSS i Sovetskogo pravitel'stva ob okhrane zdorov'ia naroda* (Moskva: MEDGIZ, 1958), 264–265.

69. GARF f. 8009, op. 1, d. 497, ll. 176–177.

70. There are no accurate statistics on underground abortion. The TsSU statistics on illegal abortion reflected the number of botched abortion cases that ended up in hospitals and were reported by doctors. Whether the case would be reported as self-induced abortion to the prosecutor depended on the doctor's personal decision. See Chapter 2.

71. In 1950 the Soviet government adopted stricter controls over birth registration. One of the key discussion points was how the stillborn cases should be reported to the ZAGS, especially in cases where the mother went into labor without medical personnel present. Experts in forensic medicine suggested that each case of stillbirth outside of medical institutions be reported to the militia. The discussion suggests that there was an increased concern with infanticide being registered as stillbirth. GARF f. 8009, op. 32, d. 887, ll. 1–11.

72. GARF f. 8009, op. 1, d. 497, ll. 177–178.

73. GARF f. 8009, op. 1, d. 497, ll. 164–165.

74. *Izvestiia*, January 8, 1955.

75. "O naloge na kholostiakov, odinokikh i bezdetnykh grazhdan SSSR." The *spravka* refers to the discussion prior to the 1941 law. See GARF f. 8009, op. 1, d. 497, l. 171. This wartime tax of the childless probably needs to be understood also in the context of the desperate search for state revenue in time of war. On tax collectors' practical approach to increasing state revenue after the war, see Julie Hessler, "A Postwar Perestroika? Toward a History of Private Enterprise," *Slavic Review* 57, no. 3 (Fall 1998): 526–527.

76. Khrushchev would again combine demographic considerations with a new taxation system in the late 1950s. See Chapter 6.

77. GARF f. 8009, op. 1, d. 497, l. 171.

78. New rates for more detailed categories of citizens are listed in GARF f. 8009, op. 1, d. 497, ll. 161–172.

79. In this calculation, the costs of keeping one child in an orphanage run by the NKZ was set at 2,800 rubles, while those run by Narkompros (People's Commissariat for Education) cost 2,994 rubles. GARF f. 8009, op. 1, d. 497, ll. 172–173. (Here for the first time it becomes clear that what is being compared is the cost of a single mother raising a child and that of keeping a child in "detskie uchrezhdeniia").

80. GARF f. 8009, op. 1, d. 497, l. 172.

81. GARF f. 8009, op. 1, d. 497, l. 174.

82. GARF f. 8009, op. 1, d. 497, l. 174.

83. GARF f. 8009, op. 1, d. 497, l. 165.

84. GARF f. 8009, op. 1, d. 497, l. 166.

85. See "Absconding Husbands" in Fitzpatrick, *Everyday Stalinism*, 143–147. Some mothers also left children and had to pay child support. However, in the Soviet discussion of child support, it is generally assumed that it is the father who leaves the family and is therefore responsible for child support.

86. GARF f. 8009, op. 1, d. 497, l. 166.

87. GARF f. 8009, op. 1, d. 497, l. 166.

88. GARF f. 8009, op. 1, d. 497, l. 164.

89. GARF f. 8009, op. 1, d. 497, ll. 166–167.

90. GARF f. 8009, op. 1, d. 497, l. 180.

91. GARF f. 8009, op. 1, d. 497, l. 181.

92. GARF f. 8009, op. 1, d. 497, l. 181.

93. GARF f. 8009, op. 1, d. 497, l. 182.

94. The proposed procedure was as follows: (1) submit a petition to the court about intention to divorce accompanied by a payment of 100 rubles; (2) summon spouse and witnesses to the court; (3) publish the announcement of filing a divorce in a local newspaper at the expense of the plaintiff; (4) go through a court investigation which would assign post-divorce childcare responsibilities; (5) pay 300–1,000 rubles to register the divorce at ZAGS; and (6) make a note about the divorce in both spouses' passports. GARF f. 8009, op. 1, d. 497, ll. 182–183.

95. "Document no. 15: Criticism of the Institution of the *De Facto* Marriage," in Rudolf Schlesinger, *Changing Attitudes in Soviet Russia: The Family in the USSR, Documents and Readings* (London: Routledge & Kegan Paul, 1949), 348–362.

96. GARF f. 8009, op. 1, d. 497, l. 180.

97. Schlesinger, *Changing Attitudes in Soviet Russia*, 355. The Ukrainian interpretation of common-law marriage was discussed in the context of amending the Civil Code of the USSR in 1939, which was undertaken to eliminate variations among republics such as this one and to establish a cohesive All-Union position on family issues. However, this project was interrupted by the war, as was the discussion of the legal definition of common-law marriage.

98. GARF f. 8009, op. 1, d. 497, l. 180.

99. GARF f. 8009, op. 1, d. 497, l. 181. The Soviet government promoted "strengthening" the family first in the mid-1930s. David Hoffmann argues that in the mid-1930s the rhetoric of "strengthening the family" was used to promote familial obligations, while depriving the family of autonomy. David Hoffmann, *Stalinist Values: The Cultural Notions of Soviet Modernity, 1917–1941* (Ithaca, NY: Cornell University Press, 2003), 108.

100. GARF f. 8009, op. 1, d. 497, l. 167.

101. GARF f. 8009, op. 1, d. 497, ll. 164, 166, 167, 178, 179.

102. GARF f. 8009, op. 1, d. 497, l. 185. In the draft I have found only the phrase "women who are not married (*zhenshchiny, ne sostoiashchei v brake*)"; it is used once in the context of a discussion of crimes against the dignity of mothers. GARF f. 8009, op. 1, d. 497, l. 192.

103. GARF f. 8009, op. 1, d. 497, l. 169.

104. In July 1947, S. Kruglov, minister of Internal Affairs, reported to Stalin and Molotov about the increasing number of mothers with small children in prison and pregnant women who gave birth in prison. Their children who were kept in prisons, camps, and colonies were physically weak and needed special care. Kruglov proposed to release (approximately 15,000) women with children up to four years old and pregnant women who were imprisoned for petty crimes. GARF f. 9401, op. 2, d. 170, ll. 210–212. A second round, in February 1949, led to the release of mothers with children up to seven years old. GARF f. 9401, op. 2, d. 234, ll. 187–188.

105. GARF f. 8009, op. 6, d. 1917, ll. 3–4 and GARF f. 8009, op. 1, d. 527, l. 118. The Kremlin's medical-sanitary administration acquired a maternity home in order to improve its work in gynecology and obstetrics. GARF f. 8009, op. 1, d. 526, l. 23.

106. GARF f. 8009, op. 1, d. 497, ll. 169–170.

107. On new postwar social hierarchies based on participation in the Great Patriotic War, see Amir Weiner, *Making Sense of War: The Second World War and the Fate of the Bolshevik Revolution* (Princeton, NJ: Princeton University Press, 2001); in contrast, Mark Edele's study shows that veteran privileges were hardly automatic. Mark Edele, *Soviet Veterans of the Second World War: A Popular Movement in an Authoritarian Society, 1941–1991* (Oxford: Oxford University Press, 2008).

108. GARF f. 8009, op. 1, d. 497, l. 169.

109. RGASPI f. 82, op. 2, d. 387, l. 93.

110. GARF f. 8009, op. 1, d. 497, l. 179.

111. James Smith, "The Politics of Sexual Knowledge: The Origins of Ireland's Containment Culture and the Carrigan Report (1931)," *Journal of the History of Sexuality* 13, no. 2 (April 2004): 208–233.

112. GARF f. 8009, op. 1, d. 497, l. 169.

113. See GARF f. 8009, op. 1, d. 496, ll. 45-50 and RGASPI f. 82, op. 2, d. 387, ll. 87–89. A copy of the same letter was addressed to Malenkov, secretary of the Central Committee. GARF f. 8009, op. 1, d. 493, ll. 48–49.

114. GARF f. 8009, op. 1, d. 493, l. 48.

115. Born in 1899, in the postwar period, Merkov was head of the department of medical-sanitary statistics within the NKZ USSR. He was trained as a sanitary statistician in Khar'kov, Ukraine, in the prewar period. In 1941 he was evacuated from Khar'kov to Ufa, the capital city of the Autonomous Republic of Bashkiria. During the evacuation, he studied reproduction in Bashkiria and published "The Reproduction of Population in the Bashkiria ASSR on the Eve of the Great Patriotic War." He did not continue this analysis of the Bashkir population into the postwar era because he was brought to Moscow in August 1943. In Moscow, he continued his study of population reproduction, this time, on an all-Union scale. GARF f. 603, op. 1, d. 324, l. 2.

116. RGASPI f. 82, op. 2, d.387, l. 90.

117. RGASPI f. 82, op. 2, d.387, l. 91.

118. TsMAMLS f. 218, op. 1, d. 46, ll. 74–75.

119. "O nekotorom izmenenii poriadka rassmotreniia v sudakh del o rastorzhenii braka," December 10, 1965, in *Vedomosti verkhovnogo soveta SSSR*, 1965, no. 49, and "Ob utverzhdenii osnov zakonodatel'stva Soiuza SSR i soiuznykh respublik o brake i sem'e," June 27, 1968 in *Sbornik zakonov SSSR i ukazov prezidiuma verkhovnogo soveta SSSR*, t.3 (Moscow, 1968), 269.

120. RGASPI f. 82, op. 2, d. 387, l. 92.

121. RGASPI f. 82, op. 2, d. 387, l. 92.

122. RGASPI f. 82, op. 2, d. 387, l. 93.

123. RGASPI f. 82, op. 2, d. 387, l. 93. In this report, the data are described as a "breakdown of families (*raspredelenie semei*)." However, the table shows the number not of families but persons (*chelovek*). The report does not indicate whether the totals include both adult men and women. After comparing this 1944 projection with TsSU's 1942 data on mothers with many children (as defined by the 1936 law) where the number of women with seven or eight children was 293,500, mothers with nine and ten, 49,800, and mothers with eleven or more, 1,700, it appears that

Starovskii's statistics only include women. For the 1942 data, see RGASPI f. 82, op. 2, d. 387, l. 53.

124. RGASPI f. 82, op. 2, d. 387, l. 96. It is not clear how the projection of mothers with many children was calculated.

125. Here, the monthly government subsidy for single mothers is set to be 125 rubles for the first child, 225 rubles for the second child, and 325 rubles for the third and additional children. The listed amount for the third and additional child differs from the 300 rubles indicated in Khrushchev's draft ukase. This is one of the two pieces of evidence to suggest that there was another draft prepared after the time of Miterev's submission of his comments on May 3, 1944, and before May 30, 1944, when Narkomfin's estimated project cost was issued. For more evidence, see below in the section titled "The 'Birth' of the Mother Heroine and the Maternal Status Hierarchy."

126. RGASPI f. 82, op. 2, d. 387, ll. 94–95.

127. RGASPI f. 82, op. 2, d. 387, l. 95.

128. I will use the three scenarios as the basic texts for this comparison since the May draft ukase has not been made available to me. My assumption that the May draft is almost identical with the three scenarios is based on the informational notes attached to them, which informed Stalin of the minimal changes made to the May draft. RGASPI f. 82, op. 2, d. 387, ll. 114, 131, 149.

129. RGASPI f. 82, op. 2, d. 387, l. 156.

130. RGASPI f. 82, op. 2, d. 387, ll. 152, 157.

131. RGASPI f. 82, op. 2, d. 387, l. 158.

132. RGASPI f. 82, op. 2, d. 387, l. 152.

133. RGASPI f. 82, op. 2, d. 387, l. 152.

134. RGASPI f. 82, op. 2, d. 387, l. 152. On the other hand, the new maternal "honors" were awarded for cumulative reproductive contributions, regardless of postwar activities.

135. RGASPI f. 82, op. 2, d. 387, l. 152.

136. RGASPI f. 82, op. 2, d. 387, ll. 129, 146, 164.

137. RGASPI f. 82, op. 2, d. 387, ll. 130, 148, 165.

138. RGASPI f. 82, op. 2, d. 387, ll. 114, 131, 149.

139. RGASPI f. 82, op. 2, d. 387, l. 162.

140. RGASPI f. 82, op. 2, d. 387, l. 157.

141. GARF f. 8009, op. 1, d. 497, l. 191.

142. On the use of *malodetnye* and *odnodetnye sem'i* in Khrushchev's *spravka*, see GARF f. 8009, op. 1, d. 497, ll. 171, 174. On the use of *malosemeinye* in the draft ukase medal, see RGASPI f. 82, op. 2, d. 387, l. 157.

143. GARF f. 8009, op. 1, d. 497, l. 172.

144. GARF f. 8009, op. 1, d. 497, l. 190.

145. RGASPI f. 82, op. 2, d. 387, ll. 157–158.

146. RGASPI f. 82, op. 2, d. 387, l. 98.

147. RGASPI f. 82, op. 2, d. 387, l. 98.

148. RGASPI f. 82, op. 2, d. 387, l. 110.

149. As a result, mothers with three children would receive one-time government aid of 400 rubles instead of the originally proposed 500 rubles. Mothers with four children would receive one-time aid of 1,300 rubles instead of 1,500 rubles and monthly subsidies of 80 rubles instead of 100 rubles. Mothers with five children would receive one-time aid of 1,700 rubles instead of 2,000 rubles and monthly subsidies of 120 rubles instead of 150 rubles. Mothers with six children would receive one-time aid of 2,000 rubles as in the June draft ukase, but monthly subsidies of 140 rubles instead of 150 rubles. RGASPI f. 82, op. 2, d. 387, ll. 99–101.

150. In her memoirs Mary Leder, who was working in the TASS office in the spring of 1944, remembered having discussed the "draft" with her colleagues at a general TASS meeting. A young female editor, a member of Komsomol, the Communist youth organization, expressed a criticism at this meeting calling the law "reactionary" and "against all socialist principles." Komsomol later reprimanded her. Mary Leder, *My Life in Stalinist Russia: An American Woman Looks Back* (Bloomington: Indiana University Press, 2001), 255–256.

151. Leder, *My Life in Stalinist Russia*, 255.

152. *Sbornik zakonov SSSR i ukazov Prezidiuma Verkhovnogo Soveta SSSR: 1938–1967* tom 2 (Moskva: Izdatel'stvo Izvestiia Sovetov deputatov trudiashchikhsia SSSR, 1968), 418–419.

153. For example, see the image of Shafaat Khamidova, a Mother Heroine, in *Sovetskaia zhenshchina* 6 (1946). Many examples of glorification of fertile Central Asian mothers can be found especially in the Central Asian press. For example, see "Bol'shaia sem'ia," *Pravda Vostoka*, August 6, 1944; "Mat' geroinia," *Pravda Vostoka*, October 11, 1944; "Odna sem'ia," *Pravda Vostoka*, February 7, 1945; and "Vospitaem detei patriotami Rodinu," *Pravda Vostoka*, July 8, 1949.

154. Masako Kohama, *Chugoku kingendaini okeru boshieiseiseisakuno kenkyu* (A Study of Public Health Policy toward Mothers and Children in Modern and Contemporary China), a Research Report" published as the result of a 2002~2005 project funded by the Japan Society for the Promotion of Science (March 2006), 9. In 1949 Mao wrote, "It is a good thing that China has a big population. Even if China's population multiplies many times, she is fully capable of finding a solution; the solution is production." Thomas Scharping, *Birth Control in China 1949–2000: Population Policy and Demographic Development* (Abingdon, UK: Routledge Curzon, 2005), 51.

155. Masako Kohama, *Chugoku kingendaini okeru boshieiseiseisakuno kenkyu*, 120, 124.

156. Galina gave birth in the mid-1980s. Masha Gessen, *The Future Is History: How Totalitarianism Reclaimed Russia* (New York: Riverhead Books, 2017), 43.

157. *Machekha* (1973) was based on the story written by Mariia Khalfina and directed by Oleg Bondarev.

158. *Moskva slezam ne verit* (1979), directed by Vladimir Men'shov, won the Academy Award for Foreign Language Film in 1981.

159. Kollontai considered that free love meant love and union between economically mutually independent men and women in a society where children could be reared in public institutions, so that the responsibility of childrearing did not fall solely on single women's shoulders. Barbara Clements, *Bolshevik Feminist: The*

Life of Aleksandra Kollontai (Bloomington: Indiana University Press, 1979), 58. Farnsworth suggests that the 1944 Family Law's new state support for single mothers, as well as providing mothers the option of leaving the child at a state orphanage, could indeed be understood as a realization of Kollontai's earlier ideas. Beatrice Farnsworth, *Aleksandra Kollontai: Socialism, Feminism, and the Bolshevik Revolution* (Stanford, CA: Stanford University Press, 1980), 399.

Chapter 2

1. There are many possible reasons that increased punishment was not desirable or practicable. A probable practical reason was that if imprisoned women were mothers without close relatives, their children would become orphans, and the state would need to take care of them. Also, the judicial system would be quickly overburdened by thousands of criminal abortion cases. There were also moral reasons. Many doctors felt that many women deserved to have an abortion because of difficult wartime living conditions or their weakened physical health. Moreover, by imprisoning women in their prime of life, the Soviet state would lose both reproductivity and productivity, at least for the duration of the sentence.

2. Atina Grossmann, *Reforming Sex: The German Movement for Birth Control and Abortion Reform: 1920–1950* (New York: Oxford University Press, 1995), 189–199. For a pioneering study of Soviet mass rape in Germany, see Norman Naimark, *The Russians in Germany: The History of the Soviet Zone of Occupation, 1945–1949* (Cambridge, MA: Harvard University Press, 1995), 61–140. Rape by Red Army soldiers was reported not only in Germany but also other places captured by Soviet troops at the end of the war. Norman Naimark, *Stalin and the Fate of Europe: The Postwar Struggle for Sovereignty* (Cambridge, MA: Harvard University Press, 2019), 4, 207, 233–234.

3. Takashi Kamitsubo, *Mizukono Uta* [Songs of Unborn Children] (Tokyo: Shakai shisosha, 1993); Masaharu Shimokawa, *Bokyaku no Hikiageshi: Izumi Seiichito Futsukaichi Hoyojo* [A Forgotten History of Repatriation: Izumi Seiichi and Futsukaichi Sanatorium](Fukuoka: Gen shobo, 2017); Keitaro Takeda, *Chinmokuno yonjunen: Hikiage josei kyoseichuzetsuno kiroku* [Forty Years of Silence: Records of Forced Abortions on Repatriated Women] (Tokyo: Chuokoronsha, 1985). On rape in Manchuria, see also Sakura Furukubo, "Manshuni okeru nihonjin joseino keiken [Japanese Women's Experience in Manchuria]," in *Nihonno feminizumu* [Japan's Feminism], vol. 10, *Joseishi/Jenda-shi* [Women's History and Gender History], ed. Masako Amano (Tokyo: Iwanami shoten, 2009), 1–14.

4. Miho Ogino, *Kazoku keikakueno michi: Kindai nihonno seishokuo moguru seiji* [The Road to Family Planning: The Politics of Reproduction in Modern Japan](Tokyo: Iwanami shoten, 2008), 171–175; and Grossmann, *Reforming Sex*, 194.

5. In the Soviet zone, abortion became practically legal in 1947, but it was recriminalized in September 1950. Grossmann, *Reforming Sex*, 195–198.

6. Ogino, *Kazoku keikakueno michi*, 142–175.

7. Mie Nakachi "A Postwar Sexual Liberation? The Gendered Experience of the Soviet Union's Great Patriotic War," *Cahiers du monde russe* 51 (2011–2012): 423–440.

8. An earlier version of this discussion appeared in Mie Nakachi, "'Abortion Is Killing Us': Women's Medicine and the Postwar Dilemmas of Soviet Doctors, 1944–1946," in *Soviet Medicine: Culture, Practice, and Science*, ed. Frances Bernstein, Christopher Burton, and Daniel Healey (DeKalb: Northern Illinois University Press, 2010).

9. Elena Zubkova provides the general history of wartime and postwar liberalization, followed by political tightening in the late 1940s. Elena Zubkova, *Russia after the War: Hopes, Illusions, and Disappointments, 1945–1957* (Armonk, NY: M. E. Sharpe, 1998). The KR affair is the subject of Nikolai Krementsov, *The Cure: A Story of Cancer and Politics from the Annals of the Cold War* (Chicago: University of Chicago Press, 2002).

10. Peter Solomon, *Soviet Criminal Justice under Stalin* (Cambridge: Cambridge University Press, 1996), 212, 220.

11. The list of criteria is included in GARF f. 8009, op. 1, d. 105, ll. 90–91.

12. GARF f. 8009, op. 1, d. 105, l. 67.

13. GARF f. 8009, op. 1, d. 49, ll. 27–47.

14. With the criminalization of abortion, statistics became more complex and less accurate as underground abortion often escaped the count. Data were collected in five categories: (1) total number of abortions, (2) clinical abortion, (3) non-clinical abortion, (4) criminal abortion, and (5) the number of criminal cases reported to the prosecutor. These categories were defined and tabulated as follows:

> (1) The total number of abortions included clinical abortions in addition to non-clinical abortions and miscarriages that ended with the woman's hospitalization. There was no estimate of the overall number of abortions.
>
> (2) Clinical abortion included abortions performed by a doctor with permission from an abortion committee.
>
> (3) Non-clinical abortion included both miscarriages and abortions that ended in the woman's hospitalization.
>
> (4) Criminal abortion was the number of abortions that were prosecuted.
>
> (5) The number of abortions reported to the prosecutor was the number of cases that doctors reported to the prosecutor for further investigation.

When doctors discussed problems of abortion, they referred to either (1) total number of abortions or (3) non-clinical abortion. Doctors often referred to (3) the number of non-clinical abortions as "illegal" or "criminal" abortions because they considered that only a tiny fraction of this number were "unassisted" miscarriages. In August 1945, Dr. M. K. Gesberg argued that at his hospital, of all the reported cases of non-clinical abortion, only 2 percent were miscarriages. GARF f. 8009, op. 22, d. 53, l. 3.

For an overview of the history of Soviet abortion statistics, see Alexandre Avdeev, Alain Blum, and Irina Troitskaia, "The History of Abortion Statistics in Russia and the USSR from 1900 to 1991," *Population: An English Selection* 7 (1995): 39–66. However, because no "reliable" statistics were collected between 1936 and 1955, the authors do not cover the period on which this book focuses.

15. GARF f. 8009, op. 22, d. 53, ll. 9–11.

16. GARF f. 8009, op. 22, d. 53, ll. 11–13.

17. GARF f. 8009, op. 22, d. 27, l. 22 and GARF f. 8009, op. 6, d. 1911, ll. 83–84.

18. Iu. A. Poliakov et al., *Naselenie Rossii v XX veke: Istoricheskie ocherki*, tom 2, *1940–1959* (Moscow: ROSSPEN, 2001), 25.

19. For a discussion of stigmatized demobilized women, see Svetlana A. Alexievich, *U voiny ne zhenskoe litso. Poslednie svideteli: povesti* (Moskva: Sovetskii pisatel', 1988), 85, 171; and Barbara Alpern Engel and Anastasia Posadskaya-Vanderbeck, eds., *A Revolution of Their Own: Voices of Women in Soviet History* (Boulder, CO: Westview Press, 1998), 179.

20. GARF f. 8009, op. 22, d. 15, ll. 1–3.

21. GARF f. 8009, op. 22, d. 15, l. 3.

22. GARF f. 8009, op. 22, d. 30, l. 28.

23. GARF f. 8009, op. 22, d. 27, l. 22.

24. GARF f. 8009, op. 22, d. 30, l. 16.

25. GARF f. 8009, op. 22, d. 30, l. 30. At the 1944 Joint Plenum mentioned above, Dr. Vainshtein expressed his pleasure with the 1944 law, which seemed to have adopted his idea. In reality, reduction of abortion was not the most important concern when the policymakers discussed the minimum number of children necessary for a mother to receive state aid. However, it is interesting to see that the measure to increase births per mother coincided with a measure to prevent abortion.

26. GARF f. 8009, op. 22, d. 15, l. 3.

27. GARF f. 8009, op. 22, d. 15, l. 4.

28. No initials are available. Stenograms often do not indicate first names or initials. Last names, however, often reveal gender, since Russian female surnames usually end in the letter "a."

29. GARF f. 8009, op. 22, d. 15, ll. 8–9.

30. Except for 1937 and 1947. In 1937, the recorded number of legal and illegal abortions declined from 1.24 million (1936) to 0.57 million. Between 1938 and 1940, it increased from 0.69 million to 0.81 million. There is no record for 1941–1945. In 1946, 0.66 million abortions were reported. The number went down in 1947 to 0.58 million. However, between 1948 and 1954, it soared from 0.88 million to 1.9 million. TsMAMLS f. 218, op. 1, d. 187, l.46. It should be kept in mind that from 1937 to 1945, while abortion was illegal, recorded statistics were only the tip of the iceberg. All accounts suggest that unrecorded illegal abortions were several times the recorded numbers.

31. GARF f. 8009, op. 1, d. 497, l. 175.

32. GARF f. 8009, op. 22, d. 28, ll. 18–19. When the number of incomplete abortions and prosecuted criminal abortion cases for Ukraine increased in 1945, it was welcomed because it was understood as evidence of active participation in surveillance work. Clearly, this was an achievement after NKZ Ukraine had to issue instructions five times in 1945. GARF f. 8009, op. 22, d. 70, l. 98.

33. GARF f. 8009, op. 22, d. 29, l. 67.

34. When abortion had been legal, abortariums did exist in the USSR, which, for a foreign observer in the early 1930s was particularly noteworthy in describing the progressiveness of Soviet maternity care. Fannina Halle, *Women in Soviet Russia* (London: Routledge, 1933), 140.

35. See Dr. Polubinskii's discussion in Chapter 3 of Leningrad doctors' efforts at abortion prevention.

36. For example, see GARF f. 8009, op. 22, d. 96, l. 9.

37. During World War II, due to lack of medical personnel to treat soldiers, obstetricians, gynecologists, pediatricians, and anatomists were mobilized to take a quick course in military surgery. Mark Field, *Doctor and Patient in Soviet Russia* (Cambridge, MA: Harvard University Press, 1957), 24. There were a few gynecologists who worked in their specialization in the Red Army since the medical administration of the army added gynecological care in 1942. Professor I. F. Zhordania became the first gynecologist in the Red Army. GARF f. 8009, op. 1, d. 29, ll. 26–29. Gynecologists treated women in the military and civilians. Given the fact that most women in the army were young, it was important to preserve their reproductive health. Women in the army were supposed to have regular gynecological check-ups.

38. The number of births per 1,000 population fell from 35.3 in 1940 to 11.2 in 1943. RGASPI f. 82, op. 2, d. 387, ll. 35, 90.

39. GARF f. 8009, op. 1, d. 527, l. 54.

40. GARF f. 8009, op. 22, d. 56, l. 8.

41. Toward the end of the war (1943–1945), the infant mortality rate declined from 16 percent to 11 percent of all births, because by then only strong children had survived and the drastic fall in birth rate prevented new victims from arriving. Demographers N. A. Aralovets and O. M. Verbitskaia argue that the NKZ's improved sanitary and anti-epidemic measures played a significant role as well. Their analysis appeared in "Osobennosti smertnosti gorodskogo i sel'skogo naseleniia v tylu v 1941-1945gg.," *Naselenie Rossii v XX veke: Istoricheskie ocherki, 1940–1959*, tom 2 (Moskva: ROSSPEN, 2001), 96–97. The statistics are cited on page 125.

42. GARF f. 8009, op. 22, d. 54, l. 1.

43. In the postwar period, medical administrators tried to change this attitude. GARF f. 8009, op. 22, d. 56, ll. 8–17. In particular, Kovrigina, a pediatrician by training, argued that the most essential task of Soviet maternity care was the survival of children. GARF f. 8009, op. 22, d. 32, l. 122.

44. GARF f. 8009, op. 22, d. 57, ll. 38, 39, 100, 101.

45. The fact that doctors considered the life of the mother ultimately more important than that of the child may give an important insight into the reasons that postwar pronatalist policies did not produce a discourse about the rights of the fetus in the Soviet Union. At least two postwar conditions would have justified their focus on women. First, children who lived with mothers had much better lives in general than those who were in orphanages. Doctors would have thought it more important to save the life of a mother than that of her child, especially if the mother had other children, who would have become orphans after the mother's death. Second, from the perspective of population increase, rescuing the life and health of a mother and

preserving the possibility that she would have more children in the future seemed more logical than saving the life of one child.

46. GARF f. 8009, op. 22, d. 30, ll. 61–62.

47. GARF f. 8009, op. 22, d. 43, l. 2.

48. GARF f. 8009, op. 22, d. 56, l. 25.

49. GARF f. 8009, op. 22, d. 56, ll. 112–113.

50. GARF f. 8009, op. 22, d. 56, l. 49.

51. GARF f. 8009, op. 22, d. 11, ll. 14–16.

52. GARF f. 8009, op. 22, d. 12, l. 47.

53. Taking separate records of infertile and fertile women was probably urgent since women's infertility was not universally understood to be a disease up to this point, even among the specialists. Most likely, this meant that doctors did not have separate records on the history of diseases. On this point, agreeing with his colleague, Professor Pobedinskii commented that "infertile women need to be considered ill (bol'nye) and examined as such." GARF f. 8009, op. 22, d. 57, l. 91.

54. GARF f. 8009, op. 22, d. 57, ll. 69–70.

55. GARF f. 8009, op. 22, d. 57, l. 40.

56. GARF f. 8009, op. 22, d. 57, ll. 56–59.

57. GARF f. 8009, op. 22, d. 57, l. 91.

58. GARF f. 8009, op. 22, d. 57, l. 54.

59. GARF f. 8009, op. 22, d. 57, ll. 56–59.

60. GARF f. 8009, op. 22, d. 57, ll. 56, 66.

61. GARF f. 8009, op. 22, d. 57, ll. 74–75.

62. GARF f. 8009, op. 22, d. 67, l. 2.

63. GARF f. 8009, op. 22, d. 91, ll. 53–62.

64. GARF f. 8009, op. 22, d. 107, l. 8. Only after the end of criminalized abortion did doctors openly discuss the need to provide effective contraception to prevent abortions. The first conference seems to have taken place in Kiev in May 1959. Some of the papers from the conference were published in the professional journal *Obstetrics and Gynecology*. See O. K. Nikonchik, "Problema kontratseptsii i organizatsiia bor'by s abortami v SSSR," *Akusherstvo i ginekologiia* 6 (1959): 3-6; L. G. Stepanov, "Organizatsionnye voprosy problemy kontratseptsii," *Akusherstvo i ginekologiia* 6 (1959): 6-8; and E. F. Shamrai, "Problema kontratseptsii i puti ee dal'neishego razvitiia," *Akusherstvo i ginekologiia* 6 (1959): 8-10.

65. One could argue that prophylactic and educational approaches also operated on "fear," in the sense that women were expected to fear the damage of abortion to their health. However, this fear is qualitatively different from the fear of legal punishment.

66. GARF f. 8009, op. 22, d. 53, l. 3.

67. GARF f. 8009, op. 22, d. 53, l. 2.

68. GARF f. 8009, op. 22, d. 53, l. 6.

69. GARF f. 8009, op. 22, d. 53, l. 4

70. GARF f. 8009, op. 22, d. 53, l. 5.

71. GARF f. 8009, op. 22, d. 53, l. 2.

72. GARF f. 8009, op. 22, d. 53, ll. 3–6.

73. For example, in Moscow oblast, there were 5,000 clear cases of criminal abortion reported to the prosecutor, of which 2,700 cases were examined by the court in 1944. GARF f. 8009, op. 22, d. 53, l. 4.

74. GARF f. 8009, op. 22, d. 53, l. 6.

75. GARF f. 8009, op. 22, d. 53, l. 7.

76. GARF f. 8009, op. 1, d. 49, l. 85.

77. Field, 158. The provision of cash was dangerous as it is obviously a bribe, whereas gifts could be presented as a token of gratitude. James Heinzen, *The Art of the Bribe: Corruption under Stalin, 1943–1953* (New Haven, CT: Yale University Press, 2016), 111–115.

78. Alena Ledeneva, *Russia's Economy of Favours: Blat, Networking and Informal Exchange* (Cambridge: Cambridge University Press, 1998), 29–30. See also Sheila Fitzpatrick, "Blat in Stalin's Time," in *Bribery and Blat in Russia: Negotiating Reciprocity from the Middle Ages to the 1990s*, ed. Stephen Lovell, Alena Ledeneva, and Andrei Rogachevskii (New York: St. Martin's Press, 2000).

79. GARF f. 8009, op. 22, d. 57, ll. 30–31.

80. The number of abortions used here is the sum of the registered number of miscarriages and abortions. GARF f. 8009, op. 6, d. 1919, l. 3. On counting methods, see fn. 14 above. Professor L. S. Kaminskii's "Aborty v Leningrade v 1944 g." provides detailed analysis of prewar and wartime abortion in the city. GARF f. 8009, op. 6, d. 1919, ll. 1-12.

81. GARF f. 8009, op. 22, d. 58, ll. 44–45.

82. GARF f. 8009, op. 22, d. 58, ll. 44–45.

83. GARF f. 8009, op. 22, d. 58, ll. 46–48.

84. GARF f. 8009, op. 22, d. 58, l. 48.

85. GARF f. 8009, op. 22, d. 58, ll. 48–49.

86. GARF f. 8009, op. 22, d. 53, l. 1. The number of abortions consists of the total of non-clinical (*vnebol'nichnye*) abortions plus clinical abortions. Non-clinical abortions represent the number of botched abortions and miscarriages that required hospitalization. Approximately 15 percent of non-clinical abortions were believed to be spontaneous miscarriages. TsMAMLS f. 218, op. 1, d. 187, l. 48.

87. GARF f. 8009, op. 22, d. 53, l. 2.

88. GARF f. 8009, op. 22, d. 53, l. 2.

89. GARF f. 8009, op. 22, d. 53, l. 3.

90. GARF f. 8009, op. 22, d. 53, l. 3.

91. GARF f. 8009, op. 22, d. 53, l. 3.

92. GARF f. 8009, op. 22, d. 53, l. 3.

93. TsAGM f. 552, op. 3, d. 224, l. 10.

94. N. A. Semashko, "Ob etike sovetskogo vracha," *Gigiena i sanitariia*, nos. 1–2 (1945): 11–12, as cited in Christopher Burton, "Medical Welfare during Late Stalinism: A Study of Doctors and the Soviet Health System, 1945–1953" (PhD dissertation, University of Chicago, 2000), 253.

95. GARF f. 8009, op. 22, d. 53, l. 8.

96. GARF f. 8009, op. 22, d. 67, l. 4.

97. GARF f. 8009, op. 22, d. 69, ll. 34–44.

98. GARF f. 8009, op. 22, d. 76, ll. 4-5.

99. Yoram Gorlizki and Oleg Khlevniuk, *Cold Peace: Stalin and the Soviet Ruling Circle, 1945-1953* (Oxford: Oxford University Press, 2004), 32–35.

100. Professors Kliueva and Roskin publicly named the drug "KR" for the first time at a meeting of the Presidium of the Academy of Medical Sciences on March 13, 1947. It is an Russian abbreviation both for "kantseroliticheskaia reaktsiia (Cancerolitic reaction)" and "Kliueva and Roskin." V. D. Esakov and E. S. Levina, *Delo KR: Sudy chesti v ideologii i praktike poslevoennogo stalinizma* (Moskva: Institut RAN, 2001), 26–32.

101. In 1950, the MZ commission that studied Kliueva and Roskin's work concluded that "KR," the anti-cancer drug developed by them was not effective. GARF f. 8009, op. 32, d. 885, l. 150. For pathbreaking analysis of the most secret research on atomic energy, see David Holloway, *Stalin and the Bomb: The Soviet Union and Atomic Energy, 1939-1956* (New Haven, CT: Yale University Press, 1994).

102. Galina V. Zarechnak, *Academy of Medical Sciences of the USSR: History and Organization, 1944-1959*, Public Health Monograph No. 63 (US Department of Health, Education, and Welfare, 1960), 8.

103. Smith's appointment shortly thereafter as the first director of the US Central Intelligence Agency would only have confirmed Stalin's suspicions. Smith, in his 1950 memoir, *My Three Years in Moscow* (Philadelphia: Lippincott, 1950), 290–293, remembers the meeting with the "pure scientist" Roskin and the "pretty Dr. Klyueva" and half-regrets the "ignorance and impatience with official inertia" that made him push for a meeting that, in the end, only "caused trouble for two very remarkable people."

104. Efim I. Smirnov, *Meditsina i organizatsiia zdravookhraneniia* (Moskva: Meditsina, 1989), 7–9.

105. The French, American, and Spanish Academies of Medical Sciences were studied as models. GARF f. 8009, op. 1, d. 493, l. 71.

106. On details of such exchanges and the development of the KR affair, see Krementsov, *The Cure*. On the collaboration among the Soviet Union, the United Kingdom, and the United States on the development and mass production of penicillin, also see Krementsov, *The Cure*, 62–63.

107. The People's Commissariat of Health was reorganized as the Ministry of Health (MZ) in March 1946. The court of honor system was instituted in March 1947 by a decree on "the Courts of Honor in Ministries of SSSR and Central Departments" which ordered the organization of a court of honor in all ministries and central departments, beginning with the MZ, Trade, and Finance. Esakov and Levina, *Delo KR*, 130.

108. As this was the first of eighty-two Courts of Honor organized between 1947 and 1949, many representatives of local and central party and government organs reported on the event. One such example can be found in *Moskva poslevoennaia: 1945-1947* (Moskva: Mosgorarkhiv, 2000), 231–234.

109. For an example of a discussion of the Russian origin of medical knowledge, see B. I. Burde, "O prioritete russkikh akusherov-ginekologov (K istorii otechestvennoi nauki)," *Akusherstvo i ginekologiia* 6 (1949): 23–27.

110. This "purge" did not involve executions as in the Great Purges of the late 1930s. Instead, individuals were fired or demoted. An inspection of the Soviet Information Bureau (which oversaw international propaganda during World War II) by the Central Committee in the summer of 1946 found an "unacceptable concentration of Jews." (59) This finding guided the courts of honor, but rarely resulted in arrests. According to the top expert on the subject of late-Stalinist anti-Semitism, a new stage, including arrests and torture, began in 1948 and accelerated from 1949. On this, see Gennadi Kostyrchenko, *Out of the Red Shadows: Anti-Semitism in Stalin's Russia* (Amherst, NY: Prometheus Books, 1995), 59, 72, and Chapter Five "Escalation of the Anti-Jewish Purges" (179-247).

111. Smirnov's decision was motivated by Kovrigina herself, who had informed him that the institute had serious problems. Trained in military medicine, Smirnov knew little about maternity care, especially as he began his term as minister. He depended on Kovrigina on issues in this area and, consequently, she would have the fullest influence over the investigation. Smirnov states this clearly in his memoir. Smirnov, *Meditsina*, 287.

112. The final report does not indicate the date. GARF f. 8009, op. 22, d. 110, ll. 10–35.

113. GARF f. 8009, op. 1, d., 474, l. 46. *Rossiiskii nauchno-issledovatel'skii tsentr perinatologii, akusherstva, i ginekologii* (Moskva: Pressa, 1992), 8; V. I. Kulakov, V. A. Golubev, T. V. Lopatina, N. N. Malinkovskii, V. V. Chernaia, "Nauchnomu tsentru akusherstva ginekologii i perinatologii RAMN-50 let" (unpublished paper prepared for the fiftieth anniversary of the foundation of the institute, 1994), 3; and N. E. Granat and N. N. Malinkovskii, "100 letie so dnia sooruzheniia akusherskoi i ginekologicheskoi klinik v Moskve" (unpublished paper prepared for the 100th year anniversary since the organization of the first obstetric clinic in Moscow, 1989), 9–10. None of this celebratory literature mentions the incident that disgraced Malinovskii and caused his retirement as director of the institute. Malinovskii had made significant contributions to the organization of Soviet gynecological and obstetric care in the prewar period.

114. TsMAMLS f. 218, op. 1, d. 62, l. 60.

115. The leading cadre of the institute was 57 percent Russian and 36 percent Jewish. The percentage of Jewish doctors associated with the in-group in the letter (46 percent) would have been considered disproportionately high. The breakdown of personnel by nationality is provided in GARF f. 8009, op. 22, d. 111, l. 95. Regrettably, I cannot identify the nationality of T. A. Komissarova.

116. GARF f. 8009, op. 22, d. 110, l. 132.

117. GARF f. 8009, op. 22, d. 110, l. 132.

118. Of 100 patients examined by the investigators, 87 were not referred, suggesting that they came from private meetings.

119. TsMAMLS f. 218, op. 1, d. 61, l. 94.

120. All interview materials cited here are in GARF f. 8009, op. 22, d. 111, ll. 266–269. Information on the nationality of individual personnel was provided in GARF f. 8009, op. 22, d. 111, ll. 102–110.

121. GARF f. 8009. op. 22, d. 111, l. 10.

122. GARF f. 8009, op. 22, d. 111, l. 178. Some of these hand-written notes were filed in GARF f. 8009, op. 22, d. 110, ll. 3–17.

123. GARF f. 8009, op. 22, d. 111, l. 24.

124. His speech had been drafted by Smirnov, K. P. Gorshenin (Prosecutor General of the USSR), and G. F. Aleksandrov (the head of Agitprop) and further edited by Zhdanov. Krementsov, *The Cure*, 123-124.

125. GARF f. 8009, op. 22, d. 112, l. 47.

126. Compare GARF f. 8009, op. 22, d. 111, l. 95 and GARF f. 8009, op. 22, d. 112, l. 60.

127. GARF f. 8009, op. 22, d. 111, l. 95 and GARF f. 8009, op. 22, d. 112, l. 60.

128. The Finance Ministry's mid-level bureaucrats who proposed the legalization of the black market in the immediate postwar years were purged in the late 1940s. Julie Hessler, "A Postwar Perestroika? Toward a History of Private Enterprise," *Slavic Review* 57, no. 3 (Fall 1998): 516–542.

129. TsAGM f. 552, op. 3, d. 224, l. 10. This citation contrasts dramatically with Estrin's 1945 epigraph at the top of this chapter, laying out the "two options."

130. TsAGM f. 552, op. 3, d. 224, l. 10.

131. After receiving aid and guidance, in both cases, mothers ended up keeping the babies. GARF f. 8009, op. 22, d. 30, ll. 11–15.

132. TsAGM f. 552, op. 3, d. 224, l. 4.

133. TsAGM f. 552, op. 3, d. 224, l. 12.

134. GARF f. 8009, op. 22, d. 174, ll. 1–8.

Chapter 3

1. My understanding of the Russian terms discussed above comes from my interviews with elderly women who raised children in the immediate postwar era and from reading women's letters and other documents written in the 1940s and 1950s.

2. GARF f. 9492, op. 1, d. 1630, l. 180.

3. Soviet women's practice of calling a sexually involved relationship that produced offspring a "marriage" and the father a "husband" continued after 1944. On this, see Mie Nakachi, "Gender, Marriage, and Reproduction in the Postwar Soviet Union," in *Writing the Stalin Era: Sheila Fitzpatrick and Soviet Historiography*, ed. Golfo Alexopolous, Kiril Tomoff, and Julie Hessler (New York: Palgrave Macmillan, 2011), 101–116.

4. Sinel'nikova to M. Kalinin, chairman of the Presidium of the Supreme Soviet, the nominal head of the Soviet state. GARF, f. 9492, op. 1, d. 1635, l. 1.

5. Fabrice Virgili, *Shorn Women: Gender and Punishment in Liberation France*, trans. John Flower (London: Bloomsbury, , 2002), 177–217.

6. Between 1945 and 1955 the proportion of out-of-wedlock children to all births ranged between 14.5 and 19.7 percent. Since this was lower than the approximately 25 percent of postwar births predicted by the Central Statistical Administration (TsSU) in 1944, Kremlin leaders might have been somewhat disappointed with the final results, but they did not change the policy. RGAE f. 1562, op. 33, d. 2638, l. 76.

7. For the birth of the 1944 Family Law, see Chapter 1.

8. An earlier version of this discussion appeared in Nakachi, "Gender, Marriage, and Reproduction in the Postwar Soviet Union."

9. Mark Edele, *Soviet Veterans of the Second World War: A Popular Movement in an Authoritarian Society, 1941–1991* (Oxford: Oxford University Press, 2008), 73–78.

10. Barbara Alpern Engel and Anastasia Posadskaya-Vanderbeck, eds. *A Revolution of Their Own: Voices of Women in Soviet History*, trans. Sona Hoisinton (Boulder, CO: Westview Press, 1998), 179; Svetlana Alexievich, *U voiny ne zhenskoe litso: Poslednie svideteli* (Moskva: Sovetskii pisatel', 1988), 85.

11. Alexievich, *U voiny*, 171.

12. Alexievich, *U voiny*, 225.

13. Alexievich, *U voiny*, 66–67.

14. Alexievich, *U voiny*, 67.

15. This suggests that despite the formulation of the 1944 Family Law, it was possible for an unofficial wife to register a child under the name of the biological father, depending on place and time. This certainly reflects the mother's will but might also reflect bureaucratic failure or reluctance to implement the law.

16. GARF f. 8131, op. 28, d. 2566, ll. 44–77.

17. Vera Ketlinskaia, "Nastia," in *Den' prozhityi dvazhdy* (1945) cited in Lisa Kirschenbaum, *The Legacy of the Siege of Leningrad, 1941–1995: Myth, Memories, and Monuments* (Cambridge: Cambridge University Press, 2006), 108–110.

18. Interview with Irina in Moscow on November 9, 2002.

19. The rate of male plaintiffs was lowest in Moscow, where 59 percent of the selected divorce cases were filed by men. GARF f. 9492, op. 1, d. 492, l. 57. Other regions recorded 60–80 percent. GARF f. 9492, op. 1, d. 492, l. 151.

20. GARF f. 9492, op. 1, d. 491, l. 50.

21. GARF f. 9492, op. 1, d. 491, ll. 2, 50, 72.

22. In the RSFSR, the top reason was "existence of another marriage" (28.1 percent), the second, "family quarrels, squabbling, dissimilarity of characters" (26.9 percent), and the third, "infidelity" (16.9 percent). GARF f. 9492, op. 1, d. 491, l. 94. In Ukraine, the top reason was infidelity (36 percent), the second reasons were "de facto marital relationship with another woman" (28 percent), and "family quarrels and incompatible characters" (28 percent). GARF f. 9492, op. 1, d. 491, ll. 2–3.

23. GARF f. 9492, op. 1, d. 491, ll. 151–152.

24. GARF f. 9492, op. 1, d. 1630, l. 107.

25. GARF f. 9492, op. 1, d. 1630, l. 141.

26. GARF f. 9492, op. 1, d. 1630, l. 101.

27. GARF f. 9492, op. 1, d. 1630, l. 165.

28. Letter written by I. T. Avdeev, a World War II invalid, in 1944. GARF f. 9492, op. 1, d. 1630, l. 232.

29. GARF f. 9492, op. 1, d. 1630, ll. 223–224.

30. GARF f. 9492, op. 1, d. 1630, l. 205.

31. GARF f. 9492, op. 1, d. 1630, ll. 158, 16.

32. GARF f. 9492, op. 1, d. 1630, l. 234.

33. GARF f. 9492, op. 1, d. 1630, l. 232.

34. GARF f. 9492, op. 1, d. 491, l. 11.

35. GARF f. 9492, op. 1, d. 491, ll. 105–107.

36. GARF f. 9492, op. 1, d. 1635, l. 38. The archival material does not indicate whether Sychkov was granted a divorce.

37. GARF f. 9492, op. 1, d. 491, ll. 18, 108, 178. This L'vov divorce case (l. 178) serves as a clear example of guilt by infection. The wife seems to have been granted a divorce.

38. GARF f. 9492, op. 1, d. 491, l. 20. Although statistically inconclusive, the cases above suggest a special interest in fertility in Central Asia.

39. GARF f. 9492, op. 1, d. 491, l. 107.

40. GARF f. 9492, op. 1, d. 491, l. 95.

41. GARF f. 9492, op. 1, d. 491, l. 12.

42. GARF f. 9492, op. 1, d. 1630, ll. 261–262.

43. GARF f. 9492, op. 1, d. 1630, l. 137. For a similar case, see GARF f. 9492, op. 1, d. 1635, l. 1.

44. GARF f. 9492, op. 1, d. 1630, l. 188.

45. GARF f. 9492, op. 1, d. 1630, l. 172.

46. GARF f. 9492, op. 1, d. 1630, l. 182.

47. GARF f. 9492, op. 1, d. 1630, l. 180. I thank Mark Edele for pointing out that a "small screw of the grandiose government machine" is a direct quotation from Stalin's 1945 speech. "Priem v Kremle v chest' uchastnikov parada pobedy," *Pravda*, June 27, 1945, 2.

48. GARF f. 9492, op. 1, d. 1630, l. 177.

49. GARF f. 9492, op. 1, d. 1630, l. 115.

50. GARF f. 9492, op. 1, d. 1630, ll. 133–134.

51. GARF f. 9492, op. 1, d. 1630, l. 153.

52. GARF f. 9492, op. 1, d. 1630, l. 145.

53. This is likely to have been arranged privately. According to the prewar law, the child support payment for one child was 25 percent, for two children 33 percent, and for three or more children, 50 percent of salary.

54. GARF f. 9492, op. 1, d. 1630, l. 282.

55. GARF f. 9492, op. 1, d. 1630, l. 281.

56. GARF f. 9492, op. 1, d. 1630, ll. 227–228.

57. GARF f. 9492, op. 1, d. 1630, l. 226.

58. GARF f. 9492, op. 1, d. 1614, l. 117.

59. GARF f. 9492, op. 1, d. 1616, l. 1.

60. See the November 10, 1944, law, "On recognition of *de facto* conjugal relations in case of the death or 'Missing in Action at the Front' status of one of the spouses" in *Vedomosti verkhovnogo Soveta SSSR* 60 (1944), as cited in *Sbornik zakonov SSSR i ukazov prezidiuma verkhovnogo soveta SSSR (1938-iiul'-1956 gg.* (Moscow: Gosudarstvennoe izdatel'stvo Iuridicheskoi lit., 1956), 388.

61. The NKIu and the Red Army conducted a long correspondence to settle the issue of who should become responsible for establishing marital relations, while complaints from wives flooded both organs. For the details of this correspondence, see GARF

f. 9492, op. 1, d. 1614, ll. 106–119. Regarding aid and pensions for the families of soldiers and non-commissioned officers, see GARF f. 9492, op. 1, d. 1616, ll. 1–12. In the end, all wives of missing and dead soldiers became eligible for establishing the fact of prewar marriage. On this, see GARF f. 5446, op. 46, d. 2315, l. 4.

62. GASO-E f. 498, op. 1, d. 470, ll. 1–9. I am not citing family names of individuals from this archive because I was given access to court files with the understanding that in order to protect privacy rights, I would not copy down individuals' family names. For another example, see GASO-E f. 498, op. 1, d. 499, ll. 1–3.

63. GASO-E f. 498, op. 1, d. 605, ll. 1–3.

64. GASO-E f. 498, op. 1, d. 438, ll. 1–6.

65. TsAGM f. 819, op. 3, d. 32, ll. 1–116.

66. GARF f. 9492, op. 1, d. 1634, l. 88.

67. Nikolai Mikhailovich Rychkov (1897–1959) was the People's Commissar of Justice of the USSR (USSR Minister of Justice after March 1946) between January 1938 and January 1948. V. I. Ivkin, *Gosudarstvennaia vlast' SSSR: vysshie organy vlasti i upravleniia i ikh rukovoditeli, 1923–1991* (Moskva, ROSSPEN, 1999), 506–507.

68. Handwritten editing. GARF f. 9492, op. 1, d. 1634, l. 90. Article 21 stated that "the child of an unregistered marriage is registered under the mother's last name with the patronymic of her choice." *Sbornik zakonov SSSR i ukazov prezidiuma verkhovnogo soveta SSSR (1938-iiul' 1956 gg.)* (Moskva: Gosudarstvennoe izdatel'stvo iuridicheskoi literatury, 1956), 387.

69. GARF f. 9492, op. 1, d. 1634, ll. 86–90.

70. GARF f. 9492, op. 1, d. 1634, l. 93.

71. A contemporary source rumored that this law was to protect wives from wartime girlfriends. Mary Leder, *My Life in Stalinist Russia: An American Woman Looks Back* (Bloomington: Indiana University Press, 2001), 255. Similarly, it has been argued that the 1944 Family Law was a measure to "resolve the confusion over alimony before the return of demobilized soldiers from the front." Lauren Kaminsky, "Utopian Visions of Soviet Family Life in the Stalin-Era Soviet Union," *Central European History* 44 (2011): 83. However, in addition to the archival materials that delineate the background to the 1944 Family Law, as presented in Chapter 1, the issuance of supplementary NKIu instructions exactly on this issue proves conclusively that alimony was not the central concern of the drafters of the 1944 Family Law.

72. GARF f. 9492, op. 1, d. 491, l. 2.

73. GARF f. 9492, op. 1, d. 1634, ll. 93–94.

74. GARF f. 9492, op. 1, d. 491, ll. 94, 152.

75. GARF f. 9492, op. 1, d. 491, l. 96.

76. GARF f. 9492, op. 1, d. 491, l. 162.

77. GARF f. 9492, op. 1, d. 491, l. 94.

78. GARF f. 9492, op. 1, d. 1635, l. 50.

79. GARF f. 9492, op. 1, d. 491, l. 56.

80. GARF f. 9492, op. 1, d. 1635, ll. 51–55.

81. Among the civil court cases for 1944–1955 that were made available to me in the State Archive of Saratov oblast (GASO), I found 247 cases of "*alimenty* (alimony)" as

opposed to one divorce case. Because many files were destroyed (by fire, etc.) it is not clear how many of the "alimenty" cases were child support cases, but I presume that many were. GASO f. 3035, op. 1, op. 3, op. 5, op. 6, op. 8, op. 10, op. 12, op. 14, op. 16, op. 18, op. 20, op. 22. In GASO's branch in Engels, Saratov oblast, among the civil court cases for 1944–1950 made available to me, there were 19 "alimenty" cases and one divorce case. Gosudarstvennyi arkhiv Saratovskoi oblasti, filial v gorode Engel's (GASO-E), f. 1782, op. 1; f. 498, op. 1; f. 1225, op. 1.

82. GASO-E f. 498, op. 1, d. 462, ll. 1–12.

83. GASO, f. 3035, op. 3, d. 192, ll. 1–7.

84. GASO-E, f. 498, op. 1, d. 467, ll. 1–6.

85. The data for 1940, 1942, and 1943 involve urban areas of rear regions (without the Western front and occupied areas). The 1942 data include rear regions and Leningrad and Stalingrad oblasti. There was no equivalent data for 1945. Source: Iu. A. Poliakov et al., *Naselenie Rossii v XX veke: Istoricheskie ocherki tom 2. 1940–1959* (Moskva: ROSSPEN, 2001), 220–221.

86. The 1946–1955 data represent all areas of the RSFSR, except for 1946, which excludes the Far East and Far West peripheral areas of Nizhne-Amur, Kamchatka, Sakhalin, Kaliningrad oblasti and Khabarovsk krai. Source: Poliakov et al., *Naselenie Rossii*, 351.

87. Poliakov et al., *Naselenie Rossii*, 351.

88. Although social taboos and politically embarrassing results were sufficient reason to avoid this topic in the Soviet period, the way in which family policy undermined official statistics would have made (and continues to make) quantitative analysis difficult. But the qualitative contours of the problem-complex and the order of magnitude (millions/tens of millions) of those affected by these issues can now be gauged.

89. Edward Cohn's study demonstrates that party disciplining of party members' misconduct in marriage and family life began in the late 1940s and increased in number in the Khrushchev period. On the other hand, punishments were harsher under Stalin, and often included exclusion from the party. See Chapter 5 of Edward Cohn, *The High Title of a Communist: Postwar Party Discipline and the Values of the Soviet Regime* (DeKalb: Northern Illinois University Press, 2015).

90. RGASPI f. 6, op. 6, d. 4, l. 20.

91. The following examples were taken from letters listed in an NKIu report (dated September 30, 1944) examining questions addressed to M. I. Kalinin. GARF f. 9492, op. 1, d. 1635, ll. 1–2.

92. GARF f. 9492, op. 1, d. 1635, l. 1.

93. GARF f. 9492, op. 1, d. 1635, l. 1.

94. GARF f. 9492, op. 1, d. 1635, l. 2.

95. A. Abramova is probably the KPK investigator mentioned in Sheila Fitzpatrick, *Tear Off the Masks!*, 247–248. A. Abramova appears as a "journalist" who reported to Stalin and Zhdanov on May 1948 about difficult conditions among mothers and pregnant women regarding the June 4, 1947 ukase on petty theft in V. F. Zima, *Golod v SSSR 1946–1947 godov: proiskhozhdenie i posledstviia* (Moskva: Institut Rossiiskoi istorii, 1996), 117, and her specialty seems to have been the welfare of children and women. RGASPI f. 17, op. 118, d. 255, ll. 42–48.

96. RGASPI f. 17, op. 118, d. 255, l. 49. I would like to thank Hiroshi Nagao for drawing my attention to this material.

97. As with Khrushchev's *spravka*, the internal nature of the Abramova report, classified as a "special file" made it possible to openly address, within a strictly limited audience, the linkages between reproduction and illegitimacy.

98. RGASPI f. 17, op. 118, d. 255, ll. 49–50.

99. RGASPI f. 17, op. 118, d. 255, l. 53.

100. GARF f. 8009, op. 32, d. 949, ll. 23–25.

101. RGASPI f. 17, op. 118, d. 255, l. 54.

102. Both amounts were per child per year. The main expense in orphanages was personnel salaries.

103. RGASPI f. 17, op. 118, d. 255, ll. 54–55. The mortality rates were similar to those for the GULAG. In 1947, of all children held in "camps and colonies," 40.1 percent died. Poliakov et al., *Naselenie Rossii*, 196.

104. RGASPI f. 17, op. 118, d. 255, l. 55.

105. On prostitution in Imperial Russia, see Laurie Bernstein, *Sonia's Daughters: Prostitutes and Their Regulation in Imperial Russia* (Berkeley: University of California Press, 1995).

106. These statistics do not separate "single mothers" living in one-parent households from those cohabiting with new partners. According to the published procedure for state aid payment to single mothers, either the militia or house-management office could certify the eligibility for state aid in urban areas, whereas in rural areas only the executive committee could do so. "Polozhenie o poriadke naznacheniia i vyplaty gosudarstvennykh posobii i predostavlenii l'got beremennym zhenshchinam, mnogodetnym i odinokim materiam," in *Sobranie postanovlenii i rasporiazhenii pravitel'stva Soiuza Sovetskikh Sotsialisticheskikh Respublik* no. 11 (September 14, 1944), 221. However, Abramova's letter implies that militia involvement was more common than that of house-management.

107. RGASPI f. 17, op. 118, d. 255, ll. 55–56.

108. RGASPI f. 17, op. 118, d. 255, l. 56.

109. GARF f. 9492, op. 1, d. 1936, l. 19. In a later letter to the editor of *Literaturnaia gazeta*, such practitioners were labeled "khans (*ottsy-khany*)." *Literaturnaia gazeta*, August 28, 1954.

110. This report was likely to have been prepared after the Commission's January 25, 1949, meeting, where Minzdrav was ordered to prepare a detailed proposal. At this meeting, not Kovrigina, but Smirnov, the Minister of Health, represented MZ. RGASPI f. 17, op. 118, op. 255, ll. 79–81.

111. According to the 1944 Family Law, government support would be paid until the child turned 12.

112. Kovrigina's memo included a reminder that until the 1944 Family Law was issued, single mothers had received child support from the moment when pregnancy was established. Single mothers should be exempted from small-family taxes because "their material and moral situation is inferior to that of bachelors and [two-parent] families with less than three children." TsMAMLS f. 218, op. 1, d. 46, ll. 64–67.

113. TsMAMLS f. 218, op. 1, d. 46, ll. 74–75.

114. GARF f. 9474, op. 10, d. 68, l. 10.

115. Zh. Gausner, "Vot my i doma (Home again)," *Zvezda* no. 11, 1947, as cited in Vera Dunham, *In Stalin's Time: Middleclass Values in Soviet Fiction* (Durham, NC: Duke University Press, 1990), 102–103.

116. Since she went to school after coeducation had ended in 1943, her classmates were all women. Interview with Irina on November 9, 2002, in Moscow.

117. Interview with Liudmila on January 12, 2003, in Moscow. She was in Leningrad during the siege and postwar years. Interview with Lena on November 27, 2002, in Moscow.

118. The replacement of child support by state aid at comparable levels was Khrushchev's original idea, but as discussed in Chapter 1, state aid to single mothers was reduced in successive drafts of the 1944 law, and again in 1947.

119. See "O razmere gosudarstvennogo posobiia mnogodetnym i odinokim materiam" in *Vedomosti Verkhovnogo Soveta SSSR* 41 (1947), as reproduced in *Sbornik zakonov SSSR i ukazov prezidiuma verkhovnogo soveta SSSR, 1938–1967*, tom 2 (Moskva: Izdatel'stvo "Izvestiia sovetov deputatov trudiashchikhsia SSSR," 1968), 418–419.

120. The rate of illegitimacy was 15 percent in 1959 and 12.5 percent in 1966. See Poliakov, et al., *Naselenie Rossii*, 230; and D. I. Valentei, ed., *Demograficheskii analiz rozhdaemosti* (Moskva: Statistika, 1974), 55, respectively. The 1968 All-Union Basic Family Code made it possible for paternal information to be entered by unmarried mothers into children's birth certificates and ZAGS documents. Actual last names and patronymics could be used with paternal consent or by court order. Alternatively, mothers could use their own last name, in the masculine gender. In either case, no damning blanks would be immediately visible for all to see. See Chapter 6.

121. For the period from 1945 to 1966, the percentage of out-of-wedlock births in the USSR was always higher than that of France, Germany, the United Kingdom, and the United States. The Soviet data can be found in RGAE f. 1562, op. 33, d. 2638, l. 76. For the other countries' data, see Institut national d'études démographiques - Developed countries database, http://www.ined.fr/en/pop_figures/bdd_conjoncture/ (last accessed on September 11, 2020).

Chapter 4

1. These data and quote were taken from RGAE f. 1562, op. 329, d. 2634, l. 3; TsMAMLS f. 218, op. 1, d. 187, l. 46. In his magisterial *Demograficheskaia modernizatsiia Rossii, 1900–2000* (Moskva: Novoe izdatel'stvo, 2006), Anatolii Vishnevskii has a sub-chapter entitled "Why Was There No Baby Boom in Russia?" (pp. 163–69) in which the long-term culprit is Russia's continuing urbanization after the war. A table of birth rates on page 165 shows thirteen countries where birth rates rose more than 30 percent, comparing the periods 1936–1940 and 1946–1950. For the same comparison, only Russia and Ukraine fell by over 30 percent, the very opposite of a "baby boom."

2. RGASPI f. 17, op. 118, d. 255, l. 53.
3. For a detailed treatment of Soviet statisticians and their purge in the 1930s, see Alain Blum and Martine Mespoulet, *L'anarchie bureaucratique: Statistique et pouvoir sous Staline* (Paris: La Découverte, 2003). Also available in Russian translation as *Biurokraticheskaia anarkhiia: statistika i vlast' pri Staline* (Moskva: ROSSPEN, 2006).
4. Before Starovskii became director, three predecessors—N. Osinskii (V. V. Obolenskii), I. A. Kraval, and I. D. Vermenichev—were purged and killed in quick succession. V. I. Ivkin, *Gosudarstvennaia vlast' SSSR: vysshie organy vlasti i upravleniia i ikh rukovoditeli 1923–1991* (Moskva: ROSSPEN, 1999), 446–47, 365, 247; and Blum and Mespoulet, *L'anarchie bureaucratique*, 131, 181.
5. This refers to the title of Blum and Mespoulet, *L'anarchie bureaucratique*. See also M. S. Tol'ts, "Nedostupnoe izmerenie," *V chelovecheskom izmerenii*, A. N. Alekseev and A. G. Vishnevskii, eds. (Moskva: Progress, 1989), 325–42 .
6. A demographic institute had existed at Kiev within the USSR Academy of Sciences since the 1920s and in Leningrad since 1931, but both were closed in the 1930s.
7. These included V. S. Nemchinov, M. V. Ptukha, S. G. Strumilin, and B. Ts. Urlanis.
8. RGAE f.1562, op. 327, d.114, ll. 32–38.
9. Starovskii developed the method for so-called quick censuses, one-time countings, during the war, which was used for the postwar period as well. G. K. Oksenoit, "Vladimir Starovskii," *Vestnik statistiki* 12 (1988): 45.
10. RGAE f. 1562, op. 33, d. 2990, l. 49, 54.
11. Matthew Connelly, *Fatal Misconception: The Struggle to Control World Population* (Cambridge, MA: Harvard University Press, 2008), 142.
12. Connelly, *Fatal Misconception*, 127.
13. Miho Ogino, *Kazokukeikakueno michi: Kindainihonno seishokuo meguru seiji* [The Road to Family Planning: The Politics of Reproduction in Modern Japan] (Tokyo: Iwanami shoten, 2008), 139–40.
14. Rickie Solinger, "Bleeding Across Time: First Principles of US Population Policy," in *Reproductive States: Global Perspectives on the Invention and Implementation of Population Policy*, ed. Rickie Solinger and Mie Nakachi (New York: Oxford University Press, 2016), 70–73.
15. RGAE f. 1562, op. 33, d. 2638, l. 76.
16. RGASPI f. 82, op. 2, d. 538, ll. 59–64. In 1945, men and women between 16 and 54 were included. In 1948, women between 16 and 54 and men between 16 and 59 were included. Thus, the increase between these years does not fully reflect the actual increase in the number of adult males in 1948.
17. In 1950, the TsSU reported basic demographic data to Molotov on a monthly basis, including births, deaths, marriages, and divorces. RGASPI f. 82, op. 2, d. 538, ll. 75-92.
18. TsMAMLS f. 218, op. 1, d. 187, l. 46.
19. RGAE f. 1562, op. 329, d. 2634, l. 3.
20. RGASPI f. 82, op. 2, d. 538, ll. 71–72.
21. Abortion data are taken from TsMAMLS f. 218, op. 1, d. 187, l. 46. According to these statistics, there were 206,000 more abortions recorded for September–December 1948 than for the same months in 1947. Aside from the possibility that there were so

many more abortions in 1948, conscious underreporting in late 1947 and increased reporting in late 1948 are possible causes for this rise. Throughout this book, I use reported numbers not as accurate reflections of reality but as the numerical basis for future policies.

22. These data were taken from RGAE f. 1562, op. 329, d. 2634, l. 3.

23. For detailed analysis of the famine, see V. F. Zima, *Golod v SSSR, 1946–1947 godov: proiskhozhdenie i posledstviia* (Moskva: Izdatel'stvo tsentr instituta Rossiiskoi istorii RAN, 1996).

24. I thank Donald Filtzer for pointing out commonalities in the discussion of amenorrhea as the cause of low birth rate after famine. Filtzer's work points out that the post-famine fall in births took place primarily in urban areas rather than in rural areas where famine more severely affected food consumption. See Donald Filtzer, "The 1947 Food Crisis and Its Aftermath: Worker and Peasant Consumption in Non-Famine Regions of the RSFSR," in *The Dream Deferred: New Studies in Russian and Soviet Labour History*, ed. Donald Filtzer, Wendy Z. Goldman, Gijs Kessler, and Simon Pirani (Bern: Peter Lang, 2008). For discussion of postwar amenorrhea, see Mie Nakachi "'Abortion Is Killing Us': The Postwar Dilemma of Women's Medicine," *Soviet Medicine: Culture, Practice, and Science*, ed. Frances Bernstein, Christopher Burton, and Dan Healey (Dekalb: Northern Illinois University Press, 2010). V. F. Zima argues that the number of deaths in the RSFSR was highest in the summer of 1947. This would also explain the fact that in the first half year of 1948, the number of births was 28 percent less than for the same period in 1947. Zima, *Golod v SSSR*, 162–69.

25. Among Russian peasants most conceptions took place during the post-harvest months. This meant that the number of births would increase in late spring to early summer. On this, see David Ransel, *Village Mothers: Three Generations of Change in Russia and Tartaria* (Bloomington: Indiana University Press, 2000), 27 and 185. On variations of seasonality among different nationalities, see David Ransel, "Mothering, Medicine, and Infant Mortality in Russia: Some Comparisons," *Kennan Institute for Advanced Studies Occasional Paper*, no. 236 (1990).

26. RGASPI f. 82, op. 2, d. 538, l. 71. Allowing the effects of collectivization-related famine to be too visible in the 1937 census led to the suppression of both the data and the demographers who had processed it. Starovskii had learned this terrifying lesson well.

27. The data for 1949 births were taken from RGAE f. 1562, op. 33, d. 2638, l. 76. My thanks to Donald Filtzer for pointing this out to me. His data from RGAE f. 1562, op. 329, d. 3807, l. 1 show the same number of births.

28. Another important factor affecting the postwar conception rate and birth rate was mass demobilization. The rising number of abortions in 1947 must have been particularly alarming, since it would have meant a missed opportunity to continue the postwar baby boom as the final cohorts were released from military service. By the end of 1947, five of the six waves of postwar demobilization totaling at least 8.5 million men had already taken place. Mark Edele, *Soviet Veterans of the Second World War: A Popular Movement in an Authoritarian Society, 1941–1991* (Oxford: Oxford University Press, 2008), 22–23, 231.

29. Khrushchev's letter to Stalin is dated as "no earlier than September 20, 1946" in *Holod v Ukraïni, 1946-1947 : dokumenty i materialy*, ed. O.M. Veselova, et al. (Kiiv: Vidavnitstvo M. P. Kots', 1996), 64–65.

30. RGASPI f. 82, op. 2, d. 538, ll. 55–57.

31. There is evidence that a small-scale survey of illegal abortion took place at the local level as early as 1946 or 1947. For Saratov, see GARF f. 8009, op. 22, d. 223, ll. 64, 67.

32. GARF f. 8009, op. 22, d. 128, ll. 75–77. These rates were calculated based on the registered number of abortions. As doctors' discussions suggest, these were much lower numbers than the real numbers of abortion without legal authorization. The sudden increase in the registered number of underground abortions can mean either actual increase in abortion or reinforced surveillance. In the case of the 1948 rise, I believe that the sudden increase largely reflects reality, since there did not seem to be increased surveillance at that time. The 1949 increase in prosecution probably reflects the latter, an outcome of concerns, such as those of Starovskii and Abramova, expressed in 1948.

33. GARF f. 9492, op. 1a, d. 648, l. 84.

34. In the draft prikaz for June 30, 1950, "On measures for reducing abortion," one paragraph stated that the MZ SSSR had failed to do this in the past. GARF f. 8009, op. 22, d. 228, l. 98.

35. Sometime in late 1949, a document entitled "Basic Questions and Subjects of Study" was prepared. GARF f. 8009, op. 22, d. 228, ll. 209–214.

36. In each brigade, representatives of the MZ, state prosecutor, MIu, and VTsSPS were included. Each brigade would be assigned to one oblast and would be responsible for studying general conditions on the issue of abortion and the fulfillment of laws concerning protection of motherhood and childhood in the oblast capital and two other selected cities in the oblast. GARF f. 8009, op. 22, d. 228, l. 89. In the original plan, four brigades were to be formed to study four oblasts. GARF f. 8009, op. 22, d. 238, l. 240.

37. I have not been able to find documents that detail the evolution of this project and identify exactly which cities and oblasts conducted such a study and how many times. Trade Union authorities seem to have investigated women's working environment. According to the letter from A. Shabanov, Acting Minister of Health SSSR to G. M. Malenkov, Secretary of the Central Committee on July 3, 1950, analysis was based on materials from Sverdlovsk, Saratov, Ivanovo, Khar'kov, and Moscow oblasts, and some raions of Moscow city. GARF f. 8009, op. 32, d. 827, l. 3.

38. GARF f. 9492, op. 1a, d. 608, l. 233.

39. On the brigades, see GARF f. 8009, op. 22, d. 228, ll. 209-214 and also GARF f. 8009, op. 22, d. 238, l. 240.

40. The questions included age, marital status, class, profession, number of previous pregnancies, number of previous births, number of previous non-clinical abortions, number of family members, number of children in the family, the age of children, the age of youngest child, income level, primary caretaker of children, reasons for not sending children to crèche, housing conditions, primary reasons for attempting

abortion, by whom and how abortion was induced, and whether/when the pregnancy was registered.

41. Approximately 88.7 percent were non-clinical abortions, believed to include a small percentage of spontaneous miscarriages. GARF f. 9492, op. 1a, d. 648, ll. 84–87.

42. The 1948 survey result is available only for Saratov.

43. GARF f. 8009, op. 22, d. 223, ll. 59–68. The two reports had slightly different questions for certain categories, but were clearly comparable for most cases.

44. GARF f. 8009, op. 22, d. 223, ll. 61, 65.

45. GARF f. 8009, op. 22, d. 223, ll. 59, 64.

46. GARF f. 8009, op. 22, d. 223, ll. 60, 64.

47. GARF f. 8009, op. 22, d. 223, ll. 60, 65. According to Donald Filtzer's study, the average wage in all industries was 687 rubles per month. Donald Filtzer, *Soviet Workers and Late Stalinism: Labor and the Restoration of the Stalinist System after World War II* (Cambridge: Cambridge University Press, 2002), 235.

48. GARF f. 8009, op. 22, d. 223, ll. 61, 65.

49. GARF f. 8009, op. 22, d. 223, l. 61.

50. GARF f. 8009, op. 22, d. 223, l. 66.

51. Childcare in state crèches was free for single mothers, but due to lack of space, many single mothers could not take advantage of this right.

52. GARF f. 8009, op. 32, d. 827, ll. 10–16.

53. GARF f. 8009, op. 32, d. 949, ll. 23–25.

54. Infants up to age three were housed in *dom rebenka* (Home of the Infant), as opposed to *detskii dom* (Children's Home), which housed older children.

55. GARF f. 8009, op. 22, d. 238, ll. 128, 152.

56. GARF f. 8009, op. 32, d. 949, ll. 23–25.

57. GARF f. 8009, op. 22, d. 223, ll. 61, 66.

58. GARF f. 8009, op. 22, d. 223, l. 62.

59. "Relationship problems" is the total of the three relationship-driven reasons for abortion: "bad relationship with husband," "husband has second family," and "without husband."

60. The same question seems to have been asked in the 1948 survey with identical percentages, but this result was not mentioned in the 1948 report.

61. GARF f. 8009, op. 22, d. 223, l. 67.

62. GARF f. 8009, op. 22, d. 223, ll. 67–68.

63. GARF f. 8009, op. 22, d. 238, l. 126. The first and second items were combined in an undated summary report on the "dynamics of abortion," and instability of family is listed as 45.7 percent. However, in the general result of the brigade study, the two items were listed separately. GARF f. 8009, op. 22, d. 238, ll. 126, 146.

64. GARF f. 8009, op. 22, d. 227, l. 225.

65. GARF f. 8009, op. 22, d. 227, l. 316.

66. GARF f. 8009, op. 22, d. 227, l. 318. This major divergence may have been caused because the Saratov study allowed women to pick multiple reasons, while other studies probably allowed only one primary reason. The materials I have seen do not make clear how the local statistics were tabulated into "Union-wide" results.

67. Frederick J. Taussig, *Abortion, Spontaneous and Induced* (London: Henry Kimpton, 1936), 410, cited in Henry E. Sigerist, *Socialized Medicine in the Soviet Union* (London: Victor Gollancz, 1937), 267. In 1926, the number one reason (48 percent) for abortion was poverty. Wendy Goldman, *Women, the State and Revolution: Soviet Family Policy and Social Life, 1917–1936* (Cambridge: Cambridge University Press, 1993), 276.

68. GARF f. 9492, op. 1a, d. 648, ll. 8–11, 65. However, the report was alarming in that 38.1 percent were "young women (*molodezh'*)" under 25 years old, and called on public health organs to educate young women about "the harm of abortion and possible consequences." GARF f. 9492, op. 1a, d. 648, l. 57.

69. GARF f. 9492, op. 1a, d. 648, ll. 1–3.

70. GARF f. 9492, op. 1a, d. 648, ll. 10–11.

71. GARF f. 9492, op. 1a, d. 648, l. 51.

72. Sometimes, it appears, women were fined based on their confessions of previous abortions. GARF f. 9492, op. 1a, d. 648, ll. 82–83.

73. Several aging women I interviewed in 2002–2003 confessed that they had had one or more abortions in the postwar period without being caught.

74. GARF f. 9492, op. 1a, d. 648, l. 69.

75. GARF f. 9492, op. 1a, d. 648, l. 53.

76. GARF f. 9492, op. 1a, d. 648, ll. 1–3.

77. GARF f. 9492, op. 1a, d. 648, ll. 10–11.

78. GARF f. 9492, op. 1a, d. 648, l. 66.

79. GARF f. 9492, op. 1a, d. 648, l. 69. This case was cited in the general report discussed below as an example of how the husband/partner can often be the one encouraging an abortion. GARF f. 9492, op. 1a, d. 648, l. 81.

80. GARF f. 9492, op. 1a, d. 648, l. 68.

81. GARF f. 9492, op. 1a, d. 648, l. 54.

82. GARF f. 9492, op. 1a, d. 648, l. 66.

83. GARF f. 9492, op. 1a, d. 648, l. 72.

84. GARF f. 9492, op. 1a, d. 648, l. 73.

85. This discussion can be interpreted as meaning that the independent life of the fetus begins with the last trimester of the pregnancy. GARF f. 9492, op. 1a, d. 648, l. 76.

86. GARF f. 9492, op. 1a, d. 648, ll. 70–71.

87. GARF f. 9492, op. 1a, d. 648, l. 22.

88. GARF f. 9492, op. 1a, d. 648, ll. 69, 75.

89. GARF f. 9492, op. 1a, d. 648, l. 16.

90. GARF f. 8009, op. 22, d. 238, ll. 159–61.

91. GARF f. 9492, op. 1a, d. 648, ll. 77–83.

92. GARF f. 9492, op. 1a, d. 608, l. 233.

93. GARF f. 9492, op. 1a, d. 608, ll. 238–41.

94. To see how this was sometimes practiced, see Sheila Fitzpatrick "Wives' Tales," in *Tear Off the Masks! Identity and Imposture in Twentieth-Century Russia* (Princeton, NJ: Princeton University Press, 2005). Also see Edward Cohn, "Sex and the Married Communist: Family Troubles, Marital Infidelity, and

Party Discipline in the Postwar USSR, 1945-1964," *Russian Review* 68 (July 2009): 429–50.

95. GARF f. 9492, op. 1a, d. 608, ll. 246–251.
96. GARF f. 9492, op. 1a, d. 608, l. 234.
97. GARF f. 9492, op. 1a, d. 608, ll. 235–36, 254.
98. GARF f. 8009, op. 22, d. 209, l. 105.
99. GARF f. 8009, op. 22, d. 209, l. 1.
100. GARF f. 8009, op. 22, d. 209, l. 106.
101. GARF f. 8009, op. 22, d. 237, ll. 12–14.
102. GARF f. 8009, op. 22, d. 238, ll.113–22. Kovrigina became Minister of Health RSFSR in December 1950.
103. In 1949, Dmitrieva, head of the Moscow Central Abortion Committee, argued that doctors should not have to give false diagnoses in order to provide women with clinical abortions, suggesting that that was exactly what was going on. TsAGM f. 552, op. 3, d. 224, l. 12. It is likely that this kind of practice continued into the first half of the 1950s.
104. GARF f. 8009, op. 22, d. 49, l. 32.
105. GARF f. 8009, op. 22, d. 238, ll. 127, 131–37.
106. TsAGM f. 552, op. 3, d. 224, l. 13.
107. GARF f. 8009, op. 22, d. 237, l. 9.
108. TsAGM f. 552, op. 3, d. 224, l. 13.
109. GARF f. 8009, op. 22, d. 228, l. 35.
110. GARF f. 8009, op. 22, d. 238, ll. 127–31.
111. GARF f. 8009, op. 22, d. 238, ll. 91–98.
112. TsMAMLS f. 218, op. 1, d. 187, l. 46.
113. GARF f. 8009, op. 22, d. 238, ll. 91–92.
114. A minor amendment took place in 1939, when some venereal diseases were added to the list of criteria: "Contagious syphilis and female syphilis not susceptible to cure." GARF f. 8009, op. 25, d. 1, l. 12.

Chapter 5

1. In 1949 and 1950, anti-Semitic purges rolled through one institution after another. From mid-1950 the Ministry of State Security "uncovered" a plot by Western clandestine services to have Kremlin doctors mistreat and kill Soviet top leaders. Tortured suspects, mostly Jews, implicated themselves and others, also mostly Jews. This "Doctors' Plot" scenario built towards a bloody climax but was cut short by Stalin's death. The fictional plot was disavowed by the post-Stalin leadership on April 3, 1953 and all suspects were freed and rehabilitated. For a well-informed presentation, see Gennadi Kostyrchenko, *Out of the Red Shadows: Anti-Semitism in Stalin's Russia* (Amherst, NY: Prometheus Books, 1995), 248-305. Six of the nine prominent doctors arrested were Jews. Benjamin Pinkus, *The Jews of the Soviet Union: The History of a National Minority* (Cambridge: Cambridge University Press, 1988), 179.

2. The "Thaw (*ottepel'*)" originated as the title of Ilya Erenburg's novella, published in the journal *Znamia* in May 1954. The story's title became a metaphor for describing the period when more liberal policies were adopted, and more cultural freedom of expression became possible after the death of Stalin in 1953. Katerina Clark, "Rethinking the Past and Current Thaw," in *Glasnost' in Context: On the Recurrence of Liberalizations in Central and East European Literatures and Cultures*, ed. Marko Pavlyshyn (New York: St. Martin's Press, 1990), 1–2; Stephen Bittner, "Remembering the Avant-garde: Moscow Architects and the 'Rehabilitation' of Constructivism, 1961–1964," *Kritika* 2, no. 3 (2001): 575–576; Miriam Dobson, "The Post Stalin Era: Daily Life and Dissent," *Kritika* 12, no. 4 (2011), 923–924; Nancy Condee, "Cultural Codes of the Thaw," in *Nikita Khrushchev*, ed. William Taubman, Sergei Khrushchev, and Abbot Gleason (New Haven, CT: Yale University Press, 2000), 160–176. Studies that focus on the intelligentsia emphasize later endpoints. Vladislav Zubok, *Zhivago's Children: The Last Russian Intelligentsia* (Cambridge, MA: Harvard University Press, 2009); Denis Kozlov and Eleonory Gilburd, "The Thaw as an Event in Russian History," Denis Kozlov and Eleonory Gilburd, eds., *The Thaw: Soviet Society and Culture during the 1950s and 1960s* (Toronto: University of Toronto Press, 2013), 59. For contemporaries this was a period of uncertainty and instability as well as new possibilities, but later it came to be remembered primarily as a liberal moment. Stephen Bittner, *The Many Lives of Khrushchev's Thaw: Experience and Memory in Moscow's Arbat* (Ithaca, NY: Cornell University Press, 2008), 9.

3. De-Stalinization means the undoing of Stalin's "cult of personality" and policies after his death. For a definition, see Polly Jones, "Introduction: The Dilemmas of De-Stalinization," in *The Dilemmas of De-Stalinization: Negotiating Cultural and Social Change in the Khrushchev Era*, ed. Polly Jones (London: Routledge, 2006), 2–5. As Jones suggests, "de-Stalinization" and "Thaw" are largely synonymous, but the "Thaw" is used most commonly to refer to cultural and intellectual spheres whereas de-Stalinization tends to be used for reforms of Stalinist policies (such as the release of Gulag prisoners) and the liberalization of authoritarian systems. By this distinction, the legalization of abortion is clearly de-Stalinization, but reform of the 1944 Family Law does not fit comfortably into either concept. Nevertheless, the family law reform movement benefitted from the liberating atmosphere of the "Thaw" period and the passionate participation of top-level cultural figures, including Erenburg.

4. Christine Varga-Harris shows Leningraders asserting the "right to humane living conditions" in demanding better housing in the 1950s and 1960s; Soviet citizens began using this word to express their sense of entitlement. Christine Varga-Harris, "Forging Citizenship on the Home Front: Reviving the Socialist Contract and Constructing Soviet Identity during the Thaw," in *The Dilemmas of De-Stalinization*, ed. Polly Jones (London: Routledge, 2006), 103–104. The idea that Soviet citizens, particularly those who are needy and disabled, have the right to be helped by the state has roots in the post-revolutionary period. However, the Stalinist state shifted to a productionist principle, where the state provided support and reward according to citizens' contributions. See Maria Cristina Galmarini-Kabala, *The Right to Be*

Helped: Deviance, Entitlement, and the Soviet Moral Order (DeKalb: Northern Illinois University Press, 2016), chapters 3, 4, 5.

5. GARF f. 8009, op. 32, d. 827, l. 3.

6. GARF f. 8009, op. 22, d. 228, l. 215.

7. GARF f. 8009, op. 22, d. 228, ll. 89–92.

8. GARF f. 8009, op. 32, d. 1066, l. 22.

9. There must have been further correspondence between the MZ and the Sovmin in February, but documents are unavailable in MZ files. In general, files of obstetrics and gynecology at the MZ SSSR archives thin out in 1952 and few documents are available after 1953.

10. Kovrigina escaped the purges of her own ministry by taking nine months off for professional study, which began some time after July 1952. In January 1953, before the nine months was up, she was brought back to the MZ SSSR as a deputy to the new Minister A. F. Tret'iakov. Mariia Kovrigina, *V neoplatnom dolgu* (Moscow: Izd. polit. lit., 1985), 147–155.

11. GARF f. 9492, op. 1a, d. 736, ll. 15–20.

12. GARF f. 9492, op. 1a, d. 736, ll. 18–19.

13. Such events as the threatening criticisms at the 19th Party Congress and the purges associated with the "Doctors' Plot" set the tone for Stalin's difficult last year. For more, see Yoram Gorlizki and Oleg Khlevniuk, *Cold Peace: Stalin and the Soviet Ruling Circle, 1945–1953* (Oxford: Oxford University Press, 2004), particularly chapter 6. On Smirnov, see Jonathan Brent and Vladimir P. Naumov, *Stalin's Last Crime: The Plot against the Jewish Doctors, 1948–1953* (New York: Harper Collins, 2003), 267–268. Actually there had been rolling purges in one medical institution after another throughout the late 1940s and into the early 1950s. See Christopher Burton, "Soviet Medical Attestation and the Problem of Professionalisation under Late Stalinism, 1945–1953," *Europe-Asia Studies* 57, no. 8 (December 2005): 1220–1226. For one case in 1947–1948, see chapter 2.

14. Based on published sources and discussions with Soviet legal experts, Peter H. Juviler's "Family Reforms on the Road to Communism," in *Soviet Policy-Making: Studies of Communism in Transition*, ed. Peter H. Juviler and Henry W. Morton (New York: Frederick A. Praeger, 1967), provides an excellent overview of the family law reform movement in the mid-1950s to mid-1960s.

15. Elena Serebrovskaia, "Zhizn' vnosit popravku," *Literaturnaia gazeta*, January 16, 1954.

16. "Ot imeni syna" in *Literaturnaia gazeta*, August 28, 1954. The title of this article is vaguely religious in the depth of its indignation, since "in the name of the son" could be taken as an invocation of Christ's benevolent authority. KZOBS stands for *Kodeks zakonov ob opeke, brake, i sem'e* of RSFSR, promulgated in 1945 to reflect the USSR Supreme Soviet Decree, referred to as the 1944 Family Law.

17. GARF f. 9492, op. 1, d. 1936, l. 86.

18. GARF f. 9492, op. 1, d. 1936, ll. 80–83.

19. The number of births ranged between 4.2 and 5.0 million between 1948 and 1952. RGAE f. 1592, op. 33, d. 2163, l. 9.

20. TsMAMLS f. 217, op. 1, d. 187, l. 46.

21. Statistics for this period are from annual TsSU reports on natural population change. There were sometimes different versions filed for the same year. Since monthly aggregates were filed most consistently, I use them. For 1953, see RGAE f. 1562, op. 33, d. 1694. l. 1. A slightly different version was filed in RGAE f. 1562, op. 33, d. 1693. l. 1. For 1952, RGAE f. 1562, op. 20, d. 1011, l. 1.

22. It is also arguable that the comparison of 1940 and post-1944 data is not useful since the meaning of "registered marriage" had changed. Many non-registered marriages in 1940 would have been technically equivalent to "registered marriage" under the 1944 Family Law. In contrast, postwar "registered marriages" do not necessarily indicate stable families, since as discussed in Chapters 3 and 6, many registered marriages had ended de facto, while hardening divorce law did not allow their official termination.

23. RGAE f. 1562, op. 33, d. 2163, l. 7.

24. For a discussion of the rising number of divorce cases in the late 1950s and 1960s, see Deborah Field, "Irreconcilable Differences: Divorce and Conceptions of Private Life in the Khrushchev Era," *Russian Review* 57, no. 4 (October 1998): 599–613.

25. For details, see Chapter 3.

26. RGAE f. 1562, op. 33, d. 2163, ll. 7–12.

27. See Chapter 1.

28. *Prezidium TsK KPSS 1954-64* (Moscow: ROSSPEN, 2003), 766, 841.

29. RGASPI f. 82, op. 2, d. 538, ll. 95–96.

30. RGASPI f. 82, op. 2, d. 443, l. 34. See also RGAE f. 1562, op. 33, d. 2990, ll. 49–56.

31. RGASPI, f. 82, op. 2, d. 443, l. 34.

32. Kazuko Kawamoto, *Sorenno minshushugito kazoku: renpokazoku kihonho seiteikatei,1948–1968* [Soviet Democracy and the Family: Family Law Reform after the War, 1948–1968] (Tokyo: Yushindo, 2012), 88.

33. Mark Field, "The Re-legalization of Abortion in Soviet Russia," *New England Journal of Medicine* 255, no. 9 (August 30, 1956): 426; Peter Solomon, in a close analysis of the petty theft law of 1947, has shown that 1954 brought ways of softening and suspending sentences. As with abortion, 1955 would bring the full decriminalization of petty theft. Peter Solomon, *Soviet Criminal Justice under Stalin* (Cambridge: Cambridge University Press, 1996), 443.

34. TsMAMLS f. 218, op. 1, d. 187, l. 48.

35. TsMAMLS f. 218, op. 1, d. 188, ll. 3–5.

36. GARF f. 9492, op. 2, d. 111, l. 59.

37. TsMAMLS f. 218, op. 1, d. 187, ll. 33–35.

38. TsMAMLS f. 218, op. 1, d. 187, ll. 36–64.

39. The "Great Terror" refers to late 1930s mass executions and imprisonments without proper legal procedure. These repressions targetted not only Stalin's political rivals, but also military leaders, party and state officials, factory directors, and ordinary men and women. Most victims were later found innocent and legally rehabilitated. Robert Conquest wrote the first full account of this subject. Robert Conquest, *The Great Terror: Stalin's Purge of the Thirties* (New York: Macmillan, 1968). One of the contentious historiographical points was the extent to which Stalin organized and directed it. Arch Getty, *Origins of the Great Purges: The Soviet Communist Party*

Reconsidered, 1933–1938 (New York: Cambridge University Press, 1985) argued that Stalin's involvement was not as significant as previously thought. Since the opening of the archives in the 1990s, scholars have examined this from diverse perspectives and demonstrated widespread participation by ordinary people making unfounded accusations. Hiroaki Kuromiya, *The Voices of the Dead: Stalin's Great Terror in the 1930s* (New Haven: Yale University Press, 2007); Wendy Goldman, *Terror and Democracy in the Age of Stalin* (New York: Cambridge University Press, 2007); Wendy Goldman, *Inventing the Enemy: Denunciation and Terror in Stalin's Russia* (New York: Cambridge University Press, 2012); James Harris, *The Great Fear: Stalin's Terror of the 1930s* (Oxford: Oxford University Press, 2016). On terror in the Red Army, see Peter Whitewood, *The Red Army and the Great Terror: Stalin's Purge of the Soviet Military* (Lawrence: University Press of Kansas, 2015).

40. Source: TsMAMLS f. 218, op. 1, d. 187, l. 48. Demographers of maternal deaths argue that maternal deaths from abortions are often underrecorded because they are registered as death from infections or other types of diseases and injuries. I am grateful to Nancy Yinger, a specialist on maternal death in developing countries, for sharing her expert insights.

41. There is no date on the report, but given the context, I assume that this was the basis of the following proposal to the Sovmin. Kovrigina's sense of urgency can be inferred by the draft law coming out even before the new study had been fully analyzed and reported.

42. GARF f. 9492, op. 2, d. 111, ll. 59–60.

43. GARF f. 9492, op. 2, d. 111, ll. 61–62, 69–72.

44. Speech on August 23, 1955. TsMAMLS f. 218, op. 1, d. 188, l. 20.

45. GARF f. 9492, op. 2, d. 110, ll. 38–45.

46. GARF f. 9492, op. 1, d. 111, ll. 98–107.

47. "Virgin Lands" refers to Khrushchev's campaign calling for Slavic people to settle northern Kazakhstan in order to transform the vast grasslands into an agricultural belt through mechanized farming.

48. "Rech' tovarishcha N. S. Khrushcheva na sobranii komsomol'tsev i molodezhi g. Moskvy, iz'iavivshikh zhelanie poekhat' rabotat' na tselinnye zemli, 7 ianvaria 1955 goda," *Izvestiia*, January 8, 1955.

49. However, he did not mention his authorship of the 1944 Family Law.

50. *Izvestiia*, January 8, 1955.

51. GARF f. 9492, op. 1, d. 1936, l. 87.

52. GARF f. 9492, op. 1, d. 1936, ll. 38–42.

53. GARF f. 9492, op. 1, d. 1936, l. 67. Even though the law was promulgated union-wide in 1944 and became immediately effective, its provisions were not integrated into relevant republic family codes until 1945.

54. Interestingly, these letters are not in the Ministry of Health archive, but in Kovrigina's personal files at TsMAMLS f.218.

55. If these letters had not mentioned "abortion," they would have been forwarded to the MIu rather than the MZ.

56. TsMAMLS f. 218, op. 1, d. 187, ll. 5–6.

57. TsMAMLS f. 218, op. 1, d. 187, l. 3. When this was first issued is not clear.

58. TsMAMLS f. 218, op. 1, d. 187, ll. 8-11.

59. TsMAMLS f. 218, op. 1, d. 187, ll. 12-15.

60. TsMAMLS f. 218, op. 1, d. 187, ll. 16-17.

61. TsMAMLS f. 218, op. 1, d. 187, ll. 18-22.

62. TsMAMLS f. 218, op. 1, d. 187, ll. 7, 18, 23-24.

63. TsMAMLS f. 218, op. 1, d. 188, ll. 3-5.

64. No complete list of participants is available, but according to a stenogram, twenty-two participants were listed.

65. For example, see V. P. Mikhailov's view in TsMAMLS f. 218, op. 1, d. 188, ll. 8-9, 75.

66. TsMAMLS f. 218, op. 1, d. 188, ll. 13-14.

67. TsMAMLS f. 218, op. 1, d. 188, l. 52.

68. TsMAMLS f. 218, op. 1, d. 188, ll. 58-59.

69. TsMAMLS f. 218, op. 1, d. 188, ll. 17-19.

70. TsMAMLS f. 218, op. 1, d. 188, ll. 34-36.

71. Susan Gross Solomon, "The Demographic Argument in Soviet Debates over the Legalization of Abortion in the 1920s," *Cahiers du monde russe et sovietique* 33, no. 1 (janvier-mars 1992): 59-82; Wendy Goldman, *Women, the State and Revolution: Soviet Family Policy and Social Life, 1917-1936* (Cambridge: Cambridge University Press, 1993), 255.

72. TsMAMLS f. 218, op. 1, d. 188, ll. 7, 49-50.

73. TsMAMLS f. 218, op. 1, d. 188, ll. 34-35.

74. TsMAMLS f. 218, op. 1, d. 188, ll. 19, 36.

75. TsMAMLS f. 218, op. 1, d. 188, l. 77.

76. TsMAMLS f. 218, op. 1, d. 188, l. 45. After receiving her personal copy of the meeting stenogram, Kovrigina underlined this sentence that she herself had spoken at the event, suggesting that this was an important conclusion for her. She was not the only speaker at the meeting to use the Russian word for right (pravo).

77. TsMAMLS f. 218, op. 1, d. 188, l. 31.

78. TsMAMLS f. 218, op. 1, d. 188, l. 24.

79. TsMAMLS f. 218, op. 1, d. 188, l. 11.

80. TsMAMLS f. 218, op. 1, d. 188, ll. 90-91.

81. "Decree on the Legalization of Abortions of November 18, 1920," in N. A. Semashko, *Health Protection in the USSR* (London: Gollansz, 1934), 82-84 as it appeared in Rudolf Schlesinger ed., *The Family in the USSR: Documents and Readings* (London: Routledge and Kegan Paul, 1949), 44.

82. "O zapreshchenii abortov, . . ." *Pravda*, June 28, 1936.

83. TsMAMLS f. 218, op. 1, d. 188, l. 90.

84. RGASPI f. 82, op. 2, d. 443, l. 162.

85. N. Kovaleva, A. Korotkov, S. Mel'chin, et al., eds., *Molotov, Malenkov, Kaganovich. 1957: Stenogramma iiun'skogo plenuma TsK KPSS i drugie dokumenty* (Moskva: Demokratiia, 1998), 755.

86. "Ob otmene zapreshcheniia abortov ukaz ot 23 noiabria 1955," in *Sbornik zakonov SSSR i ukazov prezidiuma verkhovnogo soveta SSSR, 1938-iiul' -1956gg* (Moskva: Gosudarstvennoe izdatel'stvo iuridicheskoi lieratury, 1956), 402.

87. Alexandre Avdeev, Alain Blum, and Irina Troitskaia, "The History of Abortion Statistics in Russia and the USSR from 1900 to 1991," *Population: An English Selection* 7 (1995): 58–60.

88. Amy Randall convincingly argued that legalization allowed medical professionals to gain more control over and knowledge of women's reproductive health than under criminalized abortion. Amy Randall, "'Abortion Will Deprive You of Happiness!' Soviet Reproductive Politics in the Post-Stalin Era," *Journal of Women's History* 23, no. 3 (2011): 30–31.

89. Magali Barbieri, Alain Blum, Elena Dolkigh, and Amon Ergashev, "Nuptiality, Fertility, Use of Contraception, and Family Policies in Uzbekistan," *Population Studies* 50, no. 1 (March, 1996): 81. This analysis focuses on the changing reproductive practice of women of non-European origin, clarifying the growing number of abortions for the purpose of fertility control among Uzbek women.

90. Victor Agadjanian, "Is 'Abortion Culture' Fading in the Former Soviet Union? Views about Abortion and Contraception in Kazakhstan," *Studies in Family Planning* 33, no. 3 (September 2002): 239.

91. The UN 2007 abortion rate data come from various years for various countries depending on availability. Former socialist republics are well represented. http:// data.un.org/Data.aspx?d=GenderStat&f=inID%3A12 (accessed on May 24, 2020). The abortion rates for 2010 show similar trends, except that the rates for former Soviet republics generally went down. https://www.un.org/en/development/desa/population/publications/pdf/policy/WorldAbortionPolicies2013/ WorldAbortionPolicies2013_WallChart.pdf. United Nations Department of Economic and Social Affairs Population Division, *Abortion Policies and Reproductive Health around the World* (New York: United Nations, 2014), 5, shows the map of the world for 1996 and 2013, rating countries from most restrictive to least restrictive abortion policies. Former Soviet republics all fall into the least restrictive for both years. Muslim countries with severe restrictions do not provide abortion statistics, but former Soviet republics have long-standing systems for taking abortion statistics.

92. Great Britain (with the exception of Northern Ireland) practically legalized abortion in 1967. Judith Orr, *Abortion Wars: The Fight for Reproductive Rights* (Bristol: Policy Press, 2017), 20, 67. Finland legalized abortion in 1970. Miina Keski-Petäjä, "Abortion Wishes and Abortion Prevention: Women Seeking Legal Termination of Pregnancy during the 1950s and 1960s in Finland," *Finnish Yearbook of Population Research* (April 2012): 132. Sweden introduced abortion on request in 1975. Lena Lennerhed, "Troubled Women: Abortion and Psychiatry in Sweden in the 1940s and 1950s," in *Transcending Borders: Abortion in the Past and Present*, ed. Shannon Stettner, Katrina Ackerman, Kristin Burnett, and Travis Hay (Cham, Switzerland: Palgrave Macmillan, 2017), 100. In the United States, the right to abortion was recognized

in 1973. Linda Gordon, *The Moral Property of Women: A History of Birth Control Politics in America* (Urbana: University of Illinois Press, 2007), 301–302.

93. Henry David, *Family Planning and Abortion in the Socialist Countries of Central and Eastern Europe: A Compendium of Observations and Readings* (New York: Population Council, 1970), 19. Among the countries that did not follow Soviet legalization were Albania, Yugoslavia, and East Germany. Albania never introduced a less restrictive abortion policy. Yugoslavia began to relax restrictions on abortion in 1952. Thomas Frejka, "Induced Abortion and Fertility: A Quarter Century of Experience in Eastern Europe," *Population and Development Review* 9, no. 3 (September 1983): 495.

94. The first and only communist family planning association was formed in 1957 with a claim that Polish fertility was too high. John Besemeres, *Socialist Population Politics: The Political Implications of Demographic Trends in the USSR and Eastern Europe* (White Plains, NY: M. E. Sharpe, 1980),123.

95. On the Romanian tragedy, see Gail Kligman, *The Politics of Duplicity: Controlling Reproduction in Ceausescu's Romania* (Berkeley: University of California Press, 1998).

96. Early universal marriage and few women without children are additional traits. See Sergei Zakharov, "Russian Federation: From the First to Second Demographic Transition," *Demographic Research* 19, no. 24 (2008): 916–918.

97. Tyrene White, *China's Longest Campaign: Birth Planning in the People's Republic, 1949–2005* (Ithaca, NY: Cornell University Press, 2006), 35; Masako Kohama, "*Chugoku kingendaini okeru boshieiseiseisakuno kenkyu* [A Study of Public Health Policy toward Mothers and Children in Modern and Contemporary China], A Research Report," published as the result of a 2002~2005 project funded by the Japan Society for the Promotion of Science (March 2006), 12–15.

98. Susan Greenhalgh and Edwin Winckler, *Governing China's Population: From Leninist to Neoliberal Biopolitics* (Palo Alto, CA: Stanford University Press, 2005), 64–74. This was certainly the prevailing attitude in the Chinese village with which Mao identified.

99. Susan Greenhalgh, *Just One Child: Science and Policy in Deng's China* (Berkeley: University of California Press, 2008), 70.

100. Donna Harsch, "Society, the State, and Abortion in East Germany, 1950–1972," *American Historical Review* (February 1997): 58–63; Josie McLellan, *Love in the Time of Communism: Intimacy and Sexuality in the GDR* (Cambridge: Cambridge University Press, 2011), 62. On wartime and postwar abortion policy in Germany, see Atina Grossmann, *Reforming Sex: The German Movement for Birth Control and Abortion Reform, 1920–1950* (New York: Oxford University Press, 1995).

101. McLellan, *Love in the Time of Communism*, 55–61.

102. McLellan, *Love in the Time of Communism*, 66.

103. Peter Quint, "The Unification of Abortion Law," chapter 12 in *The Imperfect Union: Constitutional Structures of Germany Unification* (Princeton, NJ: Princeton University Press, 2012).

Chapter 6

1. See Natasha Maltseva, "The Other Side of the Coin," in *Women and Russia: Feminist Writings from the Soviet Union*, ed. Tatyana Mamonova (Oxford: Blackwell, 1984), 114–116; Igor Kon, *Sexual Revolution in Russia: From the Age of the Czars to Today* (New York: Free Press, 1995), 182–183.

2. Amy Randall, "'Abortion Will Deprive You of Happiness!' Soviet Reproductive Politics in the Post-Stalin Era," *Journal of Women's History* 23, no. 3 (2011): 13–38.

3. Alexandre Avdeev, Alain Blum, and Irina Troitskaia, "The History of Abortion Statistics in Russia and the USSR from 1900 to 1991," *Population: An English Selection*, 7 (1995): 64.

4. Avdeev, Blum, and Troitskaia, "The History of Abortion Statistics," 60.

5. The registered number of maternal deaths resulting from non-clinical abortions between 1949 and 1954 was around 4,000. TsMAMLS f. 218, op. 1, d. 187, l. 48. This number fell by half almost immediately after abortion was legalized. Anatolii Vishnevskii, Viktoriia Sakevich, and Boris Denisov, "Zapret aborta: osvezhite vashu pamiat'," *Demoskop Weekly* no. 707–708 (28 noiabria-11 dekabria 2016).

6. The leveling off of abortions from the 1970s has also been attributed to the aging of the reproductive cohort and an overall decline in fertility. For this argument, see Larissa Remennick, "Epidemiology and Determinants of Induced Abortion in the USSR," *Social Science and Medicine* 33, no. 7 (1991), 842. Some specialists of Soviet demography also argue that the stability of abortion statistics since the mid-1960s demonstrates the accurate and complete registration of these statistics. They also suggest that the registered number of non-clinical abortions mostly represented miscarriages. Avdeev, Blum, and Troitskaia, "The History of Abortion Statistics," 58–60.

7. On the anti-abortion campaign that targeted men, see Randall, "'Abortion Will Deprive You of Happiness,'" 26–30. Contents of this campaign reflected pre-legalization criticisms against men among medical professionals. This message, however, would have difficulty reaching men, as unlike expectant mothers, men, especially irresponsible ones, were much less likely to visit women's consultation clinics, the designated institution for dissemination of anti-abortion information.

8. On the rebirth of demography, see Murray Feshbach, *The Soviet Population Policy Debate: Actors and Issues: A Rand Note* (December 1986), 4–7. On sociology, see Liah Greenfeld, "Soviet Sociology and Sociology in the Soviet Union," *Annual Review of Sociology*.14 (1988): 99–123.

9. Constance Sorrentino, "International Comparisons of Labor Force Participation, 1960–1981," *Monthly Labor Review* (February 1983): 23–36.

10. "Ob uvelichenii prodolzhitel'nosti otpuskov po beremennosti i rodam," in *Postanovleniia KPSS i Sovetskogo pravitel'stva ob okhrane zdorov'ia naroda* (Medgiz: Moskva, 1958), 334.

11. "O dal'neishikh merakh pomoshchi zhenshchinam-materiam, rabotaiushchim na predpriiatiiakh i v uchrezhdeniiakh," in *Postanovleniia KPSS i Sovetskogo pravitel'stva ob okhrane zdorov'ia naroda* (Moskva: Medgiz, 1958), 334–335.

12. "O dopolnitel'nykh l'gotakh po nalogu na kholostiakov, odinokikh i malosemeinykh grazhdan SSSR dlia otdel'nykh grupp platel'shchikov, ukaz ot 10 fevralia 1954," in *Sbornik zakonov SSSR, 1938–1975,* tom 1 (Moskva: Izd. Izvestiia Sovetov Deputatov Trudiashchikhsia SSSR, 1975), 581.

13. "O povyshenii razmera ne oblagaemogo nalogami minimuma zarabotnoi platy rabochikh i sluzhashchikh," in *Sbornik zakonov SSSR,* tom 1, 582. For another example of tax reduction, see "Ob otmene nalogov s zarabotnoi platy rabochikh i sluzhashchikh, zakon ot 7 maia 1960 g," in *Sbornik zakonov SSSR,* tom 1, 586–588.

14. The published law specified "single women without children," but a commission report to the Central Committee clearly indicated "single women (unmarried and widows) without children." For the published law, see "Ob otmene vzimaniia naloga na kholostiakov, odinokikh i malosemeinykh grazhdan SSSR . . ." For the report, see RGANI f. 5, op. 30, d. 222, l. 219.

15. Based on an abortion study conducted in the late 1950s, Sadvokasova showed that urban women most often began regulating fertility after having one child, while rural women began regulating fertility after having two children. Sadvokasova, 150.

16. RGANI f. 5, op. 30, d. 222, ll. 216–217.

17. RGANI f. 5, op. 30, d. 222, l. 200.

18. Without records from the detailed discussions, it is not possible to understand whether the anti-alcohol campaign was already on the agenda before the Ministry of Finance had proposed the price increase as a fiscal measure. Nevertheless, for Khrushchev, the price increase on alcohol was remembered as part of his anti-alcohol campaign. N. S. Khrushchev, *Khrushchev Remembers: The Last Testament* (Boston: Little, Brown, 1974), 145. See also Vladimir G. Treml, "Alcohol in the USSR: A Fiscal Dilemma," *Soviet Studies* 27, no. 2 (April 1975): 167. The state use of revenue from alcohol sale for socially beneficial use has a historical precedent in imperial Russia, where the State Vodka Monopoly was created in 1894. In 1895 the Ministry of Finance set up the Guardianship of Public Sobriety with the mission of providing entertainment and education as a way to divert people from drinking. See Patricia Herlihy, *The Alcoholic Empire: Vodka and Politics in Late Imperial Russia* (New York: Oxford University Press, 2002).

19. For details, see I. R. Takala, *Veselie Rusi* (Sankt Peterburg: Zhurnal Neva, 2002), 251–252.

20. See, for example, the August 18, 1954, Ministry of Health prikaz "On Measures for Anti-Alcohol Propaganda," in RGANI f. 5, op. 30, d. 59, ll. 88–91.

21. The commission considered it necessary for the TsSU to conduct a poll of limited scale, involving 3 to 5 percent of the working population in order to obtain necessary statistics for policy assessment. RGANI f. 5, op. 30, d. 222, l. 218.

22. This law would pay 12 rubles per month per child to poor families (income per family member under 50 rubles) until the child was 8 years old. "O vvedenii posobii na detei maloobespechennym sem'iam," ukaz ot 25 sentiabria 1974, *Vedomosti Verkhovnogo Soveta SSSR* 40 (1974): 663.

23. The first account of the reform of the 1944 Family Law was written by Peter Juviler. Peter Juviler, "Family Reforms on the Road to Communism," in *Soviet*

Policy-Making: Studies of Communism in Transition, ed. Peter H. Juviler and Henry W. Morton (New York: Frederick A. Praeger, 1967), 30–55.

24. Kazuko Kawamoto, Sorenno minshushugito kazoku: renpokazoku kihonho seiteikatei, 1948-1968 [Soviet Democracy and the Family: The Process of Making the All-Union Soviet Family Law, 1948-1968] (Tokyo: Yushindo kobunsha, 2012), 101.

25. Samuil Iakovlevich Marshak (1887–1964) is famous both for his original poetry, much of it for children, and for his translations into Russian from both English (Shakespeare, Coleridge) and Scottish (Burns). Marshak would not live to see the law reformed. A. E. Vaksberg, Moia zhizn' v zhizni tom 2 (Moscow: Terra-Sport, 2000), 137. Georgii Nestorovich Speranskii (1873–1969) was the founding father of Soviet pediatrics.

26. Juviler, "Family Reforms on the Road to Communism," 39; Kawamoto, Sorenno minshushugito kazoku, 117–118. Kawamoto, who has conducted the closest study of MIu and Sovmin archives on family law searched, but did not find any documents revealing the reasons for the inexplicable delays of 1961 and 1964. Kawamoto, 118-119, 140-142.

27. V. I. Ivkin, Gosudarstvennaia vlast' SSSR: vysshie organy vlasti i upravleniia i ikh rukovoditeli 1923-1991 (Moskva: ROSSPEN, 1999), 578.

28. Veniamin Aleksandrovich Kaverin (1902–1989) was an author of war stories in many genres (newspaper, novel) and had just finished a history of microbiology.

29. Vaksberg, Moia zhizn' v zhizni, 137–139, 144–145.

30. Juviler, "Family Reforms on the Road to Communism," 40–41; Kawamoto, Sorenno minshushugito kazoku, 127.

31. Kawamoto, Sorenno minshushugito kazoku, 127–128. Peter Juviler's anonymous informants, some of whom were among the draft authors, also told him in 1963 that the reform would soon appear. Juviler, "Family Reforms on the Road to Communism," 40–41.

32. N. S. Khrushchev was removed from power at a Presidium meeting on October 13, 1964. Prezidium TsK KPSS, 1954-1964 t. 1: Chernovye protokol'nye zapisi zasedanii. Stenogrammy (Moskva: ROSSPEN, 2004), 862. Less than two months after Khrushchev's ouster, on December 8, 1964, Vorobiev told a joint meeting of the two commissions for legislative preparation of the Supreme Soviet that "for reasons which have nothing to do with the work of commissions," the preparations for the publication of the draft all-union family law had stopped until recently, but could now resume. In fact, in January 1965 the draft was submitted to the Presidium of the Supreme Soviet and the Central Committee. Kawamoto, Sorennno minshushugito kazoku, 128.

33. The Russian name is Osnovy zakonodatel'stva soiuza SSR i soiuznykh respublik o brake i sem'e.

34. "Proekt osnovy zakonodatel'stva Soiuza SSR i Soiuznykh respublik o brake i sem'e," Literaturnaia gazeta, April 10, 1968.

35. "Zakon, kotorogo zhdut," Literaturnaia gazeta, April 17, 1968.

36. "Zakon, kotorogo zhdut," Literaturnaia gazeta, April 17, 1968.

37. Clearly, there were many out-of-wedlock children born in stable relationships that were not marriage. This often happened as the result of difficulty in getting a divorce

from a previous marriage. Thus, the simplification of divorce in 1965 would help decrease the number of out-of-wedlock children. On this, see P. Kalistratova and T. Mal'tsman, "Suprugi razvodiatsia . . ." *Literaturnaia gazeta*, May 15, 1968.

38. "Ravenstvo pered zakonom" *Literaturnaia gazeta*, May 8, 1968.

39. "Dolg pered sem'ei," *Literaturnaia gazeta*, May 15, 1968.

40. "Rozhdenie zakona," *Literaturnaia gazeta*, June 19, 1968.

41. "Schast'e i zabota - deti!" *Literaturnaia gazeta,* May 8, 1968.

42. "Ob utverzhdenii osnov zakonodatel'stva Soiuza SSR i Soiuznykh respublik o brake i sem'e" zakon ot 27 iiunia 1968, *Vedomosti verkhovnogo Soveta SSR,* 1968, no. 27, p. 241.

43. A. G. Kharchev, *Brak i sem'ia v SSSR: opyt sotsiologicheskogo issledovaniia* (Moskva: Mysl', 1964), 212.

44. The number of divorces shot up after simplification in 1965, a factor for shrinking the size of the family. In 1965, the number of divorces per 1,000 was 1.6. It grew to 2.6 per 1,000 in 1970, and to 3.4 in 1974. As a comparison, in 1975, the number of registered divorces per 1,000 population was 3.1 in the Soviet Union and 4.8 in the United States. Gail W. Lapidus, *Women in Soviet Society: Equality, Development, and Social Change* (Berkeley: University of California Press, 1978), 251. In Baltic and Slavic republics, the divorce rate was around 4 per 1,000, whereas in Muslim republics, it was less than 2. Shiokawa Nobuaki, "Kyusoren no kazoku to shakai," in *Surabu no shakai: Koza surabu no sekai,* vol. 4 (Tokyo: Kobundo, 1994), 229.

45. Wesley Andrew Fisher, *The Soviet Marriage Market: Mate-Selection in Russia and the USSR* (New York: Praeger, 1980), 149.

46. V. I. Perevedentsev, "Neobkhodimo stimulirovat' rost naseleniia v nashei strane," *Voprosy filosofii* 11 (1974): 91. Jennifer Utrata, *Women without Men: Single Mothers and Family Change in the New Russia* (Ithaca, NY: Cornell University Press, 2015), 35.

47. Andrea Chandler, *Democracy, Gender, and Social Policy in Russia: A Wayward Society* (New York: Palgrave Macmillan, 2013), 52.

48. Some argued that single motherhood should not be considered the result of dissolute lives but rather a "demographic disease," suggesting that the common understanding in the late 1970s was still similar to that of the late 1960s. "Liubov' i demografiia," *Literaturnaia gazeta*, May 4, 1977.

49. For example, an unmarried mother, A. P., went out with her boss (married, age 38) for ten years and gave birth to her son, Nikita. She felt that when people found out about her never-married status, men regarded her contemptuously and women looked on her with pity. Her son found out that the mother of his friend told her that she should not play with him because his mother was weak and loose. "Khotim byt' schastlivym," *Literaturnaia gazeta*, May 4, 1977.

50. E. A. Sadvokasova, *Sotsial'no-gigienicheskie aspekty regulirovaniia razmerov sem'i* (Moskva: Izdatel'stvo Meditsina, 1969), 6.

51. Sadvokasova, *Sotsial'no-gigienicheskie aspekty,* 120–122.

52. Sadvokasova, *Sotsial'no-gigienicheskie aspekty,* 144.

53. Sadvokasova, *Sotsial'no-gigienicheskie aspekty,* 152–163.

54. Sadvokasova, *Sotsial'no-gigienicheskie aspekty,* 143–149.

55. V. L. Krasnenkov, "Nekotorye sotsial'no-gigienicheskie aspekty kriminal'nykh abortov sredi zhenshchin g. Kalinina," *Zdravookhranenie Rossiiskoi Federatsii* 5 (1977): 20–21; A. A. Popov, "Mediko-demograficheskie i sotsial'no-gigienicheskie prichiny i faktory iskusstvennogo aborta (obzor literatury)," *Zdravookhranenie Rossiiskoi Federatsii* (Hereafter *ZRF*) 9 (1980): 28.

56. Sadvokasova, *Sotsial'no-gigienicheskie aspekty,* 147. Harmful effects on the next fetus or child among those who terminated their first pregnancy was pointed out, for example, in M. Ia. Podluzhnaia, "O roli meditsinskoi demografii v sotsial'no-gigienicheskom izuchenii zdorov'ia naseleniia," *ZRF* 8 (1978): 12.

57. In the rural areas, typically this began after the birth of the second child. Sadvokasova, *Sotsial'no-gigienicheskie aspekty,* 175.

58. Sadvokasova, *Sotsial'no-gigienicheskie aspekty,* 179-180.

59. The percentage of women married before age 20 increased from 12.9 percent in 1962 to 20.6 percent in 1965. Sadvokasova, *Sotsial'no-gigienicheskie aspekty,* 170.

60. N. A. Shneiderman, "Dinamika i regional'nye osobennosti rozhdaemosti v RSFSR," *ZRF* 11 (1979): 24. It is likely that underground abortion was still fairly common, particularly in big cities, as many women wanted to avoid being suspected of getting an abortion by missing the three days off from work required to complete the official abortion procedure in the hospital or specialized clinic. Carola Hansson and Karin Liden, *Moscow Women: Thirteen Interviews,* trans. Gerry Bothmer, George Blecher, and Lone Blecher (New York: Pantheon Books, 1983), 147.

61. A. B. Karnov and I. A. Danilov, *Aktual'nye voprosy akusherstva i ginekologii* (Barnaul, 1975), 53–54, as cited in A. A. Popov, "O chastote i prichinakh vne-bol'nichnykh abortov (Obzor literatury)," *ZRF* 6 (1982): 27.

62. Shneiderman, "Dinamika i regional'nye osobennosti," 27.

63. Sadvokasova, *Sotsial'no-gigienicheskie aspekty,* 125.

64. Sadvokasova, *Sotsial'no-gigienicheskie aspekty,* 6, 125–128.

65. O. K. Nikonchik, "Problema kontratseptsii i organizatsiia bor'by s abortami v SSSR," *Akusherstvo i ginekologiia* 6 (1959): 5. Other substances whose contraceptive properties were studied around this time were polyphenol and galascorbine. For example, see R. P. Tel'nova, "Kontratseptivnye svoistva nekotorykh polifenolov," *Akusherstvo i ginekologiia* 6 (1959): 11–13; and L. Ia. Gorpinenko, "Mikroflora vlagalishcha i sheiki matki u zhenshchin pri mestnom primenenii galaskorbina kak protivozachatochnogo sredstva," *Akusherstvo i ginekologiia* 6 (1959): 13–15.

66. Sadvokasova, *Sotsial'no-gigienicheskie aspekty,* 135.

67. Josie McLellan, *Love in the Time of Communism: Intimacy and Sexuality in the GDR* (Cambridge: Cambridge University Press, 2011), 61. East Germany acquired the formula from West Germany. Donna Harsch's book review of Annette Leo and Christian Konig, *Die 'Wunschkindpille'. Weibliche Erfahrung und Staatliche Geburtenpolitik in der DDR* (Gottingen: Wallstein Verlag, 2015), in *German History* 34, no. 2 (1 June 2016): 358–359, refers to the Stasi's involvement in recruiting the spy who stole information on the production of the pill from the West German company Schering.

68. A USSR Ministry of Health report on this symposium was cited in A. A. Popov, A. P. Visser, and E. Ketting, "Contraceptive Knowledge, Attitudes, and Practice in Russia during the 1980s," *Studies in Family Planning* 24, no. 4 (July–August 1993): 235.

69. L. S. Persianinov and I. A. Manuilova, "O rasshirennoi programme VOZ [WHO] po reproduktsii cheloveka," *Akusherstvo i ginekologiia* 6 (June 1975): 1–3; and L. S. Persianinov and I. A. Manuilova, "Sostoianie i perspektivy nauchnykh issledovanii v Moskovskom nauchno-metodicheskom tsentre VOZ po reproduktsii cheloveka," *Akusherstvo i ginekologiia* 6 (June 1975): 3–7.

70. For contemporary criticism of the pill in the United States, see Barbara Seaman, *The Doctors: Case against the Pill* (New York: Peter H. Wyden, 1969); Morton Mintz, *The Pill: An Alarming Report* (Boston: Beacon Press, 1970); Jules Saltman, *The Pill: Its Effects, Its Dangers, Its Future* (New York: Grosset and Dunlap, 1970). For a very useful analysis of the politics of oral contraception involving scientists, the pharmaceutical industry, physicians, and women, see Elizabeth Siegel Watkins, *On the Pill: A Social History of Oral Contraceptives, 1950–1970* (Baltimore, MD: Johns Hopkins University Press, 1998).

71. Trials took place in the late 1950s in Puerto Rico and Haiti. Watkins, *On the Pill,* 31–32.

72. The East German case shows that after the 1965 introduction of the pill, women initially hesitated to use it, fearing weight gain and loss of sensation. However, by the end of the 1970s, the pill was the main contraceptive choice for women. McLellan, *Love in the Time of Communism,* 61.

73. The data here refer to women in RFSFR. The "period total fertility" looks at five-year intervals and measures the average number of children a woman had over her whole reproductive life. From 4.74 (in 1936–1940), it fell to 2.03 (in 1966–1970), and further decreased to 1.93 (in 1976–1980). Sergei Zakharov "Russian Federation: From the First to Second Demographic Transition," *Demographic Research* 19 (July 2008): 955.

74. Feshbach, *The Soviet Population Policy Debate,* 3–40.

75. Ellen Mickiewicz, ed., *Handbook of Soviet Social Science Data* (New York: Free Press, 1973), 54.

76. Lapidus, *Women in Soviet Society,* 166.

77. Andrei Markevich, "Soviet Urban Households and the Road to Universal Employment, from the End of the 1930s to the End of the 1960s," *Continuity and Change* 20, no. 3 (2005): 449.

78. Feshbach, *The Soviet Population Policy Debate,* 5.

79. D. Valentei and G. Kiseleva, "Vzroslie i deti," *Literaturnaia gazeta,* March 17, 1971.

80. *O pobochnom deistvii i oslozhneniiakh pri primenenii oral'nykh kontratseptivov: inf ormatsionnoe pis'mo,* compiled by E. A. Babaian, A.S. Lopatin, and I. G. Lavretskii (Moscow: USSR Ministry of Public Health, 1974) as cited in Popov, Visser, and Ketting, "Contraceptive Knowledge, Attitudes, and Practice," 232.

81. A number of articles appeared in *Akusherstvo i ginekologiia* that addressed serious side effects of the pills. This was generally used as a caution against long-term use. For a discussion of oral contraception, see I. A. Manuilova, "O mekhanizme deistviia gormonal'nykh kontratseptivov," *Akusherstvo i ginekologiia* 2 (1971): 3–8.

Significantly, Manuilova, on page 7 of the article, accurately noted that many women in the West prefer the pill to other forms of contraception despite the known side-effects. She was one of the editors of the 1983 Ministry of Health report that cautioned against the long-term use of hormonal pills.

Side effects of IUDs were also discussed. The major difference between the discussions of these two kinds of contraception was that doctors considering the pill's potential effect on the fetus not fully established. For a discussion of IUDs, see Z. N. Iakubova, R. Kh. Amirov, V. G. Zil'berkan, and L. K. Krivonogov, "Opyt primeneniia vnutrimatochnykh kontratseptivov," *Akusherstvo i ginekologiia* 2 (1971): 16–18; and B. L. Gurmovoi "Vnutrimatochnaia kontratseptsiia," *Akusherstvo i ginekologiia* 2 (1971): 54–58. On harmful effects for the fetus, see, for example, the book review written by A. P. Kiriushchenkov, of K. Rothe's *Methoden der Empfängnisverhütung* (Jena: Gustav Fischer, 1973) in *Akusherstvo i ginekologiia* 7 (1974): 75.

In the mid-1980s, a number of additional anti-pill directives were issued. S. A. Polchanova, "Popularization of Contraception," in *Fel'dsher i akusherka* 5, 38–42, as cited in Popov, Visser, and Ketting, "Contraceptive Knowledge, Attitudes, and Practice," 232.

82. A. A. Popov, "Family Planning and Induced Abortion in the USSR: Basic Health and Demographic Characteristics," *Studies in Family Planning* 22, no. 6 (November–December 1991): 374.

83. A. A. Popov, "Induced Abortions in the USSR at the End of the 1980s: The Basis for the National Model of Family Planning," a paper presented at the Annual Meeting of the Population Association of America in 1992 in Denver, Colorado, 21. I am grateful to the late Murray Feshbach for drawing my attention to this paper.

84. The likeliness of contraceptive use is directly correlated to the following factors: educational level, age, the number of years of marriage, the number of previous abortions, and willingness of the husband to use contraception. Popov, "Medikodemograficheskie i sotsial'no-gigienicheskie prichiny i faktory iskusstvennogo aborta (obzor literatury)," *ZRF* 9 (1980): 30.

85. Popov, "Family Planning and Induced Abortion," 373-374.

86. Popov, "Induced Abortion in the USSR," 33–34.

87. Popov, "Induced Abortions in the USSR," 12–13.

88. This was part of the Soviet absorption of American modernization theory. One of the most influential works that presented this theme was A. G. Vishnevskii's *Demograficheskaia revoliutsiia* (Moskva: Statistika, 1976), which adapted the idea of demographic revolution from Landry, but others also discussed how urbanization and industrialization produced small families, including A. G. Volkov, "Vliianie urbanizatsii na demograficheskie protsessy v SSSR," *Problemy sovremennoi urbanizatsii* (Moskva, 1972); I. V. Arutiunian, *Sotsial'naia struktura sel'skogo naseleniia* (Moskva: Mysl', 1971); and V. A. Belova, *Chislo detei v sem'e* (Moskva: Statistika, 1975). The idea that the form of the family and marriage was a part of this "revolution" or "transformation" became influential for later Soviet and Russian scholarship. For example, see S. I. Golod, "Transformatsiia sem'i: sut' i problemy," in *Sovremennye problemy vosproizvodstva naseleniia*, ed. P. P. Zvidrin'sh (Riga: LGU, 1980). This was

the case not only for late Soviet demographers, but also for demographers of the post-socialist period. V. B. Zhiromskaia has expressed a critical concern that advocates of demographic transition theory have paid insufficient attention to particularities of Russian demographic modernization. V. B. Zhiromskaia, *Zhiznennyi potentsial poslevoennykh pokolenii v Rossii, 1946–1960* (Moskva: RGGU, 2009).

89. For a discussion of the original form of transition theory, see Simon Szreter, "The Idea of Demographic Transition and the Study of Fertility Change: A Critical Intellectual History," *Population and Development Review* 19, no. 4 (December 1993): 668. However, the revived profession of demography did not simply argue that Soviet demographic development was the same as capitalist development. Having argued the parallel between socialist development and capitalistic development, Vishnevskii emphasized the qualitative difference of socialist development as possibly providing the "most favorable" alternative to capitalist development. He also acknowledged some differences between the USSR and capitalist development, for example, that there was no tendency in Russia to postpone marriage. However, no explanation was suggested as to why this was the case. Vishnevskii, *Demograficheskaia revoliutsiia*, 48, 176.

90. Lapidus, *Women in Soviet Society,* 244.

91. The Moscow exhibition included a "modern" American kitchen to demonstrate the technological superiority of a capitalist home, but its purpose could be seen, from the socialist point of view, as the professionalization of housewives, trapped in their gilded cage. The simpler Soviet kitchen provided labor-saving technology for working women in order to emancipate them. Susan Reid, "'Our Kitchen Is Just as Good': Soviet Responses to the American Kitchen," in *Cold War Kitchen: Americanization, Technology, and European Users* (Cambridge, MA: Massachusetts Institute of Technology Press, 2009), 83–105.

92. Michele Rivkin-Fish's very insightful post-socialist study of a maternity hospital in St. Petersburg argues that the socialist health care system was made to put care providers and patients in systemic conflict. Doctors (predominantly women) considered patients irresponsible and ignorant of their health, while women expected doctors to cure all of their health problems. However, doctors were frustrated with the fact that they were not given enough resources to provide the best care possible. They were also poorly paid. Patients considered doctors part of the bureaucratic state system, abusing authority and indifferent to individual women's health. Both sides tried to make the system more personal and meaningful by establishing *blat*, exchange of favors, yet various strategies of *blat* did not always work. Michele Rivkin-Fish, *Women's Health in Post-Soviet Russia: The Politics of Intervention* (Bloomington: Indiana University Press, 2005), 123–178.

93. *Naselenie Rossii v XX veke: Istoricheskie ocherki* t. 3 (Moskva: ROSSPEN, 2005), 144.

94. Hansson and Liden, *Moscow Women,* 44, 161.

95. Natal'ia Baranskaia, "Nedelia kak nedelia," *Novyi mir*, no. 11 (1969): 23–55.

96. Vera Golubeva, "In the Northern Provinces," in *Women and Russia: Feminist Writings from the Soviet Union*, ed. Tatyana Mamonova (Boston: Beacon Press, 1984), 27.

97. V. A. Belova and L. E. Darskii, *Statistika mnenii v izuchenii rozhdaemosti* (Moskva: Statistika, 1972), 121–122.

98. Utrata, *Women without Men,* 47–50.

99. Sergey Afontsev, Gijis Kessler, Andrei Markevich, Victoria Tyazhelnikova, and Timur Valetov, "The Urban Household in Russia and the Soviet Union, 1900–2000: Patterns of Family Formation in a Turbulent Century," *History of the Family* 13 (2008): 192.

100. B. Urlanis, "Babushka v sem'e," *Literaturnaia gazeta,* March 3, 1971.

101. From Natal'ia Baranskaia, "Nedelia kak nedelia," trans. Emily Lehrman, *Massachusetts Review* 15, no. 4 (Autumn 1974): 671.

102. K. K. Bazdyrev, *Prostoe uravnenie: muzh + zhena= sem'ia* (Moskva: Statistika, 1981), 46–47.

103. Vishnevskii, *Demograficheskaia modernizatsiia,* 121. My interviewee Anna also articulated this point. Interview with Anna (born in 1967) on October 16, 2016. Jennifer Utrata's interviews conducted in the early 2000s showed that women in the late Soviet period considered that they had to marry by age 25. Utrata, *Women without Men,* 54–57.

104. Belova and Darskii, *Statistika mnenii,* 121–122.

105. Belova and Darskii, *Statistika mnenii,* 122–125.

106. Bazdyrev, *Prostoe uravnenie,* 49.

107. The relationship factor did not show up here, probably because the survey participants were all currently married women with two children, who had given birth to the second child despite all the fears and obstacles. But the authors' commentary here on the one-child family does not seem to be based completely on the married women with two children, but also on another survey involving married men and women. Bazdyrev, *Prostoe uravnenie* 45–49.

108. Lapidus, *Women in Soviet Society,* 305–306.

109. Feshbach, *The Soviet Population Policy Debate,* 5.

110. Lapidus, *Women in Soviet Society,* 286.

111. Bazdyrev, *Prostoe uravnenie* 52–53.

112. Working and student mothers received 50 rubles for the first child, 100 rubles for the second and third child. Non-working mothers received 30 rubles for the first, second, and third child. "Ob utverzhdenii polozheniia o poriadke naznacheniia i vyplati posobii beremennym zhenshchinam, mnogodetnym i odinokim materiam" August 12, 1970, *Svod zakonov SSSR* tom 2 (Moskva: Izvestiia, 1984), 725.

113. If the child was in school, the aid was extended until the child was 18. *Svod zakonov SSSR* tom 2, 720.

114. Ukaz Prezidiuma Verkhovnogo Soveta SSSR "O vvedenii posobii na deti maloobespechennym sem'iam," in *Svod zakonov SSSR,* tom 2 (Moskva: Izvestiia, 1984), 728–729.

115. Ukaz Prezidiuma Verkhovnogo Soveta SSSR, "O vnesenii izmenenii v nekotorye zakonodatel'nye akty SSSR," 18 iiulia 1980, *Vedomosti Verkhovnogo Soveta Soiuza Sovetskikh sotsialisticheskikh respublik* 30 (July 1980), 633–635.

116. *Odnazhdy dvadtsat' let spustia* (1980), directed by Iurii Egorov.

117. Postanovlenie Tsentral'nogo Komiteta KPSS i Soveta Ministrov SSSR, "O merakh po usileniiu gosudarstvennoi pomoshchi sem'iam, imeiushchim detei," ot 22 ianvaria 1981, *Svod zakonov SSSR* tom 2 (Moskva: Izvestiia, 1984), 678–684.

118. For example, M. B. Tatimov, a Kazakh demographer, criticized differentiation policy in his 1978 book, *Razvitie narodonaseleniia i demograficheskaia politika* (Alma-Ata: Izd. Nauka, 1978), 74, as cited in Feshbach, *The Soviet Population Policy Debate*, 28.

119. Lapidus, *Women in Soviet Society*, 325.

120. Lapidus, *Women in Soviet Society*, 327; Michele Rivkin-Fish, "From 'Demographic Crisis' to 'Dying Nation,': The Politics of Language and Reproduction in Russia," in *Gender and National Identity in Twentieth-Century Russian Culture*, ed. Helen Goscilo and Andrea Lanoux (DeKalb: Northern Illinois University Press, 2006), 156–157; Michele Rivkin-Fish, "Pronatalism, Gender Politics, and the Renewal of Family Support in Russia: Toward a Feminist Anthropology of 'Maternity Capital,'" *Slavic Review* 69, no. 3 (Fall 2010): 708.

121. Lynne Attwood, *The New Soviet Man and Woman: Sex-Role Socialization in the USSR* (London: Macmillan, 1990), 165–182.

122. Attwood, 184–191. In 1983, K. K. Bazdyrev published a popularizing book called *Only Child*, with a print run of 50,000 going to "a broad group of readers, demographers, sociologists, and economists" to caution against the phenomenon. K. K. Bazdyrev, *Edinstvennyi rebenok* (Moskva: Finansy i statistika, 1983). Interestingly, this was exactly at the height of the one-child campaign in China.

123. Markevich, "Soviet Urban Households," 466.

124. Mikhail Gorbachev, *Perestroika: New Thinking for Our Country and the World* (New York: Harper and Row, 1987), 116–118.

125. Diane Sainsbury, *Gender, Equality, and Welfare States* (Cambridge: Cambridge University Press, 1996), 49–103. Ann S. Orloff, "Gender and the Social Rights of Citizenship: The Comparative Analysis of Gender Relations and Welfare States," *American Sociological Review* 58 (June1993): 313.

126. Sainsbury, *Gender, Equality, and Welfare States*, 173–197.

127. Esping-Andersen calls this type a conservative or corporatist welfare regime. Gøsta Esping-Andersen, *Social Foundations of Postindustrial Economies* (New York: Oxford University Press, 1999), 81–83.

128. Gøsta Esping-Andersen categorizes welfare regimes into familialism/familialistic and de-familializing. The former means to assign "a maximum of welfare obligations to the household," while the latter means to actively shift welfare obligations outside the family, typically to the market or the welfare state. Esping-Andersen, *Social Foundations*, 45–46.

129. Esping-Andersen, *Social Foundations*, 45–46.

130. For a discussion of the three types of welfare regimes and their arrangement of care work, see Gøsta Esping-Andersen, *The Three Worlds of Welfare Capitalism* (Cambridge: Policy Press, 1990), 26–32; and Esping-Andersen, *Social Foundations*, 74–86.

131. Esping-Andersen, *Social Foundations*, 67–70.

132. Gøsta Esping-Andersen, *The Incomplete Revolution: Adapting to Women's New Roles* (Cambridge: Polity Press, 2009), 82–83, 99–100.

133. As Linda Cook has argued the Soviet welfare state does not fit into Esping-Andersen's welfare models, but his analytical concepts are useful to characterize socialist tendencies. Linda Cook, *Postcommunist Welfare States: Reform Politics in Russia and Eastern Europe* (Ithaca, NY: Cornell University Press, 2007), 37-39.

134. N. G. Iurkevich, *Sovetskaia sem'ia: Funktsii i usloviia stabil'nosti* (Minsk: Izdatel'stvo BGU im. V. I. Lenina, 1970), 192.

135. A. G. Zdravomyslov, V. P. Rozhin, and V. A. Iadov, *Chelovek i ego rabota: Sotsiologicheskoe issledovaniie* (Moskva: Izdatel'stvo 'Mysl', 1967), 311–312.

136. K. K. Bazdyrev, *Prostoe uravnenie: muzh + zhena= sem'ia* (Moskva: Statistika, 1981), 60.

137. Mark Edele, "Veterans and the Welfare State: World War II in the Soviet Context," *Comparativ: Zeitschrift fur Globalgeschichte und Vergleichende Gesellschaftsforschung* 20 (2010): 796; Mark Edele, *The Soviet Union: A Short History* (Hoboken, NJ: Wiley Blackwell, 2019), 179–182.

138. Bazdyrov, *Prostoe uravnenie*, 61.

139. Vishnevskii, ed., *Demograficheskaia modernizatsiia Rossii 1900-2000* (Moskva: Novoe Izdatel'stvo, 2006), 170-173. Zakharov, "Russian Federation," 922. Total fertility rate is the average total number of births per woman.

140. A. I. Antonov and S. A. Sorokin, *Sud'ba sem'i v Rossii XXI veka: Razmyshlenie o semeinoi politike o vozmozhnosti protivodeistviia upadki sem'i i depopuliatsii* (Moskva: Izd. Dom Graal', 2000), 334–339.

Epilogue

1. Ekaterina Lakhova, a trained pediatrician in Sverdlovsk, was one of the founding leaders for the "Women of Russia" Party. She became Yeltsin's advisor on issues related to women, children, and family. Andrea Chandler, *Democracy, Gender and Social Policy in Russia: A Wayward Society* (Houndsmills, UK: Palgrave Macmillan, 2013), 49-51. In the 1993 elections, twenty three members of the Party were elected. Mary Buckley, "Adaptation of the Soviet Women's Committee: Deputies' Voices from 'Women of Russia," in *Post-Soviet Women: From the Baltic to Central Asia*, ed. Mary Buckley (Cambridge: Cambridge University Press, 1997), 166.

2. Viktoriia Sakevich, "Abort-krivoe zerkalo demograficheskoi politiki," *Demoskop Weekly* 123-124 (August 25 —September 7, 2003), http://www.demoscope.ru/weekly/2003/0123/tema01.php.(last accessed on September 10, 2020).

3. Viktoriia Sakevich, "Problema aborta v sovremennoi Rossii," in *Zdorov'e i doverie: Gendernyi podkhod k reproduktivnoi meditsine*, ed. Elena Zdravomyslova and Anna Temkina (Sankt-Peterburg: Izdatel'stvo Evropeiskogo universiteta v Sankt-Peterburge, 2009), 145.

4. According to the Federal Service of Government Statistics (Rosstat) data, the absolute number of abortions went down from 4.1 million (1990) to 2.1 million (2000), and

the number of abortions per 1,000 women aged between 15 and 49 declined from 113.9 (1990) to 54.2 (2000). Maternal deaths declined from 943 (1990) to 503 (2000). This analysis and data are provided in a very informative article by Viktoriia Sakevich and Boris Denisov, "Pereidet li Rossiia ot aborta k planirovaniiu sem'i?" in *Demoskop Weekly*, 465–466 (May 2–22, 2011), http://www.demoscope.ru/weekly/2011/0465/ tema02.php. Rosstat, "Svedeniia o preryvanii beremennosti," https://www.gks.ru/ folder/13721 (last accessed August 29, 2020).

5. Victoria Sakevich and Maria Lipman, "Abortion in Russia: How Has the Situation Changed since the Soviet Era?" *PONARS Eurasia*, February 12, 2019, www. ponarseurasia.org/point-counter/article/abortion-russia-how-has-situation-changed-soviet-era (last accessed August 29, 2020).

6. Russian abortion data (2007) ranked the highest compared to data from sixty other countries at http://data.un.org/Data.aspx?q=abortions&d=GenderStat&f=in ID%3a12 (last accessed May 7, 2020). Analyzing 2008 data, a 2012 global study of abortions continued to find that Eastern Europe had much higher abortion rates than Western Europe. Guttmacher Institute "Facts on Induced Abortions Worldwide," https://www.who.int/reproductivehealth/publications/unsafe_abortion/induced_ abortion_2012.pdf?ua=1 (last accessed August 30, 2020).

7. Chandler, *Democracy, Gender and Social Policy in Russia*, 54.

8. From the excerpt of a press release by the Russian Government on September 8, 1995, at the Fourth World Conference on Women, http://www.un.org/womenwatch/daw/ beijing/govstatements.html (last accessed August 29, 2020). Chandler points out how, oddly, Russian statements primarily concerned women as mothers. Chandler, *Democracy, Gender and Social Policy*, 49.

9. For a comprehensive study of postcommunist welfare states, see Linda Cook, *Postcommunist Welfare States: Reform Politics in Russia and Eastern Europe*, (Ithaca, NY: Cornell University Press, 2007). Russian women's labor participation fell from near 100 percent at the end of the Soviet period to 82.7 percent in 1994, and 79.1 percent in 2001. Tatyana Teplova, "Welfare State Transformation, Childcare, and Women's Work in Russia," *Journal of Social Politics* 14, no. 3 (2007): 302–303. The number of childcare institutions fell by 40 percent between 1990 and 2000. Teplova, "Welfare State Transformation," 291–292. Among women with children under 7 years old, the percentage of women staying home increased from 17.1 percent in 1994 to 23.8 percent in 2001. Teplova, "Welfare State Transformation," 310. The percentage of women among the unemployed was 72.2 percent in 1992 and 64 percent in 1998. The period of unemployment among women was typically longer than that of men. Teplova, "Welfare State Transformation," 302–305.

10. One study showed that only 2.1 percent of Moscow women used babysitting services in 2004. Toshimi Murachi, "Gendai roshiano nyuuyoujino seikatsuto hoiku," *Yurashia kenkyu* 43, no.11 (2010): 47.

11. Tokuko Igarashi "Kyusorenno kyouwakokude tairyouno sengyoshufuwa tanjousurunoka" *Hikakukeizaikenkyu* 46, no. 1 (2009): 27.

12. Childlessness in Russia is one of the lowest in Europe. Tomáš Sobotka, "Childlessness in Europe: Reconstructing Long-Term Trends among Women Born in 1900–1972," in

Childlessness in Europe: Contexts, Causes, and Consequences, ed. Michaela Kreyenfeld, and Dirk Konietzka, Demographic Research Monographs, DOI 10.1007/978-3-319-44667-7_2.

Russia's divorce rate is by far the highest among the developed nations, well above the rate in the United States since 2000. Data from the Organisation for Economic Co-operation and Development (OECD) on marriage and divorce rates are available at http://www.oecd.org/els/family/database.htm; for the Russian divorce rate, see Rosstat https://www.gks.ru/folder/12781 (last accessed August 29, 2020). For example, the number of divorces per 1,000 people in 2017 was 4.2 in Russia, and 2.9 in the United States.

Sociologist Jennifer Utrata's study of single mothers demonstrates how both married and single mothers feel that they are raising children without men, albeit to different degrees. Jennifer Utrata, *Women without Men: Single Mothers and Family Change in the New Russia* (Ithaca, NY: Cornell University Press, 2015), 151–178.

13. The number gradually grew until 2015 and has been declining since. In 2019, the number was 1.504. Data taken from Rosstat at https://rosstat.gov.ru/folder/12781 (last accessed August 29, 20209).

14. Data provided by L'Institut national d'études démographiques (INED), https://www.ined.fr/devision2/dv_ExtractorGuide-rpc.php?cmd=PlotGraph&layout=Line&c%5b%5d=52&i%5b0%5d=33&i%5b1%5d=&doLabels=Y (last accessed Aubust 29, 2020).

15. Vladimir Popov, "Mortality and Life Expectancy in Post-Communist Countries," https://doc-research.org/2018/06/mortality-life-expectancy-post-communist/ (last accessed August 29, 2020); and Kazuhiro Kumo, *Roshiano jinko no rekishi to genzai* (Tokyo: Iwanami Shoten, 2014), 44.

16. For the 1989 Population of the USSR (census) and US (official estimates), see http://data.un.org/Data.aspx?q=Former+Soviet+Union&d=GenderStat&f=inID%3a5%3bcrID%3a140%2c157%2c159%2c198%2c205%2c35%2c83 (last accessed August 29, 2020).

17. Rosstat, "Chislenost' naseleniia," https://www.gks.ru/folder/12781 (last accessed August 29, 2020). Japan's population in 2020 was 126 million. https://www.stat.go.jp/data/jinsui/new.html (last accessed August 29, 2020). The US population as of 2020, was 330 million. See https://www.census.gov/popclock/ (last accessed on August 29, 2020).

18. Michele Rivkin-Fish, *Women's Health in Post-Soviet Russia: The Politics of Intervention* (Bloomington: Indiana University Press, 2005), 5–6, 100–102.

19. The government and the church also continue to attack LGBTQ citizens considering their presence a threat to "traditional" Russian sexuality and family. Dan Healey, *Russian Homophobia from Stalin to Sochi* (London: Bloomsbury Academic, 2018).

20. Vishnevskii, *Demograficheskaia modernizatsiia*, 175. Sergei Zakharov, "Russian Federation: From the First to Second Demographic Transition," *Demographic Research* 19, article 24 (July 2008): 907–972. The second demographic transition is a term coined in 1986 that provides a framework for understanding such phenomena observed in Western Europe since the 1970s as delayed marriage and first

birth, formation of family in cohabitation, rise in single motherhood, below replacement fertility, and diverse forms of family. A succinct formulation can be found in Ron Lesthaeghe, "The Second Demographic Transition: A Concise Overview of Its Development," *Proceedings of the National Academy of Sciences of the United States of America* 111, no. 51 (2014): 18112–18115.

21. Sakevich and Denisov, "Pereidet li Rossiia ot aborta."

22. "V Rossii uzhestochaiutsia trebovaniia k reklame abortov," *Rossiiskaia gazeta*, July 14, 2011.

23. "Zakonoproekt no. 381372-6, O vnesenii izmeneniia v stat'iu 35 Federal'nogo zakona 'Ob obiazatel'nom meditsinskom strakhovanii v Rossiiskoi Federatsii,'" cited in "Obshchestvennaia diskussiia legitimnosti aborta v Rossii prodolzhaetsia," *Demoskop Weekly*, 577–578 (December 2–25, 2013).

24. Sakevich, "Problema aborta v sovremennoi Rossii," 145–146.

25. This was approximately USD 10,000 in 2007. The amount is indexed to inflation and could be used for the child's education, toward housing, or toward the mother's pension savings. Men who adopt the second and more number of child(ren) after January 1, 2007, were also eligible. "Federal'nyi zakon Rossiiskoi Federatsii ot 29 dekabria 2006 g. N256-FZ O dopolnitel'nykh merakh gosudarstvennoi podderzhki semei, imeiushchikh detei," in *Rossiiskaia Gazeta*, 31 dekabria 2006. After a couple of extensions, on January 15, 2020, Putin announced that motherhood capital would continue at least through 2026, providing aid starting with the first child. "Putin Proposed to Pay Motherhood Capital with the Birth of the First Child," https://tass.ru/obshchestvo/7523749 (last accessed August 30, 2020).

26. For a gender analysis of pronatalist discourse in this period, see Michele Rivkin-Fish, "Pronatalism, Gender Politics, and Family Support in Russia: Toward a Feminist Anthropology of 'Maternity Capital,'" *Slavic Review* 69, no. 3 (Fall 2010): 712–716.

27. In 2012, as one of his two biggest achievements during 2008–11, Putin named stabilizing Russia's demographic slide by increasing the birth rate. (The other was overcoming the global financial crisis of 2008.) Artem Krechetnikov, "Putin ochertil 'dorozhnuiu kartu' tret'ego sroka," *BBC*, 11 aprelia 2012. https://www.bbc.com/russian/mobile/russia/2012/04/120411_putin_duma_constitution.shtml (last accessed August 30, 2020).

28. Both the number of births and the rate of births per thousand women declined between 2015 and 2019, according to the most recent Rosstat data. See Rosstat "Rozhdaemost', smertnost', i estestvennyi prirost naseleniia," https://www.gks.ru/folder/12781 (last accessed August 30, 2020).

29. Ekaterina Borozdina, Anna Rotkirch, Anna Temkina, and Elena Zdravomyslova, "Using Maternity Capital," *European Journal of Women's Studies* 23, no.1 (2016): 63,73.

30. "'Deti rozhdaiutsia ne iz-za deneg': Kak materinskii kapital privodit k obnishchaniiu rossiian," *Lenta*, 3 aprelia 2017. https://lenta.ru/articles/2017/04/03/malevamatcap/ (last accessed on August 30, 2020).

31. Borozdina et al. "Using Maternity Capital," 64 .

32. The extramarital birth rate has been steadily declining since 2005. In 2018, the percentage of extramarital births of all births was 21.2 percent. The figures were taken

from "Vnebrachnaia rozhdaemost' po sub"ektam Rossiiskoi Federatsii, 2002-2018," *Demoskop Weekly*, 865-866 (August 1-30, 2020), http://www.demoscope.ru/weekly/ssp/rus_exmar_reg.php?year=2018 (last accessed on August 30, 2020).

33. Utrata, *Women without Men*, 123–150.

34. The actual celebration is publicized as having a religious basis. July 8 is the date on which in the thirteenth century the legendary couple, Peter and Fevronia of Murom, died. Having prayed to die on the same day, they did and were canonized in the Orthodox Church in the sixteenth century.

35. http://www.fondsci.ru/ (last accessed August 30, 2020).

36. Sakevich, "V 2017 godu Gosduma otklonila chetyre zakonoproekta Mizulinoi, kasaiushchiesia abortov," *Demoskop Weekly*, 753–754 (December 18–31, 2017), http://www.demoscope.ru/weekly/2017/0753/reprod02.php(last accessed on August 30, 2020). Sakevich's article also discusses a series of proposed bills to restrict women's access to contraception, initiated by the conservative politician E. B. Mizulina, who argued that the idea of reproductive choice goes against Russia's "traditional Christian values." A number of other women politicians supported some of her proposals, including Ekaterina Lakhova, who supported the bill to prohibit the sale of abortion pills in retail stores.

37. Until 2013 total fertility rates had been low among former socialist countries in Europe. Since then, they have been rising particularly in the Baltic states, Czech Republic, Slovakia, and Romania. Albania's birth rate continues to fall. "Total fertility rate," Eurostat, https://appsso.eurostat.ec.europa.eu/nui/submitViewTableAction.do (last accessed on September 10, 2020).

38. Agnieszka Król and Paula Pustułka, "Women on Strike: Mobilizing against Reproductive Injustice in Poland," *International Feminist Journal of Politics* 20, 3 (2018): 369-378; Julia Kubisa and Katarzyna Rakowska, "Was it a Strike?: Notes on the Polish Women's Strike and the Strike of Parents of Persons with Disabilities," *Praktyka Teoretyszna* 4, 30 (2018): 20-24.

39. Gøsta Esping-Andersen, *The Incomplete Revolution: Adapting to Women's New Roles* (Cambridge: Polity Press, 2009), 44–49, 89.

40. Kumo, *Roshiano jinko no rekishi to genzai*, 56-64.

41. "Poslanie Prezidenta Federal'nomu Sobraniiu," Dec. 12, 2012. http://kremlin.ru/events/president/news/17118 (last accessed October 25, 2020).

Bibliography

Russian Archives

Central Archives
The Russian State Archive of Contemporary History (RGANI)
The Russian State Archive of Socio-Political History (RGASPI)
The Russian State Archive of the Economy (RGAE)
The State Archive of the Russian Federation (GARF)
    f. r-8009 Ministry of Health
    f. r-8131 Prosecutor's Office
    f. r-9401 Ministry of Internal Affairs
    f. r-9474 Supreme Court
    f. r-9492 Ministry of Justice

Local Archives
The Central Archives of Moscow (TsAGM)
The Central Moscow Archive-Museum Personal Collections (TsMAMLS)
The State Archive of Contemporary History of Saratov Oblast (GANISO)
The State Archive of Saratov Oblast (GASO)
The State Archive of Saratov Oblast-Engels' Branch (GASO-E)

Document Collections

Holod v Ukraïni, 1946–1947: dokumenty i materialy. Edited by O.M. Veselova, et al. Kiiv: Vidavnitstvo M. P. Kots', 1996.

Kovaleva, N. A., A. Korotkov, S. Mel'chin, et al., eds. *Molotov, Malenkov, Kaganovich. 1957: Stenogramma iiun'skogo plenuma TsK KPSS i drugie dokumenty.* Moskva: Mezhdunarodnyi fond "Demokratiia," 1998.

Lenin, V. I. *Polnoe sobranie sochinenii* tom 23. Moskva: Gos. Izd-vo politicheskoi literatury, 1961.

Livshin, A. Ia., and I. B. Orlov, compilers. *Pis'ma vo vlast', 1917–1927: Zaiavleniia, zhaloby, donosy, pis'ma v gosudarstvennye struktury i bol'shevistskim vozhdiam.* Moskva: ROSSPEN, 1998.

Marks, K., i F. Engel's. *Sochineniia,* tom 20. 2nd ed. Moskva: Politizdat, 1961.

Marks, K., i F. Engel's. *Sochineniia,* tom 26, chast' 2. 2nd ed. Moskva: Politizdat, 1963.

Marx, Karl, and Frederick Engels. *Collected Works* vol. 35. New York: International Publishers, 1975.

Marx, Karl, and Frederick Engels. *Collected Works,* vol. 41. Moscow: Progress Publishers, 1985.

Moskva poslevoennaia: 1945–1947. Moskva: Mosgorarkhiv, 2000.

Moskva voennaia 1941/1945: Memuary i arkhivnye dokumenty. Moskva: Izdatel'stvo ob'edineniia Mosgorarkhiv, 1995.

Postanovleniia KPSS i Sovetskogo pravitel'stva ob okhrane zdorov'ia naroda. Moskva: MEDGIZ, 1958.

Prezidium TsK KPSS 1954–64. Moskva: ROSSPEN, 2003.

Sbornik zakonov SSSR, 1938–1975, tom 1. Moskva: Izd. Izvestiia Sovetov Deputatov Trudiashchikhsia SSSR, 1975.

Sbornik zakonov SSSR i ukazov prezidiuma verkhovnogo soveta SSSR, tom 3. Moskva: Izvestiia sovetov deputatov trudiashchikhsia SSSR, 1968.

Sbornik zakonov SSSR i ukazov prezidiuma verkhovnogo soveta SSSR (1938-iiul' 1956 gg.). Moskva: Gosudarstvennoe izdatel'stvo iuridicheskoi literatury, 1956.

Schlesinger, Rudolf, ed. *The Family in the USSR: Documents and Readings*. London: Routledge and Kegan Paul, 1949.

Stalin, I. V. *Sochineniia*, tom 1 [XIV] 1934–1940. Edited by Robert H. McNeal. Stanford, CA: Hoover Institution on War, Revolution, and Peace, 1967.

Svod zakonov SSSR, tom 2. Moskva: Izvestiia, 1984.

Zhenshchiny i deti v SSSR: Statisticheskii sbornik. Moskva: Gosstatizdat, 1963.

Soviet Periodicals and Serial Publications

Akusherstvo i ginekologiia
Demoskop Weekly
Fel'dsher i akusherka
Izvestiia
Literaturnaia gazeta
Pravda
Pravda Vostoka
Sobranie postanovlenii i rasporiazhenii pravitel'stva Soiuza Sovetskikh Sotsialisticheskikh Respublik
Sotsialisticheskaia zakonnost'
Sovetskaia zhenshchina
Sovetskoe gosudarstvo i pravo
Vedomosti Verkhovnogo Soveta SSSR
Vestnik statistiki
Voprosy filosofii
Zdravookhranenie Rossiiskoi Federatsii

Interviewees cited
by pseudonym, year of birth, and interview date

Liudmila (b. 1923), January 12, 2003
Lena (b. 1925), November 27, 2002
Irina (b. 1929) on November 9, 2002
Anna (b. 1967) on October 16, 2016

Other Interview

Dr. O. G. Frolova, head of the Department of Socio-Medical analysis at the Research Center for Obstetrics, Gynecology, and Perinatology in Moscow, interviewed on May 23, 2003

Russian Publications

Aleksievich, Svetlana. *U voiny ne zhenskoe litso: Poslednie svideteli*. Moskva: Sovetskii pisatel', 1988.

Antonov, A. I., and S. A. Sorokin. *Sud'ba sem' i v Rossii XXI veka: Razmyshlenie o semeinoi politike o vozmozhnosti protivodeistviia upadki sem'i i depopuliatsii*. Moskva: Izd. Dom Graal', 2000.

Arutiunian, I. V. *Sotsial'naia struktura sel'skogo naseleniia*. Moskva: Mysl', 1971.

Babaian, E. A., A. S. Lopatin, and I. G. Lavretskii. *O pobochnom deistvii i oslozhneniiakh pri primenenii oral'nykh kontratseptivov: informatsionnoe pis'mo*. Moskva: SSSR Ministerstvo zdravookhranenii, 1974.

Baranskaia, Natal'ia. "Nedelia kak nedelia." *Novyi mir*, no. 11 (1969): 23–55.

Bazdyrev, K. K. *Edinstvennyi rebenok*. Moskva: Finansy i statistika, 1983.

Bazdyrev, K. K. *Prostoe uravnenie: muzh + zhena= sem'ia*. Moskva: Statistika, 1981.

Belova, V. A. *Chislo detei v sem'e*. Moskva: Statistika, 1975.

Belova, V. A., and L. E. Darskii. *Statistika mnenii v izuchenii rozhdaemosti*. Moskva: Statistika, 1972.

Blium, Alain. *Rodit'sia, zhit' i umeret' v SSSR*. Moskva: Novoe izdatel'stvo, 2005. [Translation of *Naitre, vivre et mourir en URSS: 1917–1991*. Paris: Plon, 1994].

Bodrova, V. V. *Narodonaselenie evropeiskikh sotsialisticheskikh stran*. Moskva: Statistika, 1976.

Bogdan, Valentina. *Mimikriia v SSSR, Vospominaniia inzhenera, 1935–1942 gody*. Frankfurt: Polyglott-Druck GmbH, 1981.

Budnitskii, Oleg. "Muzhchiny i zhenshchiny v Krasnoi armii (1941–1945)." *Cahiers du monde russe* 52, no. 2–3 (avril-septembre 2011): 405–422.

Burde, B. I. "O prioritete russkikh akusherov-ginekologov (K istorii otechestvennoi nauki)." *Akusherstvo i ginekologiia* 6 (1949): 23–27.

Darskii, L. E., ed. *Rozhdaemost': Problemy izucheniia: Sbornik statei*. Moskva: Statistika, 1976.

Demograficheskaia entsiklopediia. Moskva: Izd. Entsiklopeidiia, 2013.

Demograficheskie aspekty zaniatosti. Moskva: Statistika, 1975.

Esakov, V. D., and E. S. Levina. *Delo KR.: Sudy chesti v ideologii i praktike poslevoennogo stalinizma*. Moskva: Institut RAN, 2001.

Golod, S. I. "Transformatsiia sem'i: sut' i problem." In *Sovremennye problemy vosproizvodstva naseleniia*. Edited by P. P. Zvidrin'sh. Riga: LGU, 1980.

Gorpinenko, L. Ia. "Mikroflora vlagalishcha i sheiki matki u zhenshchin pri mestnom primenenii galaskorbina kak protivozachatochnogo sredstva." *Akusherstvo i ginekologiia* 6 (1959): 13–15.

Granat, N. E., and N. N. Malinkovskii. "100 letie so dnia sooruzheniia akusherskoi i ginekologicheskoi klinik v Moskve." Unpublished paper prepared for the 100th year anniversary since the organization of the first obstetric clinic in Moscow, 1989.

Gurmovoi, B. L. "Vnutrimatochnaia kontratseptiia." *Akusherstvo i ginekologiia* 2 (1971): 54–58.

Iakubova, Z. N., R. Kh. Amirov, V. G. Zil'berkan, and L. K. Krivonogov. "Opyt primeneniia vnutrimatochnykh kontratseptivov." *Akusherstvo i ginekologiia* 2 (1971): 16–18.

Iakunin, V. I. et al. *Gosudarstvennaia politika vyvoda Rossii iz demograficheskogo krizisa*. Moskva: Ekonomika, 2007.

Institut Marksizma-Leninizma pre TsK KPSS. *Predmetnyi ukazatel' ko vtoromu izdaniiu Sochinenii K. Marksa i F. Engel'sa*, part I (A-M). Moskva: 1978.

Iurkevich, N. G. *Sovetskaia sem'ia: Funktsii i usloviia stabil'nosti*. Minsk: Izdatel'stvo BGU im. V. I. Lenina, 1970.

Ivanova, Iu. N. *Khrabreishie iz prekrasnykh: Zhenshchiny Rossii v voinakh*. Moskva: ROSSPEN, 2002.

Ivkin, V. I. *Gosudarstvennaia vlast' SSSR: vysshie organy vlasti i upravleniia i ikh rukovoditeli 1923–1991*. Moskva: ROSSPEN, 1999.

Karnov A. B., and Danilov I. A. *Aktual'nye voprosy akusherstva i ginekologii*. Barnaul, 1975.

Kharchev, A. G. *Brak i sem'ia v SSSR: opyt sotsiologicheskogo issledovaniia*. Moskva: Mysl', 1964.

Khrushchev, N. S. "Rech' tovarishcha N. S. Khrushcheva na sobranii komsomol'tsev i molodezhi g. Moskvy, iz'iavivshikh zhelanie poekhat' rabotat' na tselinnye zemli, 7 ianvaria 1955 goda." *Izvestiia*, January 8, 1955.

Kovrigina, M. D. *V neoplatnom dolgu*. Moscow: Izd. polit. lit., 1985.

Krivosheev, G. F., ed. *Grif sekretnosti sniat: Poteri Vooruzhennykh Sil SSSR v voinakh, boevykh deistviiakh i voennykh konfliktakh*. Moskva: Voenizdat, 1993.

Kulakov, V. I., V. A. Golubev, T. V. Lopatina, N. N. Malinkovskii, and V. V. Chernaia. "Nauchnomu tsentru akusherstva ginekologii i perinatologii RAMN-50 let." Unpublished paper prepared for the fiftieth anniversary of the foundation of the institute, 1994.

Kumanev, G. A. "Evakuatsiia naseleniia SSSR: dostignutye rezul'taty i poteri." In *Liudskie poteri SSSR v Velikoi otechestvennoi voine*. Edited by R. B. Evdokimov. St. Petersburg: Russko-Baltiiskii informatsionnyi tsentr, 1995.

Manuilova, I. A. "O mekhanizme deistviia gormonal'nykh kontratseptivov," *Akusherstvo i ginekologiia* 2 (1971): 3–8.

Maslov, P. P. "Sotsial'nye modeli." In *Sotsiologiia v SSSR*, tom. 2. Moskva: Mysl', 1965.

Nikonchik, O. K. "Problema kontratseptsii i organizatsiia bor'by s abortami v SSSR." *Akusherstvo i ginekologiia* 6 (1959): 3–6.

Opyt sovetskoi meditsiny v velikoi otechestvennoi voine 1941–1945. Moskva: Medgiz, 1951.

Perevedentsev, V. I. "Neobkhodimo stimulirovat' rost naseleniia v nashei strane," *Voprosy filosofii* 11 (1974): 88–92.

Persianinov, L. S., and I. A. Manuikova. "O rasshirennoi programme VOZ [WHO] po reproduktsii cheloveka." *Akusherstvo i ginekologiia* 6 (June 1975): 1–3.

Persianinov, L. S., and I. A. Manuikova. "Sostoianie i perspektivy nauchnykh issledovanii v Moskovskom nauchno-metodicheskom tsentre VOZ po reproduktsii cheloveka." *Akusherstvo i ginekologiia* 6 (June 1975): 3–7.

Poliakov, Iu. A. et al. *Naselenie Rossii v XX vek: istoricheskie ocherki, 1900–1939*, tom 1. Moskva: ROSSPEN, 2000.

Poliakov, Iu. A. et al. *Naselenie Rossii v XX veke: Istoricheskie ocherki, 1940–1959 gg.* tom 2. Moskva: ROSSPEN, 2001.

Poliakov, Iu. A. et al. *Naselenie Rossii v XX veke: Istoricheskie ocherki*, tom 3. Moskva: ROSSPEN, 2005.

Popovskii, Mark. *Tretii lishnii: On, ona i sovetskii rezhim*. London: Overseas Publications Interchange, 1985.

Ptukha, M. V. *Ocherki po statistike naseleniia*. Moskva: Gosstatizdat TsSU SSSR, 1960.

Pyzhikov, A.V. "Sovetskoe poslevoennoe obshchestvo i predposylki khrushchevskikh reform." *Voprosy istorii*, 2 (2002): 33–43.

Riabushkin, T. V. et al., eds. *Sovetskaia demografiia za 70 let*. Moskva: Nauka, 1987.

Rossiiskii nauchno-issledovatel'skii tsentr perinatologii, akusherstva, i ginekologii. Moskva: Pressa, 1992.

Sadvokasova, E. A. *Sotsial'no-gigienicheskie aspekty regulirovaniia razmerov sem'i.* Moskva: Meditsina, 1969.

Sakevich, Viktoriia. "Problema aborta v sovremennoi Rossii." In *Zdorov'e i doverie: Gendernyi podkhod k reproduktivnoi meditsine.* Edited by Elena Zdravomyslova and Anna Temkina. Sankt-Peterburg: Izdatel'stvo Evropeiskogo universiteta v Sankt-Peterburge, 2009.

Sakevich, Victoria, and Maria Lipman. "Abortion in Russia: How Has the Situation Changed since the Soviet Era?" *PONARS Eurasia*, February 12, 2019.

Serebrovskaia, Elena. "Zhizn' vnosit popravku." *Literaturnaia gazeta*, January 16.

Shamrai, E. F. "Problema kontraseptsii i puti ee dal'neishego razvitiiаю" *Akusherstvo i ginekologiia* 6 (1959): 8–10.

Shikheeva-Gaister, Inna. *Semeinaia khronika vremen kul'ta lichnosti 1925–1953, Pamiati nashikh roditelei i mladshei sestrenki posviashchaetsia.* Moskva: Niudiamed-AO, 1998.

Sifman, R. I. *Dinamika rozhdaemosti v SSSR.* Moskva: Statistika, 1974.

Smirnov, Efim I. *Meditsina i organizatsiia zdravookhraneniia.* Moskva: Meditsina, 1989.

Sovetskaia Ukraina v gody Velikoi Otechestvennoi Voiny, 1941–1945: Ukrainskaia SSR v period korennogo pereloma v khode Velikoi Otechestvennoi voiny. Kiev: Naukova Dumka, 1985.

Starovskii, V. N. "Metodika issledovaniia elementov rosta narodonaseleniia." In *Sotsiologiia v SSSR*, tom 1. Moscow: Mysl', 1965.

Stepanov, L. G. "Organizatsionnye voprosy problemy kontraseptsii." *Akusherstvo i ginekologiia* 6 (1959): 6-8.

Strumilin, S. G. *Izbrannye proizvedeniia* tom 1. Moskva: Nauka, 1963.

Strumilin, S. G. *Izbrannye proizvedeniia* tom 3. Moskva: Nauka, 1964.

Strumilin, S. G. *Ocherki sovetskoi ekonomiki: resursy i perspektivy.* Moskva: Gos. izd-vo, 1930.

Takala, I. R. *Veselie Rusi.* Sankt Peterburg: Zhurnal Neva, 2002.

Tatimov, M. B. *Razvitie narodonaseleniia i demograficheskaia politika.* Alma-Ata: Nauka, 1978.

Tel'nova, R. P. "Kontratseptivnye svoistva nekotorykh polifenolov," *Akusherstvo i ginekologiia* 6 (1959): 11–13.

Tol'ts, M. S. "Nedostupnoe izmerenie." *V chelovecheskom izmerenii.* Edited by A. N. Alekseev and A. G. Vishnevskii. Moskva: Progress, 1989.

Tol'ts, M. S. "Skol'ko zhe nas togda bylo?" *Ogonek*, no. 51 (1987).

Ulitskaia, Liudmila. *Kazus Kukotskogo.* Moskva: Eksmo, 2000.

Urlanis, B. Ts. *Rozhdaemost' i prodolzhitel'nost' zhizni v SSSR.* Moscow: Gostatizdat, 1963.

Vaksberg, A. E. *Moia zhizn' v zhizni*, tom 2. Moscow: Terra-Sport, 2000.

Valentei, D. I., ed. *Demograficheskii analiz rozhdaemosti.* Moskva: Statistika, 1974.

Vishnevskii, A. G., ed. *Demograficheskaia modernizatsiia Rossii, 1900–2000.* Moskva: Novoe Izdatel'stvo, 2006.

Vishnevskii, A. G. *Demograficheskaia revoliutsiia.* Moskva: Statistika, 1976.

Vishnevskii, A. G. "Sud'ba odnogo demografa: portret na fone epokhi." *Cahiers du monde russe et sovietique* 34, no. 4 (1993): 577–629.

Vishnevskii, A. G. *Vosproizvodstvo naseleniia i obshchestvo: istoriia, sovremennost', vzgliad v budushchee.* Moscow: Finansy i statistika, 1982.

Vishnevskii, A. G., Viktoriia Sakevich, and Boris Denisov. "Zapret aborta: osvezhite vashu pamiat." *Demoskop Weekly* no. 707–708 (28 noiabria-11 dekabria 2016).

Volkov, A. G. *Sem'ia—ob'ekt demografii.* Moskva: Mysl, 1986.

Volkov, A. G. "Vliianie urbanizatsii na demograficheskie protsessy v SSSR." *Problemy sovremennoi urbanizatsii.* Moskva: Statistika, 1972.

Vorob'ev, N. Ia. *Vsesoiuznaia perepis' naseleniia 1926g.* Moskva: Gosstatizdat, 1957.

Zdravomyslov, A. G., V. P. Rozhin, and V. A. Iadov. *Chelovek i ego rabota: Sotsiologicheskoe issledovaniie.* Moskva: Izdatel'stvo Mysl', 1967.

Zdravomyslova, Elena. "Gendernoe grazhdanstvo i abortnaia kul'tura." In *Zdorov'e i doverie: Gendernyi podkhod k reproduktivnoi meditsine.* Edited by Elena Zdravomyslova and Anna Temkina. St. Peterburg: Evropeiskii universitet v Sankt-Peterburge, 2009.

Zhiromskaia, V. B. *Zhiznennyi potentsial poslevoennykh pokolenii v Rossii, 1946–1960.* Moskva: RGGU, 2009.

Zima, V. F. *Golod v SSSR 1946–1947 godov: Proiskhozhdeniie i posledstviia.* Moskva: Institut Rossiiskoi istorii RAN, 1996.

Zubkova, Elena. "Preodolenie voiny-preodolenie pobedy: Sovetskaia povsednevnost' i strategii vyzhivaniia (1945–1953)." In *Pobediteli i pobezhdennye: Ot voiny k miru: SSSR, Frantsiia, Velikobritaniia, Germaniia, SShA (1941–1950).* Edited by B. Fizeler and N. Muan. Moskva: ROSSPEN, 2010.

Non-Russian Publications

Afontsev, Sergey, Gijis Kessler, Andrei Markevich, Victoria Tyazhelnikova, and Timur Valetov. "The Urban Household in Russia and the Soviet Union, 1900–2000: Patterns of Family Formation in a Turbulent Century." *History of the Family* 13 (2008): 178–194.

Agadjanian, Victor. "Is 'Abortion Culture' Fading in the Former Soviet Union? Views about Abortion and Contraception in Kazakhstan." *Studies in Family Planning,* 33, no. 3 (September 2002): 237–48.

Alexopoulos, Golfo. *Stalin's Outcasts: Aliens, Citizens, and the Soviet State, 1926–1936.* Ithaca, NY: Cornell University Press, 2003.

Anderson, Barbara A., and Brian D. Silver. "Demographic Consequences of World War II on the Non-Russian Nationalities of the USSR." In *The Impact of World War II on the Soviet Union.* Edited by Susan Linz. Totowa, NJ: Rowman and Allanheld, 1985.

Anderson, Barbara A., and Brian D. Silver. "Infant Mortality in the Soviet Union: Regional Differences and Measurement Issues." *Population and Development Review* 12, no. 4 (1986): 705–738.

Attwood, Lynne. *Creating the New Soviet Woman: Women's Magazines as Engineers of Female Identity, 1922–1953.* New York: St. Martin's Press, 1999.

Attwood, Lynne. *The New Soviet Man and Woman: Sex-Role Socialization in the USSR.* London: Macmillan, 1990.

Avdeev, Alexandre, Alain Blum, and Irina Troitskaia. "The History of Abortion Statistics in Russia and the USSR from 1900 to 1991." *Population: An English Selection* 7 (1995): 39–66.

Avdeev, Alexandre, and Alain Monnier. "A Survey of Modern Russian Fertility." *Population: An English Selection* 7 (1995): 1–38.

Bailes, Kendall. *Technology and Society under Lenin and Stalin: Origins of the Soviet Technical Intelligentsia, 1917–1941.* Princeton, NJ: Princeton University Press, 1978.

Ball, Alan. *And Now My Soul Is Hardened: Abandoned Children in Soviet Russia, 1918–1930*. Berkeley: University of California Press, 1994.

Baranskaia, Natal'ia. "Nedelia kak nedelia." Translated as "A Week Like Any Other Week" by Emily Lehrman. *Massachusetts Review* 15, no. 4 (Autumn 1974): 657–703.

Barbieri, Magali, Alain Blum, Elena Dolkigh, and Amon Ergashev. "Nuptiality, Fertility, Use of Contraception, and Family Policies in Uzbekistan." *Population Studies*, 50, no. 1 (March 1996): 69–88.

Bebel, August. *Woman in the Past, Present, and Future*. Translated from *Die Frau in der Vergangenheit, Gegenwart und Zukunft* by H. B. Adams Walther. London: William Reeves, 1893.

Berkhoff, Karel C. *Harvest of Despair: Life and Death in Ukraine under Nazi Rule*. Cambridge, MA: Belknap Press of Harvard University Press, 2004.

Bernstein, Frances. *The Dictatorship of Sex: Lifestyle Advice for the Soviet Masses*. DeKalb: Northern Illinois University Press, 2007.

Bernstein, Laurie. *Sonia's Daughters: Prostitutes and Their Regulation in Imperial Russia*. Berkeley: University of California Press, 1995.

Besemeres, John. *Socialist Population Politics: The Political Implications of Demographic Trends in the USSR and Eastern Europe*. White Plains, NY: M. E. Sharpe, 1980.

Bittner, Stephen. *The Many Lives of Khrushchev's Thaw: Experience and Memory in Moscow's Arbat*. Ithaca, NY: Cornell University Press, 2008.

Bittner, Stephen. "Remembering the Avant-garde: Moscow Architects and the 'Rehabilitation' of Constructivism, 1961–1964." *Kritika* 2: 3 (2001): 553–576.

Blum, Alain, and Martine Mespoulet. *L'anarchie bureaucratique: Statistique et pouvoir sous Staline*. Paris: La Découverte, 2003 [*Biurokraticheskaia anarkhiia: statistika i vlast' pri Staline*. Moskva: ROSSPEN, 2006].

Bonnell, Victoria. *Iconography of Power: Soviet Political Posters under Lenin and Stalin*. Berkeley: University of California Press, 1997.

Borozdina, Ekaterina, Anna Rotkirch, Anna Temkina, and Elena Zdravomyslova. "Using Maternity Capital." *European Journal of Women's Studies* 23 no. 1 (July 2014): 60–75.

Brent, Jonathan, and Vladimir P. Naumov. *Stalin's Last Crime: The Plot against the Jewish Doctors, 1948–1953*. New York: Harper Collins, 2003.

Brooks, Jeffrey. *Thank You, Comrade Stalin! Soviet Public Culture from Revolution to Cold War*. Princeton, NJ: Princeton University Press, 2000.

Buchanan, Ann, and Anna Rotkirch. *Fertility Rates and Population Decline: No Time for Children?* Houndmills: Palgrave Macmillan, 2013.

Bucher, Greta. *Women, the Bureaucracy and Daily Life in Postwar Moscow, 1945–1953*. Boulder, CO: East European Monographs, distributed by Columbia University Press, 2006.

Buckley, Mary. "Adaptation of the Soviet Women's Committee: Deputies' Voices from 'Women of Russia.'" In *Post-Soviet Women: From the Baltic to Central Asia*. Edited by Mary Buckley. Cambridge: Cambridge University Press, 1997.

Burton, Christopher. "Medical Welfare during Late Stalinism: A Study of Doctors and the Soviet Health System, 1945–53." PhD dissertation, University of Chicago, 2000.

Burton, Christopher. "Minzdrav, Soviet Doctors, and the Policing of Reproduction in the Late Stalinist Years." *Russian History* 27, no 2 (Summer 2000): 197–221.

Burton, Christopher. "Soviet Medical Attestation and the Problem of Professionalisation under Late Stalinism, 1945–1953." *Europe-Asia Studies* 57, no. 8 (December 2005): 1211–1229.

Chandler, Andrea. *Democracy, Gender, and Social Policy in Russia: A Wayward Society.* New York: Palgrave Macmillan, 2013.

Chatterjee, Choi. *Celebrating Women: Gender, Festival Culture, and Bolshevik Ideology, 1910–1939.* Pittsburgh, PA: University of Pittsburgh Press, 2002.

Clark, Katerina. "Rethinking the Past and Current Thaw." In *Glasnost' in Context: On the Recurrence of Liberalizations in Central and East European Literatures and Cultures.* Edited by Marko Pavlyshyn. New York: St. Martin's Press, 1990.

Clements, Barbara. *Bolshevik Feminist: The Life of Aleksandra Kollontai.* Bloomington: Indiana University Press, 1979.

Clements, Barbara. "The Effects of the Civil War on Women and Family Relations." In *Party, State, and Society in the Russian Civil War: Explorations in Social History.* Edited by Diane Koenker, William Rosenberg, and Ronald Suny. Bloomington: Indiana University Press, 1989.

Coale, Ansley, Barbara A. Anderson, and Erna Harm. *Human Fertility in Russia since the Nineteenth Century.* Princeton, NJ: Princeton University Press, 1979.

Cohn, Edward. *The High Title of a Communist: Postwar Party Discipline and the Values of the Soviet Regime.* DeKalb: Northern Illinois University Press, 2015.

Cohn, Edward. "Sex and the Married Communist: Family Troubles, Marital Infidelity, and Party Discipline in the Postwar USSR, 1945–1964." *Russian Review* 68 (July 2009): 429–450.

Cole, Joshua. *The Power of Large Numbers: Population, Politics, and Gender in Nineteenth-Century France.* Ithaca, NY: Cornell University Press, 2000.

Condee, Nancy. "Cultural Codes of the Thaw." *Nikita Khrushchev.* Edited by William Taubman, Sergei Khrushchev, and Abbot Gleason. New Haven, CT: Yale University Press, 2000.

Connelly, Matthew. *Fatal Misconception: The Struggle to Control World Population.* Cambridge, MA: Harvard University Press, 2008.

Conquest, Robert. *The Great Terror: Stalin's Purge of the Thirties.* New York: Macmillan, 1968.

Cook, Linda. "Eastern Europe and Russia." In *The Oxford Handbook of the Welfare State.* Edited by Francis Castles et al. New York: Oxford University Press, 2010.

Cook, Linda. *Postcommunist Welfare States: Reform Politics in Russia and Eastern Europe.* Ithaca, NY: Cornell University Press, 2007.

Cottam, K. Jean. "Soviet Women in Combat in World War II: The Rear Services, Resistance behind Enemy Lines and Military Political Workers." *International Journal of Women's Studies* 5, no. 4 (1982): 363–378.

Cottam, K. Jean. "Soviet Women in World War II: The Ground Forces and the Navy." *International Journal of Women's Studies* 3, no. 4 (1980): 345–357.

David, Henry. *Family Planning and Abortion in the Socialist Countries of Central and Eastern Europe: A Compendium of Observations and Readings.* New York: Population Council, 1970.

Davis, Christopher, and Murray Feshbach. *Rising Infant Mortality in the U.S.S.R. in the 1970's.* Washington, DC: US Dept. of Commerce, Bureau of the Census: [Supt. of Docs., US GPO, distributor], 1980.

DeWitt, Nicholas. *Education and Professional Employment in the USSR.* Washington, DC: National Science Foundation, 1961.

Djilas, Milovan. *Conversations with Stalin.* Translated by Michael B. Petrovich. San Diego: Harcourt Brace, 1962.

Dobson, Miriam. "The Post Stalin Era, Daily Life and Dissent." *Kritika* 12, no. 4 (2011): 905–924.

Dunham, Vera. *In Stalin's Time: Middleclass Values in Soviet Fiction*. Durham, NC: Duke University Press, 1990.

Edele, Mark. "The Soviet Culture of Victory." *Journal of Contemporary History* 54, no. 4 (October 2019), 780–798.

Edele, Mark. *The Soviet Union: A Short History*. Hoboken, NJ: Wiley Blackwell, 2019.

Edele, Mark. *Soviet Veterans of the Second World War: A Popular Movement in an Authoritarian Society, 1941–1991*. Oxford: Oxford University Press, 2008.

Edele, Mark. "Veterans and the Village: The Impact of Red Army Demobilization on Soviet Urbanization, 1945–1955." *Russian History* 36 (2009): 159–182.

Edele, Mark. "Veterans and the Welfare State: World War II in the Soviet Context." *Comparativ: Zeitschrift fur Globalgeschichte und Vergleichende Gesellschaftsforschung* 20 (2010): 18–33.

Ehrenburg, Ilya. *The War 1941–1945*. Translated by Tatiana Shebunina. London: MacGibbon and Kee, 1964.

Ellman, Michael, and S. Maksudov. "Soviet Deaths in the Great Patriotic War: A Note." *Europe-Asia Studies* 46, no. 4 (1994): 671–680.

Engel, Barbara Alpern, and Anastasia Posadskaya-Vanderbeck, eds. *A Revolution of Their Own: Voices of Women in Soviet History*. Translated by Sona Hoisinton. Boulder, CO: Westview Press, 1998.

Engelstein, Laura. "Abortion and the Civic Order: The Legal and Medical Debates." In *Russia's Women: Accommodation, Resistance, Transformation*. Edited by Barbara E. Clements, Barbara Alpern Engel, and Christine D. Worobec. Berkeley: University of California Press, 1991.

Engelstein, Laura. *The Keys to Happiness: Sex and the Search for Modernity in Fin-de-Siècle Russia*. Ithaca, NY: Cornell University Press, 1992.

Erickson, John. "Soviet Women at War." In *World War II and the Soviet People: Selected Papers from the Fourth World Congress for Soviet and East European Studies* (Harrogate 1990). Edited by John and Carol Garrard. New York: St. Martin's Press, 1993.

Esping-Andersen, Gøsta. *The Incomplete Revolution: Adapting to Women's New Roles* Cambridge: Polity Press, 2009.

Esping-Andersen, Gøsta. *Social Foundations of Postindustrial Economies*. New York: Oxford University Press, 1999.

Esping-Andersen, Gøsta. *The Three Worlds of Welfare Capitalism*. Cambridge: Policy Press, 1990.

Farnsworth, Beatrice. *Aleksandra Kollontai: Socialism, Feminism, and the Bolshevik Revolution*. Stanford, CA: Stanford University Press, 1980.

Feshbach, Murray. "Russia's Health and Demographic Crises: Policy Implications and Consequences." *Health and National Security Series* (Washington, DC: Chemical and Biological Arms Control Institute, April 2003).

Feshbach, Murray. *The Soviet Population Policy Debate: Actors and Issues*. Santa Monica, CA: Rand Corporation, December 1986.

Feshbach, Murray. *The Soviet Statistical System: Labor Force Recordkeeping and Reporting*. [Washington, DC:] US Department of Commerce, Bureau of the Census, 1960.

Field, Deborah. "Irreconcilable Differences: Divorce and Conceptions of Private Life in the Khrushchev Era." *Russian Review* 57, no. 4 (October 1998): 599–613.

Field, Deborah. *Private Life and Communist Morality in Khrushchev's Russia.* New York: Peter Lang, 2007.

Field, Mark. *Doctor and Patient in Soviet Russia.* Cambridge, MA: Harvard University Press, 1957.

Field, Mark. "The Re-legalization of Abortion in Soviet Russia." *New England Journal of Medicine* 255, no. 9 (August 30, 1956): 421–427.

Fieseler, Beate. "The Bitter Legacy of the 'Great Patriotic War': Red Army Disabled Soldiers under Late Stalinism." In *Late Stalinist Russia: Society between Reconstruction and Reinvention.* Edited by Juliane Fürst. London: Routledge, 2006.

Filtzer, Donald. *The Hazards of Urban Life in Late Stalinist Russia: Health, Hygiene, and Living Standards, 1943–1953.* Cambridge: Cambridge University Press, 2010.

Filtzer, Donald. "The 1947 Food Crisis and Its Aftermath: Worker and Peasant Consumption in Non-Famine Regions of the RSFSR." In *The Dream Deferred: New Studies in Russian and Soviet Labour History.* Edited by Donald Filtzer, Wendy Z. Goldman, Gijs Kessler, and Simon Pirani. Bern: Peter Lang, 2008.

Filtzer, Donald. *Soviet Workers and De-Stalinization: The Consolidation of the Modern System of Soviet Production Relations, 1953–1964.* Cambridge: Cambridge University Press, 1992.

Filtzer, Donald. *Soviet Workers and Late Stalinism: Labour and the Restoration of the Stalinist System after World War II.* Cambridge: Cambridge University Press, 2002.

Fisher, Wesley Andrew. *The Soviet Marriage Market: Mate-Selection in Russia and the USSR.* New York: Praeger, 1980.

Fitzpatrick, Sheila. "Blat in Stalin's Time." In *Bribery and Blat in Russia: Negotiating Reciprocity from the Middle Ages to the 1990s.* Edited by Stephen Lovell, Alena Ledeneva, and Andrei Rogachevskii. New York: St. Martin's Press, 2000.

Fitzpatrick, Sheila. *The Cultural Front: Power and Culture in Revolutionary Russia.* Ithaca, NY: Cornell University Press, 1992.

Fitzpatrick, Sheila. *Education and Social Mobility in the Soviet Union, 1921–1934.* Cambridge: Cambridge University Press, 1979.

Fitzpatrick, Sheila. *Everyday Stalinism: Ordinary Life in Extraordinary Times, Soviet Russia in the 1930s.* New York: Oxford University Press, 1999.

Fitzpatrick, Sheila. *Stalin's Peasants: Resistance and Survival in the Russian Village after Collectivization.* New York: Oxford University Press, 1994.

Fitzpatrick, Sheila. *Tear off the Masks!: Identity and Imposture in Twentieth-Century Russia.* Princeton, NJ: Princeton University Press, 2005.

Fitzpatrick, Sheila, and Yuri Slezkine, eds. *In the Shadow of Revolution: Life Stories of Russian Women from 1917 to the Second World War.* Princeton, NJ: Princeton University Press, 2000.

Foucault, Michel. *The Essential Foucault: Selections from Essential Works of Foucault, 1954-1984.* Edited by Paul Rabinow and Nikolas Rose. New York: New Press, 2003.

Foucault, Michel. "Governmentality." In *The Foucault Effect: Studies in Governmentality with Two Lectures by and an Interview with Michel Foucault.* Edited by Graham Burchell et al. Chicago: University of Chicago Press, 1991.

Frejka, Thomas. "Induced Abortion and Fertility: A Quarter Century of Experience in Eastern Europe." *Population and Development Review* 9, no. 3 (September 1983): 494–520.

Furukubo, Sakura. "Manshuni okeru nihonjin joseino keiken [Japanese Women's Experience in Manchuria]." *Nihonno feminizumu* [Japan's Feminism] *vol. 10: Joseishi/*

Jenda-shi [Women's History and Gender History]. Edited by Masako Amano. Tokyo: Iwanami shoten, 2009.

Gal, Susan. "Between Speech and Silence: The Problematics of Research on Language and Gender." In *Gender at the Crossroads of Knowledge: Feminist Anthropology in the Postmodern Era*. Edited by Micaela di Leonardo. Berkeley: University of California Press, 1991.

Gal, Susan, and Gail Kligman. *The Politics of Gender after Socialism: A Comparative Historical Essay*. Princeton, NJ: Princeton University Press, 2000.

Gallagher, Catherine. "The Body versus the Social Body in the Works of Thomas Malthus and Henry Mayhew." In *The Making of the Modern Body: Sexuality and Society in the Nineteenth Century*. Edited by Catherine Gallagher and Thomas Laqueur. Berkeley: University of California Press, 1987.

Galmarini-Kabala, Maria Cristina. *The Right to Be Helped: Deviance, Entitlement, and the Soviet Moral Order*. DeKalb: Northern Illinois University Press, 2016.

Geiger, Kent H. *The Family in Soviet Russia*. Cambridge, MA: Harvard University Press, 1968.

Gessen, Masha. *The Future Is History: How Totalitarianism Reclaimed Russia*. New York: Riverhead Books, 2017.

Getty, Arch. *Origins of the Great Purges: The Soviet Communist Party Reconsidered, 1933–1938*. New York: Cambridge University Press, 1985.

Giles, Wenona, and Jennifer Hyndman, eds. *Sites of Violence: Gender and Conflict Zones*. Berkeley: University of California, 2004.

Ginsburg, Faye, and Rayna Rapp. "The Politics of Reproduction." *Annual Review of Anthropology* 20 (1990).

Ginsburg, Faye, and Rayna Rapp, eds. *Conceiving the New World Order: The Global Politics of Reproduction*. Berkeley: University of California Press, 1995.

Goldman, Wendy. "Industrial Politics, Peasant Rebellion and the Death of the Proletarian Women's Movement in the USSR." *Slavic Review* 55, no. 1 (Spring 1996): 46–77.

Goldman, Wendy. *Inventing the Enemy: Denunciation and Terror in Stalin's Russia*. New York: Cambridge University Press, 2012.

Goldman, Wendy. *Terror and Democracy in the Age of Stalin*. New York: Cambridge University Press, 2007.

Goldman, Wendy. *Women at the Gates: Gender and Industry in Stalin's Russia*. Cambridge: Cambridge University Press, 2002.

Goldman, Wendy. *Women, the State and Revolution: Soviet Family Policy and Social Life, 1917–1936*. Cambridge: Cambridge University Press, 1993.

Goldman, Wendy, and Donald Filtzer, eds. *Hunger and War: Food Provisioning in the Soviet Union during World War II*. Bloomington: Indiana University Press, 2015.

Goldstein, Joshua. *War and Gender: How Gender Shapes the War System and Vice Versa*. Cambridge: Cambridge University Press, 2001.

Golubeva, Vera. "In the Northern Provinces." In *Women and Russia: Feminist Writings from the Soviet Union*. Edited by Tatyana Mamonova. Boston: Beacon Press, 1984.

Gorbachev, Mikhail. *Perestroika: New Thinking for Our Country and the World*. New York: Harper and Row, 1987.

Gorlizki, Yoram, and Oleg Khlevniuk. *Cold Peace: Stalin and the Soviet Ruling Circle, 1945–1953*. New York: Oxford University Press, 2004.

Gordon, Linda. *The Moral Property of Women: A History of Birth Control Politics in America*. Urbana: University of Illinois Press, 2007.

Greenfeld, Liah. "Soviet Sociology and Sociology in the Soviet Union." *Annual Review of Sociology* 14 (1988): 99–123.

Greenhalgh, Susan, and Edwin Winckler. *Governing China's Population: From Leninist to Neoliberal Biopolitics.* Stanford, CA: Stanford University Press, 2005.

Greenhalgh, Susan, and Edwin Winckler. *Just One Child: Science and Policy in Deng's China.* Berkeley: University of California Press, 2008.

Greenwood, Jeremy, Ananth Seshadri, and Guillaume Vandenbrouske. "The Baby Boom and Baby Bust." *American Economic Review* 95, no. 1 (March 2005): 183–207.

Grossmann, Atina. "A Question of Silence: The Rape of German Women by Occupation Soldiers." In *West Germany under Construction: Politics, Society, and Culture in the Adenauer Era.* Edited by Robert G. Moeller. Ann Arbor: University of Michigan Press, 1997.

Grossmann, Atina. *Reforming Sex: The German Movement for Birth Control and Abortion Reform: 1920–1950.* New York: Oxford University Press, 1995.

Grossmann, Atina. "Trauma, Memory, and Motherhood: Germans and Jewish Displaced Persons in Post-Nazi Germany, 1945–1949." *Archiv fur Sozialgeschichte* 38 (1998): 215–239.

Hachten, Charles. "Separate Yet Governed: The Representation of Soviet Property Relations in Civil Law and Public Discourses." In *Borders of Socialism: Private Spheres of Soviet Russia.* Edited by Lewis Siegelbaum. New York: Palgrave Macmillan, 2006.

Halle, Fannina. *Women in Soviet Russia.* London: Routledge, 1933.

Hansson, Carola, and Karin Liden. *Moscow Women: Thirteen Interviews.* Translated by Gerry Bothmer, George Blecher, and Lone Blecher. New York: Pantheon House, 1983.

Harris, James. *The Great Fear: Stalin's Terror of the 1930s.* Oxford: Oxford University Press, 2016.

Harris, Stephen. *Communism on Tomorrow Street: Mass Housing and Everyday Life after Stalin.* Baltimore: Woodrow Wilson Center Press and Johns Hopkins University Press, 2013.

Harsch, Donna. "Book review of Annette Leo and Christian Konig. *Die 'Wunschkindpille'. Weibliche Erfahrung und Staatliche Geburtenpolitik in der DDR* (Gottingen: Wallstein Verlag, 2015)." In *German History* 34, no. 2 (1 June 2016): 358–359.

Harsch, Donna. "Society, the State, and Abortion in East Germany, 1950–1972." *American Historical Review* (February 1997): 53–84.

Hartmann, Susan. *The Home Front and Beyond: American Women in the 1940s.* Boston: Twayne, 1982.

Healey, Dan. *Bolshevik Sexual Forensics: Diagnosing Disorder in the Clinic and Courtroom, 1917-1939.* DeKalb: Northern Illinois University Press, 2009.

Healey, Dan. *Russian Homophobia from Stalin to Sochi.* London: Bloombury Academic, 2018.

Heinzen, James. *The Art of the Bribe: Corruption under Stalin, 1943–1953.* New Haven, CT: Yale University Press, 2016.

Heitlinger, Alena. *Women and State Socialism: Sex Inequality in the Soviet Union and Czechoslovakia.* London: Macmillan, 1979.

Heer, David. "Abortion, Contraception, and Population Policy in the Soviet Union." *Soviet Studies* 17, no. 1 (July 1965): 531–539.

Heer, David. "The Demographic Transition in the Russian Empire and the Soviet Union." *Journal of Social History* 1, no. 3 (Spring 1968): 193–240.

Heer, David. "Recent Developments in Soviet Population Policy." *Studies in Family Planning* 3, no. 11 (November 1972): 257–264.

Herlihy, Patricia. *The Alcoholic Empire: Vodka and Politics in Late Imperial Russia*. New York: Oxford University Press, 2002.

Hessler, Julie. "A Postwar Perestroika?: Toward a History of Private Enterprise." *Slavic Review* 57, no. 3 (Fall 1998): 516–542.

Hoffmann, David . *Cultivating the Masses: Modern State Practices and Soviet Socialism, 1914–1939*. Ithaca, NY: Cornell University Press, 2011.

Hoffmann, David. "Mothers in the Motherland: Stalinist Pronatalism in Its Pan-European Context." *Journal of Social History* 34, no. 1 (Autumn 2000): 35–54.

Hoffmann, David. *Stalinist Values: The Cultural Norms of Soviet Modernity, 1917–1941*. Ithaca, NY: Cornell University Press, 2003.

Holloway, David. *Stalin and the Bomb: The Soviet Union and Atomic Energy, 1939–1956*. New Haven, CT: Yale University Press, 1994.

Honey, Maureen. *Creating Rosie the Riveter: Class, Gender, and Propaganda during World War II*. Amherst: University of Massachusetts Press, 1984.

Hornsby, Robert. *Protest, Reform and Repression in Khrushchev's Soviet Union*. Cambridge: Cambridge University Press, 2013.

Hyer, Janet. "Managing the Female Organism: Doctors and the Medicalization of Women's Paid Work in Soviet Russia during the 1920s." In *Women in Russia and Ukraine*. Edited by Rosalind Marsh. Cambridge: Cambridge University Press, 1996.

Igarashi, Tokuko. "Kyusorenno kyowakokude tairyono sengyoshufuwa tanjosurunoka. [Will There Be an Emergence of Many Housewives in the Former Soviet Union?"] *Hikakukeizaikenkyu* 46, no. 1 (2009): 17–34.

Issoupova, Olga. "From Duty to Pleasure? Motherhood in Soviet and Post-Soviet Russia." In *Gender, State and Society in Soviet and Post-Soviet Russia*. Edited by Sarah Ashwin. London: Routledge, 2000.

Janos, Andrew C. *The Politics of Backwardness in Hungary, 1825–1945*. Princeton, NJ: Princeton University Press, 1982

Jones, Polly, ed. *The Dilemmas of De-Stalinization: Negotiating Cultural and Social Change in the Khrushchev Era*. London: Routledge, 2006.

Juviler, Peter H. "Family Reforms on the Road to Communism." In *Soviet Policy-Making: Studies of Communism in Transition*. Edited by Peter H. Juviler and Henry W. Morton. New York: Frederick A. Praeger, 1967.

Kabo, Vladimir. *The Road to Australia, Memoirs*. Canberra: Aboriginal Studies Press, 1998.

Kaminsky, Lauren. "Utopian Visions of Family Life in the Stalin-Era Soviet Union." *Central European History* 44 (2011): 63–91.

Kamitsubo, Takashi. *Mizukono Uta* [Songs of Unborn Children]. Tokyo: Shakai shisosha, 1993.

Kawamoto, Kazuko. *Sorenno minshushugito kazoku: renpokazoku kihonho seiteikatei,1948–1968* [Soviet Democracy and the Family: The Process of Making the All-Union Soviet Family Law, 1948-1968]. Tokyo: Yushindo kobunsha, 2012.

Kay, Rebecca. "Images of an Ideal Woman: Perceptions of Russian Womanhood through the Media, Education and Women's Own Eyes." In *Post-Soviet Women: From the Baltic to Central Asia*. Edited by Mary Buckley. Cambridge: Cambridge University Press, 1997.

Keil, Sally Van Wagenen. *Those Wonderful Women in Their Flying Machines: The Unknown Heroines of World War II*. New York: Rawson, Wade, 1979.

Keski-Petäjä, Miina. "Abortion Wishes and Abortion Prevention: Women Seeking Legal Termination of Pregnancy during the 1950s and 1960s in Finland." *Finnish Yearbook of Population Research* (April 2012): 113–135.

Kessler, Gijs. "A Population under Pressure: Household Responses to Demographic and Economic Shock in the Interwar Soviet Union." In *The Dream Deferred: New Studies in Russian and Soviet Labour History*. Edited by Donald Filtzer, Wendy Goldman, Gijs Kessler, and Simon Pirani. Bern: Peter Lang, 2008.

Kharkhordin, Oleg. *The Collective and the Individual in Russia: A Study of Practices.* Berkeley: University of California Press, 1999.

Khrushchev, N. S. *Khrushchev Remembers: The Last Testament.* Boston: Little, Brown, 1974.

Kiamenetsky, Ihor. *Hitler's Occupation of Ukraine, 1941–1944.* Milwaukee, WI: Marquette University Press, 1956.

Kirschenbaum, Lisa. *The Legacy of the Siege of Leningrad, 1941–1995: Myth, Memories, and Monuments.* Cambridge: Cambridge University Press, 2006.

Kligman, Gail. *The Politics of Duplicity: Controlling Reproduction in Ceausescu's Romania.* Berkeley: University of California Press, 1998.

Koenker, Diane. "Class and Consciousness in a Socialist Society: Workers in the Printing Trades during NEP." In *Russia in the Era of NEP.* Edited by Sheila Fitzpatrick, Alexander Rabinowitch, and Richard Stites. Bloomington: University of Indiana Press, 1991.

Kohama, Masako. "*Chugoku kingendaini okeru boshieiseiseisakuno kenkyu* [A Study of Public Health Policy toward Mothers and Children in Modern and Contemporary China], A Research Report." Published as the result of a 2002~2005 project funded by the Japan Society for the Promotion of Science, March 2006.

Kon, Igor. *Sexual Revolution in Russia: From the Age of the Czars to Today.* New York: Free Press, 1995.

Kostyrchenko, Gennadi. *Out of the Red Shadows: Anti-Semitism in Stalin's Russia.* Amherst, NY: Prometheus Books, 1995.

Kotkin, Stephen. *Magnetic Mountain: Stalinism as a Civilization.* Berkeley: University of California Press, 1995.

Kozlov, Denis, and Eleonory Gilburd. "The Thaw as an Event in Russian History." In *The Thaw: Soviet Society and Culture during the 1950s and 1960s.* Edited by Denis Kozlov and Eleonory Gilburd. Toronto: University of Toronto Press, 2013.

Krawchenko, Bohdan. "Soviet Ukraine under Nazi Occupation, 1941–44." In *Ukraine: The Challenges of World War II.* Edited by Taras Hunczak and Dmytro Shtohryn. Lanham, MD: University Press of America, 2003.

Krementsov, Nikolai. *The Cure: A Story of Cancer and Politics from the Annals of the Cold War.* Chicago: University of Chicago Press, 2002.

Krylova, Anna. "'Healers of Wounded Souls': The Crisis of Private Life in Soviet Literature." *Journal of Modern History* 73, no. 2 (June 2001): 307–331.

Krylova, Anna. *Soviet Women in Combat: A History of Violence on the Eastern Front.* Cambridge: Cambridge University Press, 2010.

Kukhterin, Sergei. "Fathers and Patriarchs in Communist and Post-communist Russia." In *Gender, State and Society in Soviet and Post-Soviet Russia.* Edited by Sarah Ashwin. London: Routledge, 2000.

Kumo, Kazuhiro. *Roshiano jinko no rekishi to genzai* [Demographic History of Russia]. Tokyo: Iwanami Shoten, 2014.

Kuromiya, Hiroaki. *The Voices of the Dead: Stalin's Great Terror in the 1930s*. New Haven: Yale University Press, 2007.

Lapidus, Gail. "The Female Industrial Labor Force: Reassessment and Options." In *Industrial Labor in the USSR*. Edited by Arcadius Kahan and Blair Ruble. New York: Pergamon Press, 1979.

Lapidus, Gail. *Women in Soviet Society: Equality, Development, and Social Change*. Berkeley: University of California Press, 1978.

LaPierre, Brian. *Hooligans in Khrushchev's Russia: Defining, Policing, and Producing Deviance during the Thaw*. Madison: University of Wisconsin Press, 2012.

Ledeneva, Alena. *Russia's Economy of Favours: Blat, Networking and Informal Exchange*. Cambridge: Cambridge University Press, 1998.

Leder, Mary. *My Life in Stalinist Russia: An American Woman Looks Back*. Bloomington: Indiana University Press, 2001.

Lennerhed, Lena. "Troubled Women: Abortion and Psychiatry in Sweden in the 1940s and 1950s." In *Transcending Borders: Abortion in the Past and Present*. Edited by Shannon Stettner, Katrina Ackerman, Kristin Burnett, and Travis Hay. Cham, Switzerland: Palgrave Macmillan, 2017.

Lorimer, Frank. *The Population of the Soviet Union: History and Prospects*. Geneva: League of Nations, 1946.

Lovell, Stephen. *Summerfolk: A History of the Dacha, 1710–2000*. Ithaca, NY: Cornell University Press, 2003.

Madison, Bernice. *Social Welfare in the Soviet Union*. Stanford, CA: Stanford University Press, 1968.

Malthus, T. R. *An Essay on the Principle of Population; or A View of Its Past and Present Effects on Human Happiness; With an Inquiry into our Prospects Respecting the Future Removal or Mitigation of the Evils which It Occasions*. Selected and introduced by Donald Winch. Cambridge: Cambridge University Press, 1992 [1803].

Maltseva, Natasha. "The Other Side of the Coin." In *Women and Russia: Feminist Writings from the Soviet Union*. Edited by Tatyana Mamonova. Oxford: Blackwell, 1984.

Manley, Rebecca. *To the Tashkent Station: Evacuation and Survival in the Soviet Union at War*. Ithaca, NY: Cornell University Press, 2009.

Markevich, Andrei. "Soviet Urban Households and the Road to Universal Employment, from the End of the 1930s to the End of the 1960s." *Continuity and Change* 20, no. 3 (2005): 443–473.

Markwick, Roger, and Euridice Cardona. *Soviet Women on the Frontline in the Second World War*. New York: Palgrave Macmillan, 2012.

Martin, Terry. *The Affirmative Action Empire*. Ithaca, NY: Cornell University Press, 2001.

Massell, Gregory. *The Surrogate Proletariat: Moslem Women and Revolutionary Strategies in Soviet Central Asia, 1919–1929*. Princeton, NJ: Princeton University Press, 1974.

Mazur, Peter. "Birth Control and Regional Differentials in the Soviet Union." *Population Studies* 22, no. 3 (November 1968): 319–333.

Mazur, Peter. "Reconstruction of Fertility Trends for the Female Population of the U.S.S.R." *Population Studies* 21, no. 1 (July 1967): 33–52.

Mazur, Peter. "Social and Demographic Determinants of Abortion in Poland." *Population Studies* 29, no. 1 (March 1975): 21–35.

McLellan, Josie. *Love in the Time of Communism: Intimacy and Sexuality in the GDR*. Cambridge: Cambridge University Press, 2011.

Meek, Ronald, ed. *Marx and Engels on Malthus*. London: Lawrence and Wishart, 1953.

Merridale, Catherine. *Ivan's War: Life and Death in the Red Army, 1939–1945*. New York: Metropolitan Books, 2006.

Michaels, Paula. *Curative Powers: Medicine and Empire in Stalin's Central Asia*. Pittsburgh: University of Pittsburgh Press, 2003.

Michaels, Paula. *Lamaze: An International History*. New York: Oxford University Press, 2014.

Michaels, Paula. "Motherhood, Patriotism, and Ethnicity: Soviet Kazakhstan and the 1936 Abortion Ban." *Feminist Studies* 27, no. 2 (Summer 2001): 307–333.

Mickiewicz, Ellen, ed. *Handbook of Soviet Social Science Data*. New York: Free Press, 1973.

Mintz, Morton, *The Pill: An Alarming Report*. Boston: Beacon Press, 1970.

Moeller, Robert. *Protecting Motherhood: Women and the Family in the Politics of Postwar Germany*. Berkeley: University of California Press, 1993.

Mouton, Michelle. *From Nurturing the Nation to Purifying the Volk: Weimar and Nazi Family Policy, 1918–1945*. Cambridge: Cambridge University Press, 2007.

M. S. Khrushchov i Ukraina. Kiiv: Natsionalna akademiia nauk Ukrainy, In-t istorii Ukrainy, 1995.

Murachi, Toshimi. "Gendai roshiano nyuyojino seikatsuto hoiku. [Infants and Childcare in Today's Russia]." *Yurashia kenkyu* 43, no.11 (2010): 45–50.

Naiman, Eric. *Sex in Public: The Incarnation of Early Soviet Ideology*. Princeton, NJ: Princeton University Press, 1997.

Naimark, Norman. *The Russians in Germany: The History of the Soviet Zone of Occupation, 1945–1949*. Cambridge, MA: Harvard University Press, 1995.

Naimark, Norman. *Stalin and the Fate of Europe: The Postwar Struggle for Sovereignty*. Cambridge, MA: Harvard University Press, 2019.

Nakachi, Mie. "'Abortion Is Killing Us': The Postwar Dilemma of Women's Medicine." *The Science, Culture, and Practice of Soviet Medicine*. Edited by Frances Bernstein, Christopher Burton, and Daniel Healey. DeKalb: Northern Illinois University Press, 2013.

Nakachi, Mie. "Gender, Marriage, and Reproduction in the Postwar Soviet Union." In *Writing the Stalin Era: Sheila Fitzpatrick and Soviet Historiography*. Edited by Golfo Alexopolous, Kiril Tomoff, and Julie Hessler. New York: Palgrave Macmillan, 2011.

Nakachi, Mie. "Liberation without Contraception? The Rise of the Abortion Empire and Pronatalism in Socialist and Postsocialist Russia." In *Reproductive States: Global Perspectives on the Invention and Implementation of Population Policy*. Edited by Rickie Solinger and Mie Nakachi. New York: Oxford University Press, 2016.

Nakachi, Mie. "N. S. Khrushchev and the 1944 Soviet Family Law: Politics, Reproduction, and Language." *East European Politics and Societies* 20, no. 1 (February 2006): 40–68.

Nakachi, Mie. "Population, Politics and Reproduction: Late Stalinism and Its Legacy." In *Late Stalinist Russia: Society between Reconstruction and Reinvention*. Edited by Juliane Fürst. London: Routledge, 2006.

Nakachi, Mie. "A Postwar Sexual Liberation? The Gendered Experience of the Soviet Union's Great Patriotic War." *Cahiers du monde russe* 52, no. 2/3 (2011): 423–440.

Nakachi, Mie. "Roshiano fukushito jenda." In *Shin sekaino shakaifukushi 5 Kyusoren too* ["Welfare and Gender in Russia" in *Global Social Welfare*, vol. 5, *Former Soviet Union and East-Central Europe*]. Edited by Manabu Sengoku. Tokyo: Junposha, 2019.

Nye, Robert A. *Crime, Madness, and Politics in Modern France: The Medical Concept of National Decline*. Princeton, NJ: Princeton University Press, 1984.

Obinger, Herbert, and Carina Schmitt. "Guns and Butter? Regime Competition and the Welfare State during the Cold War." *World Politics* 63, no. 2 (April 2011): 246–270.

Ogino Miho. *Kazokukeikakueno michi: Kindainihonno seishokuo meguru seiji* [The Road to Family Planning: The Politics of Reproduction in Modern Japan]. Tokyo: Iwanami shoten, 2008.

Orloff, Ann S. "Gender." In *The Oxford Handbook of the Welfare State*. Edited by Francis Castles et al. New York: Oxford University Press, 2010.

Orloff, Ann S. "Gender and the Social Rights of Citizenship: The Comparative Analysis of Gender Relations and Welfare States." *American Sociological Review* 53 (June 1993): 303–328.

Orr, Judith. *Abortion Wars: The Fight for Reproductive Rights*. Bristol: Policy Press, 2017.

Pauli, Julia. "Creating Illegitimacy: Negotiating Relations and Reproduction within Christian Contexts in Northwest Namibia." *Journal of Religion in Africa* 42 (2012): 408–432.

Perelli-Harris, Brienna, and Theodore P. Gerber. "Non-marital Childbearing in Russia: Second Demographic Transition or Pattern of Disadvantage?" *Demography* 48 no. 1 (February 2011): 317–342.

Perkovskii, A. L., and S. I. Pirozhkov. "Demografichni vtrati narodonaseleniia Ukrainskoi RSR u 40-kh gg." *Ukrains'kii istorichnii zhurnal* 2 (February 1990): 15–24.

Pinkus, Benjamin. *The Jews of the Soviet Union: The History of a National Minority*. Cambridge: Cambridge University Press, 1988.

Poliakov, Iu. A. et al. "A Half Century of Silence: The 1937 Census." *Russian Studies in History* 31, no. 1 (Summer 1992): 10–98.

Polian, Pavel. *Against Their Will: The History and Geography of Forced Migrations in the USSR*. Budapest: Central European University Press, 2004.

Popov, A. A. "Family Planning and Induced Abortion in the USSR: Basic Health and Demographic Characteristics." *Studies in Family Planning* 22, no. 6 (November–December 1991): 368–377.

Popov, A. A. "Induced Abortions in the USSR at the End of the 1980s: The Basis for the National Model of Family Planning." A paper presented at the Annual Meeting of the Population Association of America in Denver, Colorado, 1992.

Popov, A. A., A. P. Visser, and E. Ketting. "Contraceptive Knowledge, Attitudes, and Practice in Russia during the 1980s." *Studies in Family Planning* 24, no. 4 (July–August 1993): 227–235.

Quint, Peter. "The Unification of Abortion Law." In *The Imperfect Union: Constitutional Structures of Germany Unification*. Princeton, NJ: Princeton University Press, 2012.

Rabinow, Paul, and Nikolas Rose, eds. *The Essential Foucault: Selections from Essential Works of Foucault, 1954–1984*. New York: New Press, 2003.

Raeff, Marc. "The Well-Ordered Police State and the Development of Modernity in Seventeenth and Eighteenth-Century Europe: An Attempt at a Comparative Approach." *The American Historical Review* 80, no. 5 (Dec. 1975): 1221-1243.

Randall, Amy. "'Abortion Will Deprive You of Happiness!' Soviet Reproductive Politics in the Post-Stalin Era." *Journal of Women's History* 23, no. 3 (2011): 13–38.

Ransel, David. "Mothering, Medicine, and Infant Mortality in Russia: Some Comparisons." *Kennan Institute for Advanced Studies Occasional Paper*, no. 236 (1990).

Ransel, David. *Village Mothers: Three Generations of Change in Russia and Tataria*. Bloomington: Indiana University Press, 2000.

Reese, Roger. *Why Stalin's Soldiers Fought: The Red Army's Military Effectiveness in World War II*. Lawrence: University Press of Kansas, 2011.

Reid, Susan. "'Our Kitchen Is Just as Good': Soviet Responses to the American Kitchen." In *Cold War Kitchen: Americanization, Technology, and European Users*, 83–105. Cambridge, MA: Massachusetts Institute of Technology Press, 2009,

Remennick, Larissa. "Epidemiology and Determinants of Induced Abortion in the USSR." *Social Science and Medicine* 33, no. 7 (1991): 841–848.

Rivkin-Fish, Michele. "From 'Demographic Crisis' to 'Dying Nation': The Politics of Language and Reproduction in Russia." In *Gender and National Identity in Twentieth-Century Russian Culture*. Edited by Helen Goscilo and Andrea Lanoux. DeKalb: Northern Illinois University Press, 2006.

Rivkin-Fish, Michele. "Pronatalism, Gender Politics, and the Renewal of Family Support in Russia: Toward a Feminist Anthropology of 'Maternity Capital.'" *Slavic Review* 69, no. 3 (Fall 2010): 701–724.

Rivkin-Fish, Michele. *Women's Health in Post-Soviet Russia: The Politics of Intervention*. Bloomington: Indiana University Press, 2005.

Rosefielde, Steven. "Excess Collectivization Deaths, 1929–1933: New Demographic Evidence." *Slavic Review* 43, no. 1 (1984): 83–88.

Rosefielde, Steven. "Excess Mortality in the Soviet Union: A Reconsideration of the Demographic Consequences of Forced Industrialization, 1929–1949." *Soviet Studies* 35 (1983): 385–409.

Russell, Cheryl. *The Baby Boom: Americans Born 1946 to 1964*. Amityville, NY: New Strategist Press, 2009.

Ryabushkin, T. V. "Mikhail Vassilievitch Ptukha, 1884–1961." *Revue de l'Institut International de Statistique / Review of the International Statistical Institute* 29, no. 3 (1961): 111–112.

Sainsbury, Diane. *Gender, Equality, and Welfare States*. Cambridge: Cambridge University Press, 1996.

Saltman, Jules. *The Pill: Its Effects, Its Dangers, Its Future*. New York: Grosset and Dunlap, 1970.

Scharping, Thomas. *Birth Control in China 1949–2000: Population Policy and Demographic Development*. Abingdon, Oxfordshire, UK: Routledge Curzon, 2005.

Scherbov, Sergei, and Harrie van Vianen. "Marital and Fertility Careers of Russian Women Born between 1910 and 1934." *Population and Development Review* 25, no. 1 (March 1999): 129–143.

Schwartz, Lee. "A History of the Russian and Soviet Censuses." In *Research Guide to the Russian and Soviet Censuses*. Edited by Ralph S. Clem. Ithaca, NY: Cornell University Press, 1986.

Scott, James C. *Seeing Like a State: How Certain Schemes to Improve the Human Condition Have Failed*. New Haven: Yale University Press, 1998.

Seaman, Barbara. *The Doctors: Case against the Pill*. New York: Peter H. Wyden, 1969.

Semashko, N. A. *Health Protection in the USSR*. London: Gollansz, 1934.

Shaw, Claire L. *Deaf in the USSR: Marginality, Community, and Soviet Identity, 1917–1991*. Ithaca, NY: Cornell University Press, 2017.

Shimokawa, Masaharu. *Bokyaku no Hikiageshi: Izumi Seiichito Futsukaichi Hoyojo* [A Forgotten History of Repatriation: Izumi Seiichi and Futsukaichi Sanatorium]. Fukuoka: Gen shobo, 2017.

Shiokawa, Nobuaki, "Kyusoren no kazoku to shakai" [Family and Society in the Former Soviet Union]. In *Surabu no shakai: Koza surabu no sekai*, vol. 4. Tokyo: Kobundo, 1994.

Shtange, Galina Vladimirovna. "Remembrances." In *Intimacy and Terror, Soviet Diaries of the 1930*. Edited by Veronique Garros, Natalia Korenevskaya, and Thomas Lahusen. New York: New Press, 1995.

Sigerist, Henry E. *Socialized Medicine in the Soviet Union*. London: Victor Gollancz, 1937.

Smith, Gregory. "The Impact of World War II on Women, Family Life, and Mores in Moscow, 1941–1945." PhD dissertation, Stanford University, 1990.

Smith, James. "The Politics of Sexual Knowledge: The Origins of Ireland's Containment Culture and the Carrigan Report (1931)." *Journal of the History of Sexuality* 13, no. 2 (April 2004): 208–233.

Smith, Mark B. *Property of Communists: The Urban Housing Program from Stalin to Khrushchev*. DeKalb: Northern Illinois University Press, 2010

Smith, Mark B. "The Withering Away of the Danger Society: The Pension Reforms of 1956 and 1964 in the Soviet Union." *Social Science History* 39 (Spring 2015): 129–148.

Smith, Walter Bedell. *My Three Years in Moscow*. Philadelphia: Lippincott, 1950.

Snyder, Timothy, *Bloodlands: Europe between Hitler and Stalin*. London: Vintage, 2011.

Sobotka, Tomas. "Childlessness in Europe: Reconstructing Long-Term Trends among Women Born in 1900–1972." In *Childlessness in Europe: Contexts, Causes, and Consequences*. Edited by Michaela Kreyenfeld and Dirk Konietzka. Rostock, Germany: Demographic Research Monographs, 2017.

Sobotka, Tomas. "Fertility in Central and Eastern Europe after 1989: Collapse and Gradual Recovery." *Historical Social Research* 36, no. 2 (2011): 246–295.

Solinger, Rickie. "Bleeding across Time: First Principles of US Population Policy." In *Reproductive States: Global Perspectives on the Invention and Implementation of Population Policy*. Edited by Rickie Solinger and Mie Nakachi. New York: Oxford University Press, 2016.

Solomon, Peter. *Soviet Criminal Justice under Stalin*. Cambridge: Cambridge University Press, 1996.

Solomon, Susan Gross. "The Demographic Argument in Soviet Debates over the Legalization of Abortion in the 1920s." *Cahiers du monde russe et sovietique*, 33, no. 1 (janvier-mars 1992): 59–81.

Solomon, Susan Gross. "The Soviet Legalization of Abortion in German Medical Discourse: A Study of the Use of Selective Perceptions in Cross-Cultural Scientific Relations." *Social Studies of Science* 22, no. 3 (1992): 455–485.

Solomon, Susan, and John Hutchinson, eds. *Health and Society in Revolutionary Russia*. Bloomington: Indiana University Press, 1990.

Sorrentino, Constance. "International Comparisons of Labor Force Participation, 1960–1981." *Monthly Labor Review* (February 1983): 23–36.

Starks, Tricia. *The Body Soviet: Propaganda, Hygiene, and the Revolutionary State*. Madison: University of Wisconsin Press, 2008.

Statiev, Alexander. *The Soviet Counterinsurgency in the Western Borderlands*. Cambridge: Cambridge University Press, 2010.

Stites, Richard. *The Women's Liberation Movement in Russia: Feminism, Nihilism and Bolshevism, 1860–1930*. Princeton, NJ: Princeton University Press, 1978.

Szreter, Simon. "The Idea of Demographic Transition and the Study of Fertility Change: A Critical Intellectual History." *Population and Development Review* 19, no. 4 (December1993): 659–701.

Takeda, Keitaro. *Chinmokuno yonjunen: Hikiage josei kyoseichuzetsuno kiroku* [Forty Years of Silence: Records of Forced Abortions on Repatriated Women]. Tokyo: Chuokoronsha, 1985.

Taubman, William. *Khrushchev: The Man and His Era.* New York: W. W. Norton, 2003.

Taussig, Frederick J. *Abortion, Spontaneous and Induced.* London: Henry Kimpton, 1936.

Teplova, Tatyana, "Welfare State Transformation, Childcare, and Women's Work in Russia." *Journal of Social Politics* 14, no. 3 (2007): 284–322.

Timasheff, Nicholas S. *The Great Retreat: The Growth and Decline of Communism in Russia.* Dutton: New York, 1946.

Tolts, Mark. "Population Trends in the Russian Federation: Reflections on the Legacy of Soviet Censorship and Distortions of Demographic Statistics." *Eurasian Geography and Economics* 49, no. 1 (2008): 87–98.

Treml, Vladimir G. "Alcohol in the USSR: A Fiscal Dilemma." *Soviet Studies* 27, no. 2 (April 1975): 161–177.

Trotsky, Leon. *The Revolution Betrayed.* 11th ed. Pathfinder: New York, 1998 (1937).

Tyler May, Elaine. *Homeward Bound: American Families in the Cold War Era.* New York: Basic Books, 1999.

United Nations Department of Economic and Social Affairs, Population Division. *Abortion Policies and Reproductive Health around the World.* New York: United Nations, 2014.

Utrata, Jennifer. *Women without Men: Single Mothers and Family Change in the New Russia.* Ithaca, NY: Cornell University Press, 2015.

Varga-Harris, Christine. "Forging Citizenship on the Home Front: Reviving the Socialist Contract and Constructing Soviet Identity during the Thaw." In *The Dilemmas of De-Stalinization.* Edited by Polly Jones. London: Routledge, 2006.

Varga-Harris, Christine. *Stories of House and Home: Soviet Apartment Life during the Khrushchev Years.* Ithaca, NY: Cornell University Press, 2015.

Ventura, Stephanie J., and Christine A. Bachrach. "Nonmarital Childbearing in the United States, 1940-1999." *National Vital Statistics Reports* 48, no. 16 (October 18, 2000): 1-39.

Virgili, Fabrice. *Shorn Women: Gender and Punishment in Liberation France.* Translated by John Flower. London: Bloomsbury, 2002.

Waters, Elizabeth. "The Female Form in Soviet Political Iconography: 1917–1932." In *Russia's Women: Accommodation, Resistance, Transformation.* Edited by Barbara Clements, Barbara Alpern Engel, and Christine Worobec. Berkeley: University of California Press, 1991.

Watkins, Elizabeth Siegel, *On the Pill: A Social History of Oral Contraceptives, 1950–1970.* Baltimore, MD: Johns Hopkins University Press, 1998.

Weiner, Amir. *Making Sense of War: The Second World War and the Fate of the Bolshevik Revolution.* Princeton, NJ: Princeton University Press, 2001.

Wheatcroft, Stephen G. "On Assessing the Size of Forced Concentration Camp Labor in the Soviet Union, 1929–1956." *Soviet Studies* 33, no. 2 (1981): 265–295.

Wheatcroft, Stephen G. "A Further Note of Clarification on the Famine, the Camps and Excess Mortality." *Europe-Asia Studies* 49, no. 3 (May 1997): 503–505.

White, Tyrene. *China's Longest Campaign: Birth Planning in the People's Republic, 1949–2005.* Ithaca, NY: Cornell University Press, 2006.

Whitewood, Peter. *The Red Army and the Great Terror: Stalin's Purge of the Soviet Military.* Lawrence: University Press of Kansas, 2015.

Williams, Christopher. "Abortion and Women's Health in Russia and the Soviet Successor States." In *Women in Russia and Ukraine*. Edited by Rosalind Marsh. Cambridge: Cambridge University Press, 1996.

Winter, Jay, and Michael Teitelbaum. *The Global Spread of Fertility Decline: Population, Fear, and Uncertainty*. New Haven, CT: Yale University Press, 2013.

Wood, Elizabeth. *The Baba and the Comrade: Gender and Politics in Revolutionary Russia*. Bloomington: Indiana University Press, 1997.

Zakharov, S. V., and E. I. Ivanova. "Fertility Decline and Recent Changes in Russia: On the Threshold of the Second Demographic Transition." In *Russia's Demographic "Crisis."* Edited by Julie DaVanzo. Santa Monica, CA: RAND, 1996.

Zakharov, S. V., and E. I. Ivanova. "Russian Federation: From the First to Second Demographic Transition." *Demographic Research* 19, article 24 (2008): 907–972.

Zarechnak, Galina V. *Academy of Medical Sciences of the USSR: History and Organization, 1944–1959*. Public Health Monograph No. 63. US Department of Health, Education, and Welfare, 1960.

Zubkova, Elena. *Russia after the War: Hopes, Illusions, and Disappointments, 1945–1957*. Armonk, NY: M. E. Sharpe, 1998.

Zubok, Vladislav. *Zhivago's Children: The Last Russian Intelligentsia*. Cambridge, MA: Harvard University Press, 2009.

Index

All organizations are Soviet unless otherwise indicated.

For the benefit of digital users, indexed terms that span two pages (e.g., 52–53) may, on occasion, appear on only one of those pages.

abortion. *See also* clinical abortion; criminal abortion; anti-abortion campaigns
  birth rate declines and, 19, 123, 124–25, 127–28, 152, 174
  curettage and, 1, 1–2n.3
  eugenics and, 57
  infertility and, 1–2, 66–67, 68, 69, 138, 144, 151, 166, 167, 197–98
  rates of, 1–2, 16, 61–62, 126–27, 160
  socialism and, 8, 16, 187–88, 203
Abramova, A.
  advocacy for increased aid to single mothers by, 117, 118–19, 162
  report (1948) on problems faced by out-of-wedlock children and single mothers by, 114, 115–19, 123, 129, 152, 194
  tax increase on single men proposed by, 118–20
abstinence, 7–8
Academy of Medical Sciences (AMS), 80–81, 84, 199–200
Akhmatova, Anna, 79–80
Akusherstvo i ginekologiia (Obstetrics and Gynecology, journal*),* 81
Alexievich, Svetlana, 11, 21, 92–93
All Union Central Council of Trade Unions (VTsSPS)
  doctors' criticisms of, 168
  interministerial abortion study of 1948-49 and, 130–31, 150–51
  orphanages and, 133–34
  proposed reforms to abortion law during 1950s and, 153–54, 168
  re-legalization of abortion (1955) and, 19

All-Union Family Law. *See* Family Law of 1968
amenorrhea, 66, 67–68, 128
anti-abortion campaigns, 5, 186–87, 202, 218, 220–21
anti-Semitism,
  Holocaust, 2, 24–25
  Doctors' Plot, 154, 155, 157, 157n.12, 158
  Purge of Moscow Institute for Gynecology and Obstetrics, 18, 81, 82n.114
Arkhangel'skii, B. A., 56, 66–67, 69, 70, 76
artificial insemination, 68–69
Australia, 188–89

babki, 73, 176
*babushka*s (grandmothers), 205–6, 214–15, 220
babyboom/ "babyboomlet", 22, 22n.4, 123, 123n.1, 127–28, 128n.28
Baranskaia, Nataliia, 204–5, 206
Bebel, August, 8
Belarus, or Belorussia 16, 21, 130–31
Bezlepkina, Liudmila, 217
birth control pill, 184, 200–2
birth rate. *See also* pronatalism
  abortion cited as reason for decline in, 19, 123, 124–25, 127–28, 152, 174
  census of 1959 and, 193
  contraception and, 148, 203–4
  declines during 1960s and 1970s in, 15, 201, 214
  ethnic differences in, 163
  famine of 1946-47 and, 127–29
  loss of traditional gender roles blamed for declines in, 210

birth rate (*cont.*)
    military strength and, 9
    postwar period (1945-55) and, 10, 17–18,
        19, 21–23, 25–27, 29, 32, 35, 40–41, 45,
        85–86, 123, 126–29, 162, 163
    prewar period and, 9
    regional differences in, 163
    reproductive health and, 58, 65, 66
    Russian Federation and, 217–18,
        219–20, 222
    socialist views of, 7–9, 188, 203
    Stalin's industrialization campaigns of
        the 1930s and, 9–10
    Ukraine and, 25–27
    welfare systems and, 16–17
    Western countries and, 188–89, 206,
        211–12, 213
    women's workforce participation and,
        16, 201, 206, 222
    World War II and, 27, 45, 63
blat, 58, 73, 204, 204n.90
Bolshevik Party, 4, 8, 13–14, 55. *See also*
    socialism
Brezhnev, Leonid, 14–15, 208
Burova, M.D., 27

Canada, 188–89, 197
Catholic Church, 43–44, 183, 221
Census
    census of 1939, 123–24
    census of 1959, 163–64, 188, 193, 201
    census of 1970, 188, 201
    census of 1989, 217–18
Central Asia, 2, 16, 25, 163, 182–83, 190,
    208–9, 210–11
Central Committee of Communist Party,
    169, 179–80, 181–82, 192–93
Central Lenin Institute for Training
    Doctors survey (1958-9), 198
Central Statistical Administration (TsSU),
    27–28, 46–47, 126–27, 163
childcare
    *babushka*s and, 205–6, 214–15, 220
    clinical abortions linked to lack of
        access to, 198
    crèches and, 13, 30, 42–43, 123, 132–33
    criminal abortions linked to lack of
        access to, 132–33, 165–66, 167

    "double burden" and, 175, 204,
        208, 210–11
    expectations of Soviet women
        regarding, 5–6, 10, 17, 22–23, 134–35,
        151, 172, 197, 205, 207, 210–11
    facilities for, 7, 9, 13–14, 30, 42–43, 116–
        17, 121–22, 123, 204, 207, 208, 217
    Family Law of 1936 and, 7, 9, 13–14, 42–43
    Family Law of 1944 and, 10, 22–23, 30,
        38–39, 40–41, 64–65, 121–22, 133–34
    legal requirements for two-parent
        families and, 38
    maternity leaves and, 12–13, 46, 156–57,
        187–88, 189, 208, 212, 214
    Narkomzdrav and, 42
    reform campaigns promoting men's
        involvement in, 213
    Russian Federation and, 217
    socialist ideals and, 7, 203–4, 213–14
    Soviet welfare system guarantees
        regarding, 12–13
    Western countries and, 212–13
    women's choice to limit family size
        linked to lack of access to, 207
    women's workforce participation and,
        133, 204
child support
    24th Party Congress (1971) and, 208
    common law marriage and, 10, 38, 39–40,
        101–3, 106–8, 112, 121
    Council of Ministers decree (1970)
        and, 208–9
    divorce provisions and, 39, 101, 110
    Family Law of 1926 and, 39–40
    Family Law of 1936 and, 7, 10, 22–23, 40
    Family Law of 1944 and, 10, 19, 30,
        37–38, 39, 45–46, 51, 53–54, 86–87,
        88–89, 90–91, 101–3, 106–8, 109,
        114, 121, 171
    Family Law of 1968 and, 193
    reform proposals during 1950s
        and, 190–91
    state support for single mothers
        and, 24, 30
    viewed as abortion-reduction strategy,
        86–87, 137
    women's postwar call for increases
        in, 36–37

China, 16, 54, 183–84
Chukovskii, Kornei, 192
clinical abortion. *See also* legalized
    abortion
  in Central Asia, 182–83
  China and, 16, 54, 183–84
  conditions encountered during, 186
  criteria for allowance of, 76–78, 79, 85,
    87, 148–50, 151–52, 157, 164, 167–68,
    174–75, 218–19
  doctor consultations prior to, 181, 186
  doctors' advocacy for, 18, 56–58, 59–60,
    65, 70, 74–75, 85, 137, 147–48, 150–
    51, 175, 182
  Eastern European socialist regimes and,
    16, 183, 184–85
  economic problems cited as reason for,
    136, 150, 174–75
  expectant mother's health cited as
    reason for, 150, 167–68, 173–74, 221
  Family Law of 1936 outlawing, 3–4, 7
  favoritism and nepotism in access to, 83
  fees for, 149, 151–52, 167
  housing problems linked to, 198
  increase following legalization (1955)
    of, 186–87
  infertility and, 197–98
  Japan and, 4–5, 57, 85–86
  lack of childcare cited as reason for, 198
  long-term side effects from, 197–98
  out-of-wedlock relationship with father
    cited as reason for, 136
  presence of other small children cited as
    reason for, 136, 167–68, 172–73
  rape cited as a reason for, 177, 221
  rates of, 20, 60, 74, 150, 186–87, 199
  reforms during 1950s designed to
    expand access to, 148–51, 153–55,
    157, 165, 168–69, 174–77, 179
  relationship problems cited as reason
    for, 149, 172, 173, 198
  Russian Federation and, 20, 216–17,
    218–19, 220–21
  subterfuge used to obtain, 58, 73, 85
  surveillance by the Soviet state and,
    14–15, 18, 57–61, 69–73, 74, 75–76,
    78–79, 81, 85, 87
  Ukraine and, 33, 64, 75

vacuum aspirations ("mini abortions")
    and, 202–3
  viability of infant cited as reason
    for, 167–68
  waiting periods as obstacle to,
    181, 218–19
  in Western countries, 197, 212–13
  women's rights and, 1, 4–5, 56, 153, 155,
    175–76, 177
Cold War, 5, 79–84, 124
collective farm, 138–39, 162, 190
Commissariat of Social Security, 13
Committee on the Question of Women's
    Labor and Improvement of the
    Protection of Motherhood and
    Childhood (1948), 119–20
common-law marriage. *See also*
    out-of-wedlock births
  child support and, 10, 38, 39–40, 101–3,
    106–8, 112, 121
  divorce and, 112, 197
  Family Law of 1926 and, 9, 39–40
  Family Law of 1944 and, 40, 101–3,
    106–8, 112, 121
  prewar registration system and, 38
  psychological disadvantages for women
    and children of, 19
  war widow pensions and, 104–5, 108
Constitution of the Soviet Union
    (1936), 12–13
contraception
  birth control pill and, 184, 200–2
  birth rate and, 148, 203–4
  China and, 54, 183–84
  doctors' advocacy for improved access
    to, 19, 70, 137, 148, 174–75, 187
  effectiveness and safety of, 200–1
  Family Law of 1936 and, 9
  Family Law of 1944 and, 32–33
  Kovrigina's advocacy for, 178
  limited availability in Eastern
    Europe of, 16
  limited availability in Soviet Union
    of, 1–2, 16, 17, 58–59, 60, 61–62,
    121, 150, 179, 187–88, 197, 200,
    201–3, 214–15
  Malthus and, 7
  pronatalism and suppression of, 148

contraception (*cont.*)
  reproductive health and, 20, 199
  Russian Federation and, 216–17, 218
  sex education and, 199
  socialism and, 8–9, 203
  viewed as means of reducing criminal
    abortion, 20, 145, 151–52, 182,
    197–98, 200, 202–3
  in Western countries, 212–13
  women's rights and, 20, 197
Council of Ministers (Sovmin)
  abortion law reform proposals in 1950s
    and, 157, 165, 168–69, 174, 179
  child support decree (1970) by, 208–9
  divorce reform proposals and, 169–70
  Family Law of 1968 and, 193
  interministerial abortion study of
    1948–49 and, 130, 150–51
Council of Obstetrics and Gynecology, 74
Council of Unions and the Council
  of Nationalities of the Supreme
  Soviet, 192–93
Court of Honor, 80, 80n.106, 81
criminal abortion
  childcare access cited as reason
    for, 132–33, 165–66, 167
  contraception viewed as means of
    reducing, 20, 145, 151–52, 182,
    197–98, 200, 202–3
  criteria for exceptions to, 76–78, 79, 85,
    87, 148–50, 151–52, 157, 164, 167
  deaths resulting from, 3, 56, 62, 141,
    151, 166, 167, 174, 181, 187
  divorce cited as a reason for, 137, 139
  doctor-patient trust viewed as means of
    reducing, 145–47
  economic conditions cited as reason for,
    77, 85–86, 132, 134–37, 139–40, 151,
    164–65, 167
  Family Law of 1936 and, 7, 9, 13–14, 33,
    58, 59, 60, 63, 148–49, 151–52, 154,
    160, 164, 165–66, 176
  Family Law of 1944 and, 14, 22, 23,
    30–31, 32–33, 36, 45–46, 51
  famine of 1946-47 and, 128, 129
  housing problems cited as reason for,
    134–36, 151, 156–57, 165
  infertility following, 1–2, 144, 150, 151,
    166, 167, 199

  late-term abortions and, 141
  married women and, 151
  medical problems resulting from, 3, 64,
    70, 73, 138–39
  out-of-wedlock relationship with father
    cited as reason for, 139–40, 144
  presence of other small children cited
    as reason for, 134–35, 138–40, 143,
    165, 167
  prosecutions for, 59, 60, 62–63, 71–73,
    130–31, 137–45, 157, 180–81
  punishments for, 59, 142, 143, 156–57
  rates of, 116–17, 130, 131, 150, 164, 166,
    187, 199
  relationship problems cited as reason
    for, 134–35, 137, 138, 139–41, 144–
    45, 151, 167
  reproductive health harmed by, 58–59,
    166, 174, 175, 176–77
  Ukraine and, 63, 130–31
  urban *versus* rural areas and,
    138–39, 199
  women soldiers in World War II and, 12
  working conditions cited as reason for,
    135–36, 147, 156–57
  World War II and, 61–64, 126
Cuba, 16

Day of Family, 220–21
demographic policy in the Soviet Union.
    See also specific laws
  24th Party Congress (1971) and, 208
  25th Party Congress (1976) and, 201
  educational campaign stressing
    traditional gender roles (1980s)
    and, 210
  ethnic groups' fertility rates and,
    203–4, 208–10
  familialism, 212–14
  preferential policies for specific regions
    and, 209–10
  research on women's choices to limit
    family size and, 206–8
  self-censorship and, 6, 124
  socialist ideals and, 203
  Stalin's purge of demographers,
    15, 123–25
Deng Xiaoping, 183–84
Deng Yingchao, 183–84

Denmark, 197
de-Stalinization, 154, 178, 183, 187
divorce
    children's interests and, 99, 100
    child support and, 39, 101, 110
    common-law marriages and, 112, 197
    criminal abortion linked to, 137, 139
    Family Law of 1918 and, 9
    Family Law of 1926 and, 9
    Family Law of 1936 and, 7, 10, 39–40
    Family Law of 1944 and, 18–19, 22, 29,
        30–31, 39, 46, 49, 50–51, 90–91, 94–
        101, 105–6, 108–12, 121, 154, 156,
        161–63, 169, 172, 191
    Family Law of 1968 and, 193, 196–97
    fees and, 39, 49
    infertility and sexual dysfunction cited
        as reason for, 97–99
    infidelity and, 95–98
    loss of traditional gender roles blamed
        for increased rates of, 210
    men as more frequent initiators of,
        95–97, 99
    people's courts and, 108–10
    postwar increase in, 12, 113
    pronatalism and, 98–99
    publication of announcements of, 111–12
    restoration of prewar families and, 111
    rural marriages and, 50–51
    "second families" as reason for, 97
    Ukase of 1965 simplifies, 46, 193, 196,
        244n.119, 278n.44
    Western countries and, 188–89
    World War II and, 88
Dmitrieva, A.I., 4–5, 85–86, 153, 176–77
doctors
    advocacy for clinical abortion among,
        18, 56–58, 59–60, 65, 70, 74–75, 85,
        137, 147–48, 150–51, 175, 182
    advocacy for contraception by, 19, 70,
        137, 148, 174–75, 187
    "Doctors' Plot" (1953) and, 19, 154, 157–58
    Jewish doctors and, 18, 84, 154
    KR Affair (1947), 58, 79–81
    punishment for performing criminal
        abortions and, 142–43, 156–57
    reproductive health prioritized by, 56,
        58, 64–66, 71, 73–75

    Soviet state's disciplining of, 18, 58,
        79–87, 154
    surveillance system for clinical
        abortions and, 6, 59–63, 69, 74, 75–76,
        78–79, 81, 85, 87
    World War II and, 6, 61–63
"double burden," 175, 204, 208, 210–11

East Germany, 56–57, 184–85, 200
Engels, Friedrich, 7–8, 184
Erenburg, Ilia, 11, 12, 24, 191–92
Estonia, 16
Estrin, A.L., 56, 71–72, 76–77, 83
Eugenic Protection Law (Japan), 57

familialism, 212–14
Family Law of 1918, 9, 22–23, 39–40, 54
Family Law of 1926, 9, 39–40
Family Law of 1936
    abortion criminalized under, 7, 9, 13–14,
        33, 58, 59, 60, 63, 148–49, 151–52,
        154, 160, 164, 165–66, 176
    childcare facilities expanded through, 7,
        9, 13–14, 42–43
    child support provisions in, 7, 10,
        22–23, 40
    contraceptive access limited under, 9
    divorce restricted under, 7, 10, 39–40
    marriage and, 10, 40
    pronatalism and, 9–10, 176
    Stalin and, 3–4, 22–23, 164
    state aid to mothers and, 9–10, 13–14,
        27–28, 49
Family Law of 1944
    abortion criminalized under, 14, 22, 23,
        30–31, 32–33, 36, 45–46, 51
    childcare and, 10, 22–23, 30, 38–39, 40–41,
        64–65, 121–22, 133–34
    child support and, 10, 19, 30, 37–38, 39,
        45–46, 51, 53–54, 86–87, 88–89, 90–
        91, 101–3, 106–8, 109, 114, 121, 171
    Committee on the Question of Women's
        Labor and Improvement of the
        Protection of Motherhood and
        Childhood and, 119–20
    common-law marriage, 40, 101–3,
        106–8, 112, 121
    contraception and, 32–33

Family Law of 1944 (*cont.*)
divorce and, 18–19, 22, 29, 30–31, 39,
46, 49, 50–51, 90–91, 94–101, 105–6,
108–12, 121, 154, 156, 161–63, 169,
172, 191
infanticide penalties in, 32–34,
36, 46, 51
Khrushchev and, 18, 21–22, 23, 28–36,
40, 42, 43–44, 45–46, 47–51, 53–54,
105–6, 122, 126–27, 154, 164, 171,
220–21, 222
legal distinctions between one-parent
and two-parent families in, 38–39,
44, 90–91
marriage and, 12, 18–19, 29, 30, 34, 39,
40–41, 91, 94–95, 101, 103–4, 105–6,
108, 161–63
maternity leave and, 46
Motherhood Glory order established by,
2–3, 47–48, 51–52, 54
Motherhood Heroine title established
by, 2–3, 47–51, 54
Motherhood Medal established by, 2–3,
51–52, 53*t*, 54
Narkomzdrav and, 45–46, 47, 49, 51, 65
out-of-wedlock births and, 17–18,
22–23, 24, 29, 30, 34, 36–42, 43–44,
45–46, 52–53, 86, 88–89, 105–6,
107–8, 109, 114–19, 122, 154, 155,
158–60, 161, 162, 191
patronymic provisions in, 30, 38, 41,
54, 115
People's Commissariat of Justice's role in
implementing, 105–13
pronatalism ideology and, 2–3, 10,
13–14, 17–18, 22–24, 28–36, 51,
52–54, 77–78, 105–7, 122, 162,
164, 196
registration of children of unmarried
mothers' surnames under, 88–
89, 100–1, 115, 117–18, 158,
159–60, 169
rest homes for single mothers and, 43
single mothers' right to leave children at
orphanages and, 37, 90, 133–34
small family taxes and, 30–31, 34–35,
36, 44, 48, 49–51, 53*t*, 143, 171,
189, 191

Stalin and, 47, 49
state aid for pregnant women and, 2,
28–30, 42, 45, 51–52, 78–79
state aid to mothers of large families
and, 42, 49, 53*t*, 54
state support for mothers and, 2–3,
10, 22, 24, 28–42, 45, 51–54, 90,
96–97, 114, 118–19, 121–22, 156,
159, 162–63
state support for rural mothers and, 47,
49, 51, 52
Family Law of 1968
child support and, 193
cohabitation and, 196
debate among Communist Party leaders
preceding, 191–93
divorce and, 193, 196–97
out-of-wedlock births and, 20,
187–88, 193–96
public discussion of, 193–94
registration of children's names
under, 195
family planning programs, 20,
216–17, 218
famine (1946-47), 124–25, 127–29
fatherless children. *See*
out-of-wedlock births
feminist, 4–5, 200–1, 212, 217
fertility. *See* birth rate; infertility
Finland, 4–5, 197
France, 89–90, 188–89, 197
free love, 8, 55

Gausner, Zh., 120
Germany. *See* East Germany; Nazi
Germany; West Germany
Gorbachev, Mikhail, 15, 211–12
Gorshenin, K. P., 143, 157, 167, 169
Gosplan (State Planning
Committee), 21–22
Gozulov, A. I., 124
Great Britain. *See* United Kingdom
Great Leap Forward (China), 183–84
Great Patriotic War. *See* World War II
(Great Patriotic War)
Great Terror/Great Purge, 2n.8, 6,
9–10n.50, 14, 26, 81n.109,
123–24, 123–24n.4, 166

Holocaust, 2, 24–25
Holodomor, 25n.16
Home Again (Gausner), 120
Honecker, Erich, 184
household work
    *babushka*s (grandmothers), 205–6,
      214–15, 220
    gender ideologies and, 211–12
    household appliances and, 208, 212–13
    men's refusal to participate in, 205,
      207, 210
    reform campaigns promoting men's
      involvement in, 213
    socialist ideals regarding, 7, 204, 214
    Western countries and, 212
housing
    clinical abortion linked to problems
      with, 198
    criminal abortion linked to problems
      with, 134–36, 151, 156–57, 165
    interministerial report of 1948–49
      and, 131
    reform and, 13n.80
    single mothers and, 116–17, 123
    Soviet shortages in, 17
    Soviet welfare system guarantees
      regarding, 12–13
    women's choice to limit family size
      linked to, 207
    World War II and, 67
Hungary, 16, 183, 191–92
Huxley, Julian, 124–25

illegal abortion. *See* criminal abortion
illegitimate/illegitimacy, see also out-
      of-wedlock births, 41–42, 43–44,
      85–86, 89, 90–91, 115, 115–16n.97,
      122n.119, 158, 160
infanticide, 32–34, 36, 43, 46, 51
infantilism, 66, 67
infant mortality rates, 45, 66, 129
infertility
    abortion and, 1–2, 66–67, 68, 69, 138,
      144, 151, 166, 167, 197–98
    artificial insemination and, 68–69
    clinical abortion and, 197–98
    criminal abortion and, 1–2, 144, 150,
      151, 166, 167, 199

divorce and, 97–99
men and, 66–67, 68–69, 98
prophylactic measures designed to
    limit, 75
venereal disease and, 67, 68, 69
World War II and, 65, 66–68
Institute for Obstetrics and Gynecology
    of the Academy of Medical Science,
    199–200
Institute of Demography (Ukraine), 26
Ireland, 43–44
Italy, 212, 221
Iurkevich, N.G., 213

Japan
    "baby boomlet" after World War II and,
      22, 85–86
    clinical abortion in, 4–5, 57, 85–86
    decolonization and, 22
    Eugenic Protection Law and, 57
    female participation in the workforce
      and, 188–89
    Manchuria during World War II
      and, 57
    pronatalism during World War II
      in, 125
    US occupation after World War II
      and, 57
Jews, *see* anti-semitism
Juviler, Peter, 21–22n.3, 158n.13, 192–93n.29,
    192–93n.30

Kaganovich, Lazar, 180n.82, 180
Kazakhstan, 16, 138, 139–40, 182–83
Kharchev, A.G., 204
Khrushchev, Nikita
    20th Party Congress (1956), 16
    anti-alcohol campaign during 1950s
      and, 190–91
    childless taxes (1941) and, 22, 26, 34,
      114, 170
    Family Law of 1944 and, 21–22, 23,
      28–36, 40, 42, 43–44, 45–46, 47–51,
      53–54, 105–6, 122, 126–27, 154, 164,
      171, 220–21, 222
    famine of 1946-47 and, 128–29
    "kitchen debate" (1959) and, 204
    as leader of the Soviet Union, 187

Khrushchev, Nikita (*cont.*)
limited scope of family law reforms
under, 14–15, 154
ouster (1964) of, 14–15, 193
out-of-wedlock births promoted by, 3,
24, 36–37, 159–60
pronatalism and, 5, 21–24, 25–27,
28–36, 43–44, 52–53, 105–6, 170,
172–73, 193
Ptukha and, 26–27
small family taxes and, 35, 50–51
Stalin denounced by, 16
on Starovskii, 163
state aid for mothers and, 28–29, 31–32,
37, 222
state aid for pregnancy and, 28–29
tax reform during 1950s and, 189, 191
Ukraine and, 17–18, 21–22, 24–27
Virgin Lands and, 170
World War II and, 21, 22, 25–26
"kitchen debate" (1959), 204
Kliachko, M.M., 71–72, 144
Kliueva, Nina G., 58, 79–80
kolkhoz, see collective farm
Kollontai, Alexandra, 8, 22–23, 55
Komissarova, T.A., 82
Komsomol, 52n.152, 170
Konstantinov, V.I., 165–68, 176, 177
Kovrigina, Mariia D.
Central Committee of Communist
Party position of, 81
Committee on the Question of Women's
Labor and Improvement of the
Protection of Motherhood and
Childhood and, 119
contraceptive access advocated by, 178
criteria for exceptions to criminal
abortion and, 79
Doctors' Plot (1953) and, 157
Family Law of 1944 and, 45
on importance of increasing birth rate
in postwar Soviet Union, 78
on infertility caused by abortions, 144
interministerial study of abortion
(1948-49) and, 125, 130, 137
legalization of abortion (1955) and,
4, 153–55, 164, 167, 174–75,
177–81, 186

on men's responsibility for abortion,
123, 143, 144, 152, 157
as minister of health, 126
Ministry of Health's history of Soviet
abortion policy and, 165–66
purge of Moscow Institute for
Gynecology and Obstetrics
and, 81–84
Social-Legal Consultation Office
and, 147
Soviet state disciplining of doctors and,
18, 79–87, 154
on subterfuge to obtain clinical
abortions, 58
surveillance system for clinical
abortions and, 69, 76, 78
woman's right to abortion and, 1, 4, 153,
155, 177
KR Affair (1947), 58, 79–81

Latvia, 16, 191
legalized abortion. *See also* clinical
abortion
advocates during early 1950s
for, 174–81
cancellation of women's criminal
responsibility (1954), 14, 144–45,
164, 171–72, 175
initial era (1920-1936) of, 3–4, 9, 166,
176, 179
re-establishment (1955) of, 3–5, 14,
15–16, 19, 180–81
Lenin, Vladimir I., 8
Leningrad, 74
Leningrad Institute for Gynecology and
Obstetrics, 84
Lithuania, 130–31
Liu Shaoqi, 183–84

Malenkov, G.M., 68, 155–56,
160–61, 171–72
Malinovskii, M.S., 65, 67, 81–84
Malthus, Thomas/anti-Malthusian, 7–8
Mao Zedong, 183–84
marriage. *See also* common-law marriage
Family Law of 1918 and, 9
Family Law of 1926 and, 9, 39–40
Family Law of 1936 and, 10, 40

Family Law of 1944 and, 12, 18–19, 29, 30, 34, 39, 40–41, 91, 94–95, 101, 103–4, 105–6, 108, 161–63
Soviet women's desire for, 5–6, 18–19
Marx, Karl, 7–8
maternity leave
    Constitution of 1936 and, 12–13
    extensions during 1970s and 80s of, 187–88, 208, 214
    Family Law of 1944 and, 46
    reform proposals during 1950s and, 156–57, 189
    Western countries and, 212
Matsepanova, O.D., 78–79
Medvedev, Dmitrii, 219
Medvedeva, Svetlana, 220–21
Merkov, A.M., 45
Mikhailov, V.P., 67–68, 83, 176–77
Mikoyan, Anastas, 180, 208–9
Mikoyan commission (1950s), 208–9
military of the Soviet Union.
    See also World War II (Great Patriotic War)
    birth rates and the long-term strength of, 9
    rapes during World War II by members of, 56–57
    romantic relationships during World War II and, 10–12, 61–62, 91–94, 96–97, 121
    Soviet victories over Nazi Germany and, 27
    taxes on members of, 35, 50
    women enlisted in, 2, 11–12, 61–62, 92–94, 121
Ministry of Health (MZ), see also People's Commissariat of Health for events prior to 1946
    clinical abortion's legalization (1955) and, 180–81
    Committee on the Question of Women's Labor and Improvement of the Protection of Motherhood and Childhood and, 119–20
    Court of Honor at, 80–81
    Doctors' Plot (1953) and, 157
    history of Soviet abortion policy reviewed (1955) by, 165–67

interministerial study of abortion (1948-49) and, 125–26, 130–31, 135–36, 137, 150–51, 152
Kliueva and Roskin trial at, 80–81
Moscow Institute and, 84
orphanage study by, 117, 134
prophylactic approach to public health emphasized during 1950s by, 145, 150–52
proposed reforms to abortion law during 1950s and, 153–55, 168, 174–77
proposed reforms to improve women's socioeconomic conditions and, 155–57, 189
Ministry of Justice (MIu), See also People's Commissariat of Justice for events prior to 1946
    abortion surveillance system and, 129, 130
    divorce reforms advocated by, 169
    interministerial study of abortion (1948-49) and, 125–26, 130–31, 150–51
    proposed reforms to abortion law during 1950s and, 153–55, 164, 168
    proposed reforms to improve women's socioeconomic conditions and, 155–56
    prosecutions for criminal abortion and, 137–45
    reforms to aid out-of-wedlock children and, 191
    reforms to Family Law of 1944 and, 150–51
    re-legalization of abortion (1955) and, 19
Ministry of Social Welfare, 157
miscarriages
    clinical abortions and later incidents of, 197–98
    famine of 1946-47 and, 128
    induced miscarriages and, 63, 140
    infantilism and, 67
    medical problems following, 73
    prophylactic measures designed to limit, 75
    World War II and, 65, 67

Miterev, Georgii, 28, 45, 66, 75–76, 79–80
Molotov, Vyacheslav, 27–28, 51, 109, 172
Mongolia, 16
morning-after pill, 221
Moscow Does not Believe in Tears
    (film), 55
Moscow Institute for Gynecology and
    Obstetrics (MIGO), 58, 81–84, 147
Mother Heroine title, 2–3, 16, 47–51,
    54, 208–9
motherhood capital law (Russia,
    2006), 219–20
Motherhood Glory order, 47–48, 51–52,
    54, 208–9
Motherhood Medal, 2–3, 51–52, 53*t*,
    54, 208–9
*The Mother's Notebook (Pamiatka
    Materi)*, 172
Muslim women in the Soviet Union,
    15–16, 182–83

Narkomfin, *see* People's Commissariat of
    Finance
Narkomiust, *see* People's Commissariat of
    Justice
Narkomzdrav, *see* People's Commissariat
    of Health
"Nastia" (Ketlinskaia), 94–95
Nazi Germany. *See also* World War II
    (Great Patriotic War)
    abortion and, 33
    forced labor and, 33
    France occupied by, 89–90
    Soviet military victory over, 27
    Soviet territories occupied by, 2, 12, 21,
        24, 25–26, 31, 33, 96–97
Nikolaev, A.P., 67, 70–71, 76, 84
Nixon, Richard, 204
NKVD, *see* People's Commissariat of
    Internal Affairs
non-clinical abortion. *See* criminal
    abortion
Norway, 197

Once, Twenty Years Later (film), 209
oral contraception, 155, 200–2
Organization of Ukrainian Nationalists
    (OUN), 25

orphanages (*dom rebenka* and *detskii dom*)
    health conditions of children at, 117,
        121–22, 134
    increased postwar population in, 133
    Ministry of Health study of, 117, 134
    single mothers' right to leave children
        at, 37, 90, 133–34
    taxes supporting, 22, 26, 34–35
    in Ukraine, 34–35
    World War II and, 24–25, 26
Orthodox Church, 218–19, 220–21
out-of-wedlock births. *See also* child
    support
    Committee on the Question of Women's
        Labor and Improvement of the
        Protection of Motherhood and
        Childhood and, 119–20
    criminal abortion linked to,
        139–40, 144
    decline following re-legalization of
        abortion (1955) in, 181
    definition of, 89
    Family Law of 1918 and, 54
    Family Law of 1944 and, 17–18, 22–23,
        24, 29, 30, 34, 36–42, 43–44, 45–46,
        52–53, 86, 88–89, 105–6, 107–8, 109,
        114–19, 122, 154, 155, 158–60, 161,
        162, 191
    Family Law of 1968 and, 20,
        187–88, 193–96
    Khrushchev's promotion of, 3, 24,
        36–37, 159–60
    physical challenges faced by children
        of, 117
    pronatalist policy encouraging, 3, 5–6
    psychological disadvantages for women
        and children of, 19, 106, 114–18,
        119–20, 122, 144, 158, 159–60, 195
    registration of, 106, 107–8
    rural regions and, 163
    Russian Federation and, 220
    Soviet rates (1945-54) of, 3
    state aid proposals regarding, 191
    statistics regarding extent of, 90,
        115–16, 122

"Parental Glory" order (2008), 219
Parin, V.V., 79–80

Party Congress
    20th Party Congress (1956), 16, 183, 189
    24th Party Congress (1971), 208
    25th Party Congress (1976), 201, 208
Party Control Commission (KPK), 114
patronymic
    Committee on the Question of Women's
        Labor and Improvement of the
        Protection of Motherhood and
        Childhood and, 119–20
    cultural representations of, 55
    Family Law of 1944 and, 30, 38, 41,
        54, 115
    Family Law of 1968, 195
    incestual relationships prevented
        by, 115
    registered marriages and, 38
    pension reform, 13n.80
People's Commissariat of Finance,
        (Narkomfin or NKFin), 28, 47
People's Commissariat of Internal Affairs
        (NKVD), 25
People's Commissariat of Justice
        (Narkomiust, NKIu)
    child support cases and, 101–3
    criminal prosecutions of abortion
        and, 59, 130–31
    divorce procedures and, 100, 108–10
    Family Law of 1944 implemented
        by, 105–13
    surveillance system for clinical
        abortions and, 75–76
People's Commissariat of Health,
        (Narkomzdrav or NKZ)
    abortion clinics and, 64
    childcare facilities and, 42
    criminal prosecutions of abortion
        and, 59, 62, 63
    Family Law of 1944 and, 45–46, 47,
        49, 51, 65
    First Joint Plenum (1944), 62, 86
    maternity leave and, 46
    pronatalism and, 27–28
    Second Plenum for the Council
        of Obstetrics and Gynecology
        (1945), 68
    state aid to mothers and, 28
    state aid to pregnant women and, 28

    surveillance system for clinical
        abortions and, 76
    working conditions for pregnant
        women and, 46
People's court, 28–29, 49, 102, 105–6,
        108–9, 110, 139, 141–42, 193
Poland, 24–25, 183, 184, 221
Popova, N.V., 167, 180
premature births
    clinical abortions and later incidents
        of, 197–98
    infantilism and, 67
    late-term abortion attempts
        and, 140–41
    prophylactic measures designed to
        limit, 75
    state aid to pregnant women as means of
        reducing, 28
    World War II and, 28, 65, 67, 74
pronatalism. See also birth rate
    Brezhnev era and, 203–15
    China and, 16, 183–84
    Cold War and, 5
    contraceptives suppressed under, 148
    definition of, 9–10n.50
    divorce and, 98–99
    Family Law of 1936 and, 7, 9–10, 176
    Family Law of 1944 and, 2–3, 10,
        13–14, 17–18, 22–24, 28–36, 51,
        52–54, 77–78, 105–7, 122, 162,
        164, 196
    Khrushchev and, 5, 21–24, 25–27,
        28–36, 43–44, 52–53, 105–6, 170,
        172–73, 193
    postwar period and, 17–18
    prewar period and, 9–10, 61
    Putin and, 20, 216, 218–19, 220–21, 222
    Russian Federation and, 20, 216, 218–19,
        220–21, 222
    Ukraine and, 17–18, 21–22
    World War II mass casualties as reason
        for, 2–3
prosecutor/state prosecutor
    abortion statistics and
        33–34n.69, 59n.11
    abortion studies of the late 1940s
        and 1950 and, 129, 130, 130n.36,
        141–42, 145

prosecutor/state prosecutor (*cont.*)
  criminalized abortion (1936) and, 59,
    60, 62, 63
  Family Law of 1944 and, 51
  Legalization of abortion (1955)
    and, 19, 155, 164
  Postwar abortion surveillance
    and, 71–73, 75–76, 79, 84
  Reform of criminalized abortion
    and, 150–51, 153–54
Ptukha, Mikhail V., 26–27
Putin, Vladimir
  Orthodox Church, 218–19
  pronatalism and, 20, 216, 218–19,
    220–21, 222
  restriction on clinical abortion and,
    218–19, 220–21
  state aid for mothers and, 219–20, 222

rape
  anti-abortion campaign in post socialist
    Poland and, 221
  as a ground for legal abortion, 77, 177
  of German women, 56–57
  of Japanese women, 57
Red Army. *See* military of the
    Soviet Union
reproductive health. *See also* infertility
  amenorrhea and, 66, 67–68, 128
  birth rate and, 58, 65, 66
  contraception viewed as means of
    improving, 20, 199
  criminalization of abortion's impact on,
    58–59, 166, 174, 175, 176–77
  doctors' prioritization of, 56, 58, 64–66,
    71, 73–75
  infantilism and, 66, 67
  infant mortality rates and, 45, 66, 129
  prophylactic approach to, 69, 74, 75,
    145, 150–52, 180
  socialist approach to, 182–85, 187–88
  World War II and, 25–26, 64–65
Romania, 16, 183
Roskin, Grigorii I., 58, 79–80
Russian Federation (post 1991)
  abortion rates in, 16
  birth rate in, 217–18, 219–20, 222
  childcare in, 217

clinical abortion in, 20, 216–17,
    218–19, 220–21
contraception and, 216–17, 218
family planning programs and,
    216–17, 218
household work and, 217
market economy and, 216–17
out-of-wedlock births and, 220
population demographics in, 217–18
pronatalism and, 20, 216, 218–19,
    220–21, 222
sex education and, 20
state aid for mothers and, 219–20
women's workforce participation
    and, 217
Rychkov, N. M., 107–8, 111, 113

Sadvokasova, E.A., 207
Sakevich, Viktoriia, 216–17
Scandinavian countries, 212–13, 221
Scientific Research Institute for Physiology
    and Pathology of Women, 199–200
Semashko, N. A., 77
Serebrovskaia, Elena
  on out-of-wedlock children, 155,
    158–60, 191
  reform efforts regarding Family Law
    of 1944 and, 19, 154, 155, 169,
    171–72, 193
sex education, 20, 199, 218
sexually transmitted diseases. *See* venereal
    disease
Shostakovich, Dmitrii, 191–92, 194
Simonov, Konstantin, 10
single mothers, *see also* unmarried
    mothers
  abortion and, 85, 86, 136, 138, 143–44,
    150–51, 156, 165
  Abramova's report on, 115–20,
    121–22n.105, 129
  access to government aid and, 121–22
  childcare and, 132–34, 132–33n.51
  Family Law of 1944 and, 2–3, 38–39,
    51–54, 55n.161, 90, 91, 114
  Family Law reform campaign (1954)
    and, 155, 158, 159–60
  Family Law reform campaign
    (1956), 195

Family Law of 1968 and, 196, 197
Khrushchev's proposal and, 24, 30, 34–35, 37, 38, 41–42, 43–44
letters written to Khrushchev by, 171
Narkomfin and, 47
NKZ and, 45
post-socialist and, 217n.11, 220
pronatalism in the 1970s and 1980s and, 208–9
reduction in government aid (1947) and, 53–54, 90, 121–22
Reform proposals of Family Law of 1944 and, 156–57, 158, 191
Revision of Khrushchev's draft proposal and, 47n.126, 48, 49, 50
Tax reform of the 1950s and, 189
TsSU and, 46, 122, 161, 162–63
Variety of paths to, 121
Slavic women in the Soviet Union, 188, 190, 193, 203–4
Smirnov, Efim I., 79–80, 81–82, 157
Smith, Walter Bedell, 79–80
socialism. *See also* Bolshevik Party
abortion and, 8, 16, 187–88, 203
birth rate and, 7–9, 188, 203
childcare and, 7, 203–4, 213–14
contraception and, 8–9, 203
Eastern European regimes and, 16
free love and, 8
gender equality ideals and, 7, 9, 13, 214–15
household work and, 7, 204, 214
Malthusianism and, 7–8
reproductive health and, 182–85, 187–88
welfare system and, 12–13
women's workforce participation and, 13, 213
social-legal consultation office, 147–48
Spain, 212, 221
Speranskii, G.N., 191–92, 194
spravka (informational note), 18, 28–44, 30n.49, 34n.75, 50, 51, 52
Stalin, I. V.
census of 1939 and, 123–24
childless tax (1941) and, 22, 26, 34, 170
classification of demographic data as state secret by, 124–25

clinical abortion criminalized (1936) by, 3–4
collectivization of agricultural sector under, 9–10
death of, 14, 16, 19, 87, 152, 154, 155, 158, 169
de-Stalinization and, 154, 178, 183, 187
Doctors' Plot under, 154, 155, 157–58
Family Law of 1936 and, 3–4, 9, 22–23, 164
Family Law of 1944 and, 47, 49
famine of 1946-47 and, 124–25, 128–29
intelligentsia targeted by, 79–80
Khrushchev's denunciation of, 16
purges of demographers under 15, 123–24
purges of Moscow Institute for Gynecology and Obstetrics under, 18, 81, 82n.114
pronatalism and, 52
welfare system of the Soviet Union and, 12–13
Starovskii, V.N.
birth rate and abortion linked by, 19, 123, 124–25, 127–28, 152
census of 1939 and, 123–24
census of 1959 and, 163–64, 188
on Family Law of 1944 and divorce, 154
famine of 1946-47 and, 124–25, 127–29
interministerial abortion study of 1948–49 and, 19
Khrushchev and, 163
"On the Increase of Registered Marriages" report (1954) by, 160–64
on out-of-wedlock births, 46–47, 154, 161, 162
on postwar birth decline, 123
postwar birth rate projections by, 46–47, 126, 193
self-censorship practiced by, 124–25, 128–29
state aid for mothers
Committee on the Question of Women's Labor and Improvement of the Protection of Motherhood and Childhood and, 119
reduction (1947) in, 53–54, 90, 121–22

state aid for mothers (*cont.*)
    Family Law of 1936 and, 9–10, 13–14, 27–28, 49
    Family Law of 1944 and, 10, 22, 24, 28–30, 31–32, 34, 37–38, 118–19, 156, 159, 162–63
    Khrushchev and, 24, 28–29, 31–32, 37, 222
Stepmother (film), 55
stillbirths, 67, 141
Strumilin, S.G. 124n.7
Sweden, 4–5, 188–89, 197

Tadzhikistan, 130–31
taxes
    Abramova's proposal regarding single men and, 118–20
    childless tax (1941) and, 22, 26, 31, 34–35, 114, 118–19, 170
    Khrushchev's reforms regarding, 189, 191
    single mothers' payment of, 118, 143, 189
    small family taxes and, 30–31, 34–35, 36, 44, 48, 49–51, 53t, 143, 171, 189, 191
    vodka excise taxes and, 190–91
Thaw, 154, 154n.1, 154n.2, 155, 178
TsSU, see Central Statistical Administration

Ukraine
    abortion rates in, 16, 33
    birth rates in, 25–27
    clinical abortions in, 33, 64, 75
    collectivization and famine during 1930s in, 26
    criminal abortions in, 63, 130–31
    divorce in, 95, 97–98, 109–10
    famine of 1946-47 and, 129
    Holocaust and, 24–25
    Holodomor, 24n.16
    independence movement during World War II in, 25–26
    infanticide in, 33–34
    Khrushchev and, 17–18, 21–22, 24–27
    Nazi occupation of, 12, 21, 24–25, 33, 63
    orphanages in, 34–35

    population demographics in, 25–27
    pronatalism and, 17–18, 21–22
    World War II casualty levels in, 24–25, 27
Umniagina, Tamara S., 11, 92
underground abortion. *See* criminal abortion
United Kingdom, 4–5, 165–66, 188–89, 197
United Nations, 16, 124–25
    Fourth World Conference on Women (1995) sponsored by, 217
United States
    "baby boom" during postwar era in, 22
    birth control pill in, 200–1
    clinical abortion in, 4–5, 197
    divorce rate in, 196–97
    Japanese occupation after World War II and, 57
    population control and attitudes toward African Americans in, 125
    women's rights movement and, 4–5
    women's workforce participation and, 188–89
unmarried mothers, *see also* single mothers
    childcare and, 133
    Family Law of 1918 and, 9
    Family Law of 1944 and, 17–18, 19, 54, 89–90, 122
    Khrushchev's proposal and, 37, 38, 41–42, 43, 53–54
    The number of, 122
    Party investigation of, 6–7
    Tax reform of the 1950s and, 190, 191
    TsSU and, 46–47
    women's avoidance of, 6, 89
Urlanis, Boris Ts., 205–6
US Agency for International Development (USAID), 216–17
Uzbekistan, 98, 182–83

Vaksberg, Arkadii E., 192
venereal disease, 57–58, 67, 68, 69, 97–99
Vietnam, 16
Virgin Lands, 170
Voroshilov, K.E., 159–60, 171–72
Voznesenskii, N.A., 27

war widow pensions, 103–5, 108
"A Week Like Any Other Week"
    (Baranskaia), 204–6
welfare state, 12–13, 12–13n.76, 16–17,
    211–12, 212n.126, 214–15
West Germany, 56–57, 184–85, 188–89,
    197, 212
Women's Department (*Zhenotdel*), 13–14
women's rights,
    language of, 175
    the 1920 legalization of abortion and, 4
    the 1955 legalization of abortion and, 4,
        5, 5n.22, 174, 178–79, 181–82
    outside the USSR, 4–5, 4–5n.21,
        188–89, 206
    woman's right *vs*, 4–5, 175
women's workforce participation
    birth rates and, 16, 201, 206, 222
    childcare and, 133, 204
    "double burden" and, 5–6, 175, 204,
        208, 210–11
    Gorbachev and, 15
    during industrialization drives of
        1930s, 9
    Russian Federation and, 217
    socialist ideals and, 13, 213
    Soviet Union in comparative
        international perspective and, 17
    welfare system and, 16–17
    Western countries and, 188–89,
        206, 212–13
World Health Organization, 200
World War II (Great Patriotic War)
    abortions during, 33, 56, 61–64, 74
    birth rate during, 27, 45, 63
    casualty levels in, 2, 22, 24–25, 124
    divorce and, 88
    doctors and, 61–63
    family separations and, 2, 10–11, 22, 56,
        88, 94–95, 97, 100–2, 106, 111, 121
    Holocaust and, 2, 24–25
    mass mobilization for, 2
    Nazi occupation of Soviet territories
        during, 12, 21, 24–25, 33, 63
    orphanages and, 24–25, 26
    population loss and gender imbalances
        following, 2, 5–6, 20, 21, 22, 24–27,
        31, 32, 44, 52–53, 88, 91, 116, 120–21,
        164, 171
    premature births and, 28, 65, 67, 74
    prostitution during, 12
    rapes during, 56–57
    reproductive health and, 25–26, 64–65
    wartime relationships and, 10–12, 61–
        62, 91–94, 96–97, 121
    war widow pensions and, 103–5
    women soldiers in, 2, 11–12, 61–62,
        92–94, 121

Yeltsin, Boris, 216–17
Young Communist League,
    see *Komsomol*.

ZAGS (The office of marriages, births, and
    deaths), 39, 41, 49, 108, 115–16, 169
zhdanovshchina (Zhdanovism), 79–80
Zhenotdel (Women's Department in
    Bolshevik Party), 13–14
Zhiromskaia, V.B., 113
Zoshchenko, Mikhail, 79–80

Printed in the USA/Agawam, MA
September 12, 2022

798393.032